T0317472

Cosmeceuticals and Cosmetic Practice

Cosmeceuticals and Cosmetic Practice

EDITED BY

Patricia K. Farris, MD

Clinical Associate Professor
Tulane University School of Medicine
New Orleans, LA, USA

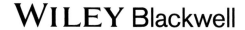

This edition first published 2014 © 2014 by John Wiley & Sons Ltd

Registered office: John Wiley & Sons, Ltd, The Atrium, Southern Gate, Chichester, West Sussex, PO19 8SQ, UK

Editorial offices: 9600 Garsington Road, Oxford, OX4 2DQ, UK
       The Atrium, Southern Gate, Chichester, West Sussex, PO19 8SQ, UK
       111 River Street, Hoboken, NJ 07030-5774, USA

For details of our global editorial offices, for customer services and for information about how to apply for permission to reuse the copyright material in this book please see our website at www.wiley.com/wiley-blackwell

Library of Congress Cataloging-in-Publication Data
Cosmeceuticals and cosmetic practice / edited by Patricia K. Farris.
   p. ; cm.
  Includes bibliographical references and index.
  ISBN 978-1-118-38483-1 (cloth : alk. paper) – ISBN 978-1-118-38479-4 (epdf) –
ISBN 978-1-118-38480-0 (epub) – ISBN 978-1-118-38481-7 (emobi) – ISBN 978-1-118-38482-4
  I. Farris, Patricia K., editor of compilation.
  [DNLM: 1. Dermatologic Agents–therapeutic use. 2. Cosmetics–therapeutic use. QV 60]
  RA778
  613′.488–dc23
                                             2013024799

A catalogue record for this book is available from the British Library.

Wiley also publishes its books in a variety of electronic formats. Some content that appears in print may not be available in electronic books.

Cover image: iStock File #22275191 © Pogonici
Cover design by Meaden Creative

Set in 9.5/13pt Meridien by Laserwords Private Limited, Chennai, India

1 2014

Contents

List of Contributors

Diane S. Berson MD, FAAD
Associate Clinical Professor Dermatology
Weill Medical College of Cornell University
New York-Presbyterian Hospital;
Private Practice
New York, NY, USA

Donald L. Bissett PhD
Retiree from The Procter & Gamble Company
Cincinnati, OH, USA

Elizabeth Bruning BS, LLB
Johnson & Johnson Consumer Companies, Inc.
Skillman, NJ, USA

Mark V. Dahl MD
Professor Emeritus
Department of Dermatology
Mayo Clinic;
Makucell, Inc.
Scottsdale, AZ, USA

Jennifer David DO, MBA
Dermatology Clinical Research Fellow
Society Hill Dermatology
Philadelphia, PA, USA

Doris Day MD, FAAD, MA
Clinical Associate Professor, Dermatology
New York University Medical Center
New York, NY, USA

Zoe Diana Draelos MD
Consulting Professor
Department of Dermatology
Duke University School of Medicine
Durham, NC, USA

Jason Emer MD
Department of Dermatology
Icahn School of Medicine at Mount Sinai
New York, NY, USA

Sung-Hwan Eom
Marine Bioprocess Research Center
Pukyong National University
Busan, Republic of Korea

Sabrina G. Fabi MD, FAAD, FAACS
Volunteer Assistant Clinical Professor
University of San Diego, California
Goldman, Butterwick, Fitzpatrick, Groff & Fabi
Cosmetic Laser Dermatology
San Diego, CA, USA

Timothy Falla PhD
VP Research & Development
Rodan & Fields, LLC
San Francisco, CA, USA

Patricia K. Farris MD
Clinical Associate Professor
Tulane University School of Medicine
New Orleans, LA, USA;
Private practice
Old Metairie Dermatology
Metairie, Louisiana, USA

Kathy Fields MD
Adjunct Clinical Assistant Professor
Stanford University
Stanford, CA, USA

Dee Anna Glaser MD
Professor and Vice-Chairman
Department of Dermatology
Professor of Internal Medicine &
    Otolaryngology
Saint Louis University School of Medicine
St Louis, MO, USA

Barbara A. Green RPh, MS
Vice President of Global Clinical & Regulatory
  Affairs
NeoStrata Company, Inc.
Princeton, NJ, USA

Tomohiro Hakozaki PhD
The Procter & Gamble Company
Cincinnati, OH, USA

Candrice R. Heath MD
Department of Dermatology
St Luke's-Roosevelt Hospital Center
New York, NY, USA

Camile L. Hexsel MD
Dermatologist, Investigator
Brazilian Center for Studies in Dermatology
Porto Alegre, RS, Brazil;
The Methodist Hospital
Houston, TX, USA

Doris Hexsel MD
Instructor, Department of Dermatology
Pontif'cia Universidade Católica do Rio Grande
  do Sul (PUC-RS);
Principal Investigator
Brazilian Center for Studies in Dermatology
Porto Alegre, RS, Brazil

Neil Houston
Research Coordinator
Clinical Unit for Research Trials and Outcomes
  in Skin (CURTIS)
Massachusetts General Hospital
Boston, MA, USA

Leah Jacob MD
Department of Dermatology
Tulane University School of Medicine
New Orleans, LA, USA

Mary B. Johnson MS
The Procter & Gamble Company
Cincinnati, OH, USA

Se-Kwon Kim PhD
Marine Bioprocess Research Center
Pukyong National University;
Marine Biochemistry Laboratory
Department of Chemistry
Pukyong National University
Busan, Republic of Korea

Alexa Boer Kimball MD, MPH
Senior Vice President, Practice Improvement,
  Mass General Physicians Organization;
Vice Chair, Department of Dermatology
Massachusetts General Hospital;
Director, Clinical Unit for Research Trials and
  Outcomes in Skin (CURTIS)
Massachusetts General Hospital;
Associate Professor
Harvard Medical School
Boston, MA, USA

Alexandra Kowcz
VP, US R&D
Beiersdorf Inc.
Wilton, CT, USA

Mary Lupo MD
Clinical Professor of Dermatology
Tulane University School of Medicine;
Private Practice
Lupo Center for Aesthetic and General
  Dermatology
New Orleans, LA, USA

Ellen Marmur MD
Icahn School of Medicine at Mount Sinai
New York, NY, USA

Adam R. Mattox DO
Department of Dermatology
Saint Louis University School of Medicine
St Louis, MO, USA

Chris Mazur BS
Senior Researcher
McDaniel Institute of Anti-Aging Research/Laser
  & Cosmetic Center
Virginia Beach, VA, USA

David H. McDaniel MD, FAAD
Director
McDaniel Institute of Anti-Aging Research/
  Laser & Cosmetic Center
Virginia Beach, VA;
Assistant Professor, Clinical Dermatology
Eastern Virginia Medical School;
Adjunct Assistant Professor, Department of
  Biological Sciences
Old Dominion University
Norfolk, VA;
Co-Director, Hampton University Skin of Color
  Research Institute
Hampton University
Hampton, VA, USA

Suzanne Micciantuono DO
Dermatology Resident
Wellington Regional Medical Center
Boca Raton, FL, USA

Adnan Nasir MD, PhD
Department of Dermatology
University of North Carolina at Chapel Hill
Chapel Hill, NC, USA

Katherine Nolan BA
Icahn School of Medicine at Mount Sinai
New York, NY, USA

John E. Oblong PhD
The Procter & Gamble Company
Cincinnati, OH, USA

Marianne N. O'Donoghue MD
Associate Professor of Dermatology
Rush University Medical Center
Chicago, IL, USA

Rosemarie Osborne PhD
The Procter & Gamble Company
Cincinnati, OH, USA

Wolfgang Pape PhD
Beiersdorf AG
Hamburg, Germany

Marta I. Rendon MD
Medical Director
The Rendon Center for Dermatology and
    Aesthetic Medicine;
Associated Clinical Professor
University of Miami
Boca Raton, FL, USA

Darrell S. Rigel MD
Clinical Professor
Department of Dermatology
New York University School of Medicine
New York, NY, USA

Katie Rodan MD
Adjunct Clinical Assistant Professor
Stanford University
Stanford, CA, USA

Nicole E. Rogers MD, FAAD
Assistant Clinical Professor
Tulane University School of Medicine
New Orleans, LA;
Private Practice
Metaire, LA, USA

Dana L. Sachs MD
Associate Professor
Department of Dermatology
University of Michigan Medical Center
Ann Arbor, MI, USA

Guenther Schneider PhD
Principal Scientist
Beiersdorf AG
Hamburg, Germany

Christina Steel PhD
Senior Researcher
McDaniel Institute of Anti-Aging Research/
    Laser & Cosmetic Center
Virginia Beach;
Department of Biological Sciences
Old Dominion University
Norfolk, VA, USA

Ying Sun PhD
Johnson & Johnson Consumer Companies, Inc.
Skillman, NJ, USA

Hema Sundaram MD, FAAD
Medical Director
Sundaram Dermatology Cosmetic & Laser
    Surgery
Rockville, MD, and Fairfax, VA, USA

Susan Taylor MD
Society Hill Dermatology, Philadelphia;
Associate Clinical Professor of Dermatology
Associate Faculty of the School of Medicine
University of Pennsylvania
Philadelphia, PA, USA

Samantha Tucker-Samaras PhD
Johnson & Johnson Consumer Companies, Inc.
Skillman, NJ, USA

Yvette Vazquez MS, PA-C
Physician Assistant
Wellington Regional Medical Center
Boca Raton, FL, USA

John J. Voorhees MD, FRCP
Duncan and Ella Poth Distinguished Professor and Chair
Department of Dermatology
University of Michigan Medical Center
Ann Arbor, MI, USA

Heidi A. Waldorf MD
Director, Laser & Cosmetic Dermatology
Mount Sinai Medical Center;
Associate Clinical Director
Icahn School of Medicine at Mount Sinai
New York, NY;
Waldorf Dermatology & Laser Associates, PC
Nanuet, NY, USA

Teresa M. Weber PhD
Director, Clinical & Scientic Affairs
Beiersdorf Inc.
Wilton, CT, USA

Susan H. Weinkle MD
Afliate Clinical Professor of Dermatology
University of South Florida
Tampa, FL;
Private Practice
Bradenton, FL, USA

Joshua A. Zeichner MD
Assistant Professor
Mount Sinai Medical Center
New York, NY, USA

Preface

The term cosmeceutical, in the US, is now a household word. It is used in magazine articles, internet postings and is even defined in the dictionary. Cosmeceuticals are a new breed of skin care products that are a hybrid between cosmetics and pharmaceuticals. The term cosmeceutical is not recognized by the Food and Drug Administration so there are no specific criteria set up for products to be included in this category. Today, we use the term cosmeceutical to refer to everything from sunscreens to prescription retinoids and almost everything in between. In fact, even simple moisturizers can technically be called cosmeceuticals as they have beneficial effects on skin physiology. In most cases, however, we reserve the use of the term cosmeceutical to refer to enhanced moisturizers containing active ingredients that provide added benefits to the skin.

The advent of cosmeceuticals represents one of the most important innovations in topical skin care. As a blend between cosmetics and pharmaceuticals, these products provide therapeutic benefits above and beyond simple cosmetics and are highly sought after by consumers. They are readily available, reasonably priced and heavily marketed, making them one of the fastest growing segments of the personal care market. Consumers turn to cosmeceuticals to treat skin aging and a myriad of skin conditions such acne, melasma and rosacea. They view these products as alternatives to medications and often try cosmeceutical products before seeking professional help. Physicians also value cosmeceuticals for their therapeutic effects. We use them in conjunction with medications to treat skin conditions and to enhance the benefits of in-office procedures.

In view of this demand, it is no surprise that cosmetic and pharmaceutical companies are focused on growing the cosmeceutical marketplace. Most major cosmetic companies have heavily invested in developing cosmeceuticals and many pharmaceutical companies are now joining in. Through basic science research these companies are working to identify potential targets for improving skin health and appearance and develop new active ingredients that can be used as interventions. They create innovative delivery systems allowing for more effective and targeted delivery of actives to the skin. Their efforts are to be commended as they have contributed significantly to the development of more effective skin care products and to our basic understanding of skin aging, moisturization and the pathogenesis of diseases.

Patients increasingly are looking to their physicians for advice on product selection. They are overwhelmed by the marketing hype that often creates unrealistic expectations and some degree of consumer confusion. They are looking for individualized skin care regimens and want to know what works and what doesn't. The aesthetic physician faces a formidable challenge to be knowledgeable about cosmeceuticals. There are few resources on the subject and the scientific studies conducted by the companies who develop these products are not always readily available. In addition, it seems as if new products and ingredients are marketed almost daily, making it impossible for us to keep up with this rapidly developing market.

This provides the rationale for this textbook. It provides you with the expertise of clinicians, researchers and industry-based cosmetic chemists from around the globe. The book is divided into three parts. Part I provides you with insight into how cosmeceuticals are developed, tested and how these science-driven skin care products are brought to market. Innovations in delivery systems and penetration enhancer will also be discussed.

Part II covers many of the key cosmeceutical ingredients including vitamin antioxidants, botanicals, growth factors, peptides and marine-based ingredients, just to name a few. Some of the newest anti-aging strategies including stem cell modulating compounds, glycation inhibitors, and ion-based anti-aging skin care are also discussed.

In Part III, clinicians who are considered leaders in the field will provide their unique and individual perspective on how cosmeceuticals can be used in clinical practice. Studies supporting the use of cosmeceuticals to treat common conditions such as acne, rosacea, hyperpigmentation, hair loss and striae are reviewed. The use of cosmeceuticals to enhance cosmetic procedures performed in the office setting such as chemical peels and laser treatments complete Part III.

Through our collective efforts, we hope to be able to provide you with a resource that will make it easier to advise your patients on product selection and give you the information you need to incorporate cosmeceuticals into your clinical practice.

I owe my deepest gratitude to my contributors who are among the leading experts in the field of topical skin care and without whom this textbook would never have been possible. I commend them for their deep commitment to professionalism and for their never-ending pursuit to put science behind cosmeceuticals. Finally, I would like to acknowledge Rachel Green and Jeffery B. Henry for all of their efforts and help in preparing this book.

Patricia K. Farris

CHAPTER 1

Cosmeceuticals and Clinical Practice

Patricia K. Farris

Tulane University School of Medicine, New Orleans, LA, USA

Definition and regulatory issues

The term cosmeceutical was coined by Albert Kligman, M.D., in 1993, referring to skin care products that are a blend of cosmetics and pharmaceuticals. This term is engrained in medical literature, the lay press, and is commonly used by consumers. There is an implied medical nature as a result of "ceutical" and an expectation of medicinal-like properties. Today cosmeceutical is generally used to refer to skin care products that contain active ingredients that are beneficial to improving skin's appearance and promoting healthy skin.

Cosmeceutical is not a legal term nor is it acknowledged by the Food and Drug Administration (FDA). The Federal Food, Drug and Cosmetic Act (FD&C Act) categorizes products as cosmetics or drugs according to their intended use. Cosmetics are defined as "articles intended to be rubbed, poured, sprinkled, or sprayed on, introduced into, or otherwise applied to the human body or any part thereof for cleansing, beautifying, promoting attractiveness, or altering the appearance." Cosmetic products include moisturizers, nail polish, lipstick, eye and facial make-up, shampoo, hair color and toothpaste. This is in contrast to a drug that is defined as "an article intended for the use in diagnosis, cure, mitigation, prevention or treatment of disease," including those intended to "affect the structure or any function of the body of man or any other animals." While the FD&C Act does not recognize the term cosmeceutical, it acknowledges that products can be both cosmetics and drugs if they have two intended uses. For example, a dandruff shampoo that is intended to clean hair and treat dandruff makes it both a cosmetic and drug. A moisturizing sunscreen that is intended to moisturize skin and protect it from sun exposure is also considered a cosmetic and drug.

It is ironic that most cosmeceuticals in the marketplace today enjoy cosmetic status in spite of the fact they contain active ingredients designed to treat, mitigate or improve skin conditions. Carefully crafted marketing and advertising campaigns avoid making any type of drug claims and limited testing prevents these ingredients from being viewed as drugs. Cosmetic status is preferred by the companies who develop and market cosmeceuticals since there is a less rigorous pre-approval process required and no new drug application (NDA) necessary. This allows companies to develop and test cosmeceuticals with far less cost than drugs and moves them quickly into the marketplace at a price point that is affordable for consumers. Recent reports suggest the FDA is considering stricter regulation over cosmeceutical skin care products but the specifics are yet to be determined.

The cosmeceutical marketplace

In spite of a lackluster economy, cosmeceutical products are maintaining a strong, significant presence in the beauty marketplace. This is due by and large to the fact that Baby Boomers, who are now in their fifties and sixties, are showing a continued interest in health and beauty products. Anti-aging products remain as top performers with consistently high increases in revenue over the past several years. Cosmeceutical sales were projected to increase 7.4% in 2012, with global sales reaching US$9.4 billion. While US cosmeceutical sales remain strong, emerging markets such as China and Brazil are expected to have significant impact on global sales. In an attempt to keep up with this demand, ingredient and end-product manufacturers are focusing their efforts on developing innovative technologies that give them unique positioning in the marketplace. Many of the latest ingredients are a blend between science and nature, making actives from botanical and marine sources among the most highly sought after in the industry.

Consumers now view cosmeceuticals as effective treatment options for a variety of skin conditions. Scientifically based marketing campaigns, celebrity and physician endorsements lend credibility to these products in the eyes of consumers. Cosmeceuticals are readily available and reasonably priced, making them an alternative to visiting a doctor and buying medications. For this reason, it is no surprise that many patients who visit our offices have tried cosmeceuticals prior to seeking cosmetic treatments. Cosmeceuticals for treating aging skin, rosacea, eczema, scars and cellulite are widely available. High end department stores promote a medical-like atmosphere going so far as to use sales persons in white coats to sell cosmeceuticals. This blurring between medicine and the mass market is unique to this category of products. And finally, there are dermatologists and plastic surgeons who market their own cosmeceutical lines. Physician lines are sold in department stores, mass retail outlets, on infomercials and home shopping channels. These lines have been widely accepted by consumers who view physician lines as more scientifically based. The success of these lines makes physicians major players in shaping the cosmeceuticals marketplace.

Cosmeceuticals in cosmetic practice

Physicians practicing aesthetic medicine have also played a role in expanding the use of cosmeceuticals. Cosmeceuticals are now a regular part of our treatment armamentarium and are used in addition to medications and procedures to improve patient outcomes. Anti-aging cosmeceuticals are among the most frequently recommended by physicians who utilize them as an integral part of a comprehensive skin rejuvenation program. Moisturizers and serums containing ingredients like vitamin C, niacinamide, retinol, peptides, growth factors and botanicals can all be used in this regard. In addition, patients undergoing cosmetic procedures such as laser resurfacing and chemical peels may be given cosmeceuticals to "prime" the skin for procedures, encourage healing and reduce complications after.

Cosmeceuticals are also recommended for patients with acne, rosacea, eczema and other skin conditions where they are commonly used in combination with prescription medications. For example, moisturizers containing anti-inflammatory botanical ingredients may be used in conjunction with prescription medications for treating rosacea. Cosmeceuticals containing soy can be used to provide added skin lightening benefits when paired with hydroquinone. This shift in treatment paradigms has placed the use of cosmeceuticals within the purview of medical practice. Now more than ever, it is imperative that physicians understand the science behind cosmeceuticals. Patients are inundated with commercial information obtained from sometimes less than reliable sources such as consumer advertising, blogs and internet websites. They turn to their physician to provide credible advice on which products to choose and which products are worth the money. Therefore, it is our responsibility to review the scientific data and clinical studies and to steer patients away from products that are not adequately tested nor have proven benefits. This can be difficult since in the realm of cosmeceuticals, well-designed clinical trials are often lacking. Thus evaluating new products and keeping informed on the rapidly changing cosmeceutical marketplace remain an ongoing challenge for physicians.

Skin care regimens based on science

It takes time and skill to develop individualized skin care regimens for patients. Physicians must fully evaluate a patient's skin type, assess the degree of photodamage and take into account any pre-existing skin conditions in order to design an appropriate regimen. It is important to consider if the patient has oily, dry or sensitive skin or if there are any pre-existing skin conditions like seborrhea, eczema, acne, and rosacea. Lifestyle considerations such as hobbies, sporting activities and occupation also play a role. A basic skin care regimen required to maintain skin health and beauty is made up of a cleanser, moisturizer and sunscreen. Toners, astringents and eye creams may also be included although these products are not considered essential. In general, regimens for cosmetic patients should include daytime products that protect the skin and nighttime products that will repair skin damage.

Cleansers are designed to remove dirt, make-up, sebum and pollutants from the skin and should be used morning and evening. Currently there are a wide variety of cleansers available, making it easy to recommend products that are appropriate for all patients. Mild cleansing products include synthetic detergent bars; these are also called syndets and lipid-free cleansers. These products have a pH that is closer to that of the skin (5.5–7) and clean the skin with little to no irritation. Syndet bars and lipid-free cleanser can be used on patients with most skin types and are especially helpful for those with dry or sensitive skin. Patients with pre-existing conditions such as eczema, rosacea and photoaging have a compromised barrier function, making gentle cleansing even more important.

Astringents and toners are used to remove any residual oils that are left on the skin after the cleansing process. Originally these products were designed to remove soap residue but today they are used primarily by patients who use cleansing creams or by those who have oily skin. Astringents and toners should be avoided in those with dry sensitive skin or in patients with a compromised barrier function. In these patients, astringents and toners may exacerbate dryness and cause burning and stinging.

Moisturizers are an essential component of a basic skin care regimen as they are necessary to hydrate the skin and to maintain barrier function. Proper moisturization can mitigate symptoms of dry skin, including itching, and improves the skin's appearance. Moisturizers are especially important for patients with conditions like rosacea and eczema where the barrier function is already compromised. Patients with oily skin and acne must also be given moisturizers since many medications used to treat acne have significant drying effects.

Photoprotection is the final essential component of the skin care regimen. Moisturizers containing sunscreens are appropriate for daily use and can be applied under make-up. Although many of these moisturizers offer good protection against ultraviolet A and ultraviolet B rays, they may not be the best choice for outdoor activities. Gel or spray-on sunscreens that are water-resistant are usually preferred by outdoor enthusiasts. Sunscreens should be selected based on skin type and personal preference.

Office dispensing

Physician-dispensed cosmeceuticals are sold in the vast majority of aesthetic practices. In 2011, dispensing lines generated US$302.9 million in sales compared to US$425 million sold in spas and salons, according to market research provided by Kline & Company. Healthcare and insurance companies frequently deny coverage for prescribed topical medications, making office dispensing a value added service for patients. As an extension to in-office dispensing, many physicians offer products for on-line purchase, making continuity easier for patients. Office-dispensed cosmeceuticals often contain higher concentrations of active ingredients than those available at mass market, making them more beneficial but also potentially more problematic. Nurses and estheticians can be helpful in instructing patients on proper product use and in providing information on how to treat complications should they arise.

While most patients view office dispensing as a value-added service, the dispensing physician must exercise extreme caution to keep the patient's best interest ahead of financial gain. Ethical conflicts occur when physicians are overly promotional, putting undue pressure on patients to buy products. It is important to dispense only products that have scientific validity, are clinically tested, and reasonably priced. Be familiar with retail alternatives should patients choose to purchase elsewhere. Private labeling has become increasingly popular with dispensing physicians and care should be taken to ensure that these products are not misrepresented as being physician developed or invented.

Efficacy and safety

Consumers seek products that are safe and effective. They prefer products that are fragrance-free, hypoallergenic, paraben-free, natural and green. They want products that are not animal-tested, favoring those with human clinical testing behind them. Responding to this demand, leading cosmetic companies are performing more extensive clinical testing than in years past although many studies do not meet rigorous scientific standards. Recently several major consumer companies have tested cosmeceuticals against leading prescription products. In these studies, achieving parity with prescription products bodes well with educated consumers and makes for strong marketing claims.

In spite of their long term safety profile, some consumers continue to have concerns about the safety of cosmeceuticals. Questions about the safety of nanoparticles, potential sensitizers and alleged carcinogens force many to seek natural and organic options. Natural cosmeceuticals refer to those with natural ingredients and are not necessarily organic. Examples of natural ingredients include aloe vera, vitamin C, soy and oatmeal. In order for a skin care product to be called organic, it must meet the new standards set by the U.S. Department of Agriculture agency in 2005. Organic skin care products must contain at least 95% organic ingredients, meaning that they were obtained from plants that were grown following organic farming guidelines. Organic crops must be grown without pesticides, hormones and chemical products, and may not plant genetically modified crops. They must also avoid any contamination during the processing of organic products. There is no scientific evidence to confirm that organic skin care products are safer or more beneficial than conventional products.

There are several excellent sources for consumers on product safety. The Cosmetic Toiletries and Fragrance Association (CTFA), now called the Personal Care Products Council, remains a trusted source on product safety. The Cosmetic Ingredient Review (CIR), a subsidiary of the Personal Care Products Council, reviews individual ingredients and determines their safety based on studies and data that are available. Information from both of these agencies is readily available on their websites and provides a valuable resource for both physicians and consumers.

Conclusion

Cosmeceuticals are now an integral part of the practice of aesthetic medicine. Physicians and their staff must be knowledgeable in order to advise patients on proper product selection and best practices. This unique category of products gives patients access to cosmetics containing beneficially active ingredients that can be used to improve the skin's appearance and treat dermatological diseases. As physicians we need to be vigilant to ensure that products recommended or sold by us are fully tested to ensure both safety and efficacy.

Further reading

Baumann L. Organic skin care. *Skin Allergy News* January 2007; 24–25.

Brandt FS, Cazzaniga A, Hann M. Cosmeceuticals: Current trends and market analysis. *Sem Cut Med Surg* 2011; **30**: 141–143.

Bruce S. Cosmeceuticals for the attenuation of extrinsic and intrinsic photoaging. *J Drugs Dermatol* 2008; **7** (2 suppl.): s 17–22.

Farris PK. Office dispensing: A responsible approach. *Sem Cut Med Surg* 2000; **19**: 195–200.

Frank NJ, Matts PJ, Ertel KD. Maintenance of healthy skin: Cleansing, moisturization and ultraviolet protection. *Journ Cosm Derm* 2007; **6**: 7–11

Ho ET, Trookman NS, Sperber BR, et al. A randomized, double-blind, controlled comparative trial of the anti-aging properties of non-prescription tri-retinol 1.1% vs. prescription tretinoin 0.025%. *Journ Drug Derm* 2012; **11**: 64–69.

Kligman AM. Why cosmeceuticals? *Cosmet Toiletries* 1993; **108**: 37–38.

Rokhsar CK, Lee S, Fitzpatrick RE. Review of photorejuvenation; devices, cosmeceuticals, or both? *Dermatol Surg* 2005; **31**; 1166–1178.

Sadick N. Cosmeceuticals: their role in dermatology practice. *Jour Drug Derm* 2003; **2**: 529–537.

U.S. Food and Drug Administration online reference of Federal Food Drug and Cosmetic Act available at: www.fda.gov.

PART I
Development, Formulation and Evaluation of Cosmeceuticals

CHAPTER 2

Bench to Beauty Counter: Development of Cosmeceuticals

Alexandra Kowcz[1], Guenther Schneider[2], Wolfgang Pape[2], and Teresa M. Weber[1]

[1]Beiersdorf Inc., Wilton, CT, USA
[2]Beiersdorf AG, Hamburg, Germany

Introduction

The development of cosmeceuticals is a complex process which involves multiple disciplines to achieve a safe, effective product that is acceptable to the consumer. Cosmeceuticals pass through many stages in the course of their development, from idea generation to final market launch. These steps are identified in Figure 2.1 and briefly outlined below.

The starting point is consumer insights and market research. This research is critical to understand consumer needs and the drivers of consumer behavior, well beyond what the consumers are able to articulate themselves. Market analysis reveals the potential demand for a new cosmeceutical product, a number of concepts are drafted to encompass the cornerstones of the idea, and the requirements profile is developed. By translating these findings into precise dermatological, chemical and physical terms, the product development team evaluates potential ingredients and product forms to create the first prototypes.

Important product characteristics of the prototype(s) are compared to the most accepted consumer product concept, and optimized for any necessary adaptations. To bring a final formulation to a fully marketable product requires a battery of stability, skin compatibility, and claim substantiation tests and the manufacturing of the final formulation.

Foundation for the development process

In-depth skin knowledge: prerequisite to cosmeceutical development

The development of cosmeceuticals is based on a deep knowledge of the skin, its biology, its chemistry, its mechanics, and how to treat various

Cosmeceuticals and Cosmetic Practice, First Edition. Edited by Patricia K. Farris.
© 2014 John Wiley & Sons, Ltd. Published 2014 by John Wiley & Sons, Ltd.

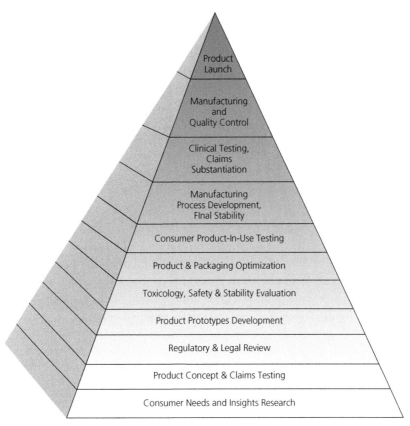

Figure 2.1 Concept to product launch process.

skin problems. Consumer characterization is an essential part of this process and covers a wide range of parameters. Skin type classification is a good starting point, with dry, oily, normal, or combination of dry and oily, as common types. Complex mechanisms influence the skin type, such as gender, age, hormonal status, and ethnic background. Skin changes over time and elderly people quite often experience very dry skin conditions. Similarly, hormonal changes, particularly in women during different stages of life, such as menopause, need to be taken into account. Ethnic background is also important, as different skin phototypes show varying sensitivity to UV light, resulting in different degrees of sunburn, tanning or photoaging, which can thus indirectly impact the efficacy of active ingredients. Finally, climate (temperature, humidity, seasonal changes), food and lifestyle have a profound, long-term influence on the skin.

From consumer insights to product idea

The changing landscape of consumer insights, leading to new product ideas, is exemplified by the sunscreen category. Originally, the predominant product forms were lotions and creams. Due to the market demand for higher SPF levels, product formulations required a higher usage of sunscreen actives, resulting in products that were often sticky, oily and unpleasant to use. The industry challenge was to launch sunscreens with both excellent protection properties and pleasant aesthetics. Existing low viscosity sunscreen lotions were perceived by consumers to have a better skin feel than the higher viscosity products. This consumer insight opened the door to a novel technology which led to the development of sprayable lotions. Although the UV filters were still the same, completely new formula bases and customized packaging had to be developed. Currently, these sprayable sunscreen products are well established, cosmetically elegant, and preferred by many consumers. This highlights the importance of translating consumer insights into an aesthetically pleasing and effective product technology.

Regulatory and legal considerations

When developing a product, there are many regulatory considerations that must be taken into account, including product composition, category (based on intended use), claims and labeling, and manufacturing. The US Food and Drug Administration (FDA) has jurisdiction over the safety, efficacy, and quality of cosmetics, drugs [Rx and OTC (Over the Counter)], medical devices and food. The Federal Trade Commission (FTC) regulates truth in advertising and marketing, and oversees business practices to protect the consumer from fraud and deception.

Cosmetics and drugs marketed in the USA must comply with the Food, Drug and Cosmetic (FDC) Act and the regulations codified in Title 21, Code of Federal Regulations. Color additives are regulated by the 1960 Color Additive Amendment to the FDC Act, and must be approved by the FDA for their specific usage.

A product's category (as cosmetic or drug) is defined by the claimed or intended uses, and in some cases, the product composition. The FDC Act defines cosmetics as

> articles intended to be rubbed, poured, sprinkled or sprayed on or introduced into or otherwise applied to the human body or any part thereof for cleansing, beautifying, promoting attractiveness or altering the appearance and articles intended for use as a component of any such articles, except that such term shall not include soap.

Drugs are defined as "articles intended for use in the diagnosis, treatment, or prevention of disease in man ... and articles intended to affect the structure or any function of the body of man."

OTC drugs have a structural and/or functional effect on the skin. The FDA has determined that the consumer is capable of diagnosing their need, and can safely treat their condition with these drugs without the direction of a physician. The FDA has published monographs that stipulate the rules and requirements for the manufacture and marketing of many OTC drug categories (e.g. Skin Protectant, Sunscreens, Acne, External Analgesics, etc.). These documents define approved active ingredients and their percentages, labeling requirements (indications, warnings, directions) and allowable claims. The regulatory requirements related to drugs are more extensive than those for cosmetics.

The differentiation of a cosmetic and a drug based on a structure/function effect was legally established in 1938 (FDC Act). Since that time, the knowledge of skin physiology and the effects of topical formulations has greatly progressed. Dr. Albert Kligman first popularized the term "cosmeceutical" in recognition of the impact that some cosmetic products may have on the skin structure and/or skin function. However, the FDA does not recognize "cosmeceuticals" and continues to regulate based on the 1938 definition.

The FDA has far-reaching authority: they can act against false, deceptive or misleading claims on labeling, deceptive packaging, adulterated and/or misbranded products, and product safety and quality issues; they can request that a company voluntarily recall drugs and cosmetic products due to concerns over safety; they can embargo imported products, and they have the authority to conduct periodic audits to monitor compliance with US statutes.

The FTC regulates the advertising of products, including claims made on websites, and those of spokespersons and testimonials included in various sponsored media channels. This regulatory body also monitors unfair competition methods, and unfair or deceptive practices affecting the consumers, and has the authority to levy fines.

Patents and trademarks

Patent protection is a basic right mentioned in the US Constitution and plays an important role in business success, serving as a strategic tool. In the USA, a patent is granted by the US Patent and Trademark Office (USPTO), and provides a means by which inventors can exclude others from using the invention described in the claims in the granted patent for a period of 20 years. Patents comprise a major part of a company's intellectual property (IP), which can be licensed and sold, and increase a company's overall value.

Patents play an integral role in the product development process and need to be carefully considered before the development process moves forward. Conducting extensive patent searches to gauge the patent landscape is critical to prevent a patent infringement lawsuit. Thus, "right to market" and "freedom to operate" are key goals for product manufacturers.

Trademarks are signs, symbols or specific indicators used to uniquely identify products or services. Registered trademarks, indicated by the ® symbol, are also approved and issued by the USPTO. The TM symbol represents a mark for which an application is pending; however, it is not yet approved and registered.

The science of formulation chemistry: product prototypes development

Actives and topical formulation bases

Many cosmetic manufacturers have extensive research programs dedicated to identifying, testing and selecting efficacious ingredients that impart a broad spectrum of skin benefits. Careful selection of active ingredients is critical to the overall product design. To fully leverage the efficacy of these actives, an appropriate formula base needs to be constructed. Actives and inactive ingredients in the formula are closely linked so that the development of a suitable base is just as important as the proper selection of the actives. This is a complicated balancing act, for many actives are difficult to incorporate into a base formula. Not only do they have to be stable in the base over a defined shelf life, but once applied on the skin, the actives need to be easily released from the formula matrix to stay on the skin surface or penetrate into the skin, depending on their function. In-depth knowledge of the human skin barrier is essential to understanding how physicochemical properties of the active can impact percutaneous absorption.

By utilizing modern delivery systems, such as microencapsulation or solubilization techniques, bioavailability and efficacy of the active can be optimized. Examples are liposomes, cyclodextrins, solid lipid nanoparticles and micro/nanoemulsions.

Some active ingredients also have the potential to irritate the skin, if not properly formulated. These undesirable side effects can lead to skin incompatibilities (e.g. redness or burning sensation), and should be minimized.

A comprehensive formulation strategy encompasses the collective knowledge of an interdisciplinary team to leverage proven methodologies, established know-how, as well as state-of-the art technology. The starting point is a technological SWOT (strength, weakness, opportunity, threat) analysis of the active with regard to the desired beneficial action on the skin. This well-known business analysis tool can help identify favorable and unfavorable factors to guide the creation of an outstanding product. For example, an oxygen-sensitive active could exhibit very good efficacy in pristine form (strength), but is rapidly degraded by oxygen (weakness). Antioxidants and an oxygen impermeable package could be used to mitigate this weakness.

The success of a cosmeceutical depends on its ability to improve a dermatological condition and is dependent on consumer compliance.

Appealing aesthetics or sophisticated textures impact how the consumer perceives the product and promotes reapplication rate, an essential factor to achieving the desired efficacy. The final product characteristics, such as color, texture, appearance, odor, viscosity and skin feel are therefore all important to the quality and consumer acceptance of a final product.

Inactive ingredients and product forms

The inactive ingredients in topical formulations have versatile functions, influencing the sensory properties of the product, their fundamental skincare properties, as well as the delivery of actives. They can be combined in different ways to achieve a variety of forms, ranging from aqueous hydrogels to water-free oils or powders, aerosols, foams, suspensions, and other colloidal systems. The most important colloidal systems for cosmeceuticals are emulsions with two predominant types: oil-in-water emulsions (o/w), where oil droplets are finely dispersed in water (water determines the main properties), and water-in-oil emulsions (w/o), where water droplets are finely dispersed in oil (oil determines the main properties).

If not properly stabilized, the incompatible phases (e.g. oil and water) of thermodynamically unstable emulsions start to separate during storage. However, when an *emulsifier* is added to the system, the droplets remain dispersed, and a stable emulsion is obtained. Typically, non-ionic or anionic emulsifiers are the stabilizers of choice. However, certain emulsion systems can be very complex (e.g. supramolecular gel structures or multi-phase systems).

Besides emulsifiers, different groups of *polymers* are employed as stabilizers or thickeners. Examples are xanthan gum, a high molecular weight polysaccharide produced by microbial fermentation, and polyacrylic acid cross-linked at different levels.

Another diverse ingredient class is *lipids*. Representatives of this class are: solid, semi-solid and liquid hydrocarbons, natural oils and waxes, fatty acid esters, partially hydrogenated or modified triglycerides, derivatives of fatty acids or fatty alcohols, and silicones. Lipids are not only important solubilizers for lipophilic actives, but also have an immediate impact on the skin feel during and after product application. The optimal combination of lipids is crucial to creating a formulation with attractive sensory properties.

Additional important *additives* in cosmeceutical products are preservatives to protect against microbial spoilage of the product, antioxidants to stabilize ingredients susceptible to oxidation, chelating agents to capture traces of certain metal ions to stop pro-oxidative effects of metal ions and prevent discolorations, and organic acids and bases to regulate the pH. Fragrances provide a pleasant scent and colors are added to enhance the product aesthetics.

Toxicology, safety and stability evaluation

In most countries, safety assessment of new finished products is a basic requirement and often has to be documented for legal purposes in a dossier, that is, the product information package which must be provided on request to certain regulatory entities.

In the USA, the FDA enforces the Food, Drug, Cosmetic Act (FDC Act) which mandates that cosmetic manufacturers must substantiate the safety of ingredients and products before they are marketed [21CFR 740.10 (a)]. In the European Union, the EU Cosmetics Directive regulates the safety of cosmetics.

Toxicological evaluation

Ideally, the starting point for the safety assessment of a cosmeceutical is the toxicological profile of each ingredient, evaluating the risk of application to healthy human skin under normal and foreseeable use conditions. The target group's age, exposure, and use conditions need to be considered carefully, in particular, if inhalative or oral exposure cannot be ruled out during or after product application.

Of central importance is to determine whether critical ingredients might become systemically available. Mechanisms of bio-availability, influenced by physical and chemical ingredient properties and metabolic processes within the skin, establish the relationship between the topical product application and the possible systemic burden. Therefore, the assessor needs to evaluate robust data about the dermal absorption of the product ingredients and their systemic burden and toxicological profile to calculate the margin of safety. These combined data serve to estimate and predict the safe use of a new product.

In many countries, expert panels review and determine the safe use of cosmetic ingredients such as UV filters, preservatives, colorants, and numerous other ingredients. Risk evaluations for these materials are published and made publicly available by these groups including the Cosmetic Ingredient Review Committee in the USA, and the European Commission Scientific Committee for Cosmetic Products in the European Union. These documents, in conjunction with a manufacturer's in-house testing data and expertise, are relied upon for the safety assessment and risk characterization of ingredients and newly developed finished products.

Safety of finished formulations

In addition to toxicological assessment, preliminary safety testing is conducted before progressing to skin tolerance and compatibility testing (which is evaluated in panels of human volunteers). In Europe, animal testing has been a topic of public discussion for many years and is legally forbidden. This has led to extensive research and development for validated and accepted alternatives throughout the world (e.g. animal-free in vitro testing methodologies) which are in use today. These methods have greatly enhanced the ability to recognize potential hazards, and to identify concentrations of ingredients that are likely not to elicit adverse dermal responses. Thus, a preliminary judgment about the tolerability of a specific composition of materials on intact healthy skin can be made, which finally needs to be confirmed by appropriate testing on human volunteers.

Skin tolerance and compatibility testing

Testing on human volunteers is subsequently conducted to assess skin tolerance after a single application and also after repeated applications. For this purpose, human patch tests, using standardized protocols, are often employed. In brief, a specific volume of product is applied to an occlusive or semi-occlusive patch which is then usually applied to the back. After a specified time, the patch is removed, the skin site is clinically graded for objective irritation (e.g. erythema, papules, pustules, bullae, weeping, etc.), and a subsequent patch is applied to the same site. The most commonly employed protocols are designed to evaluate the potential for cumulative contact irritancy, allergic sensitization, and the potential for photo-toxic responses or sun-induced allergic sensitization. They differ in the frequency and number of patch applications, and whether UV exposure is incorporated into the protocol. Variants of these patch tests and controlled use tolerability testing are also often conducted to evaluate other indicators of product mildness and acceptability for the general population and/or specific subpopulations.

Microbiology

Many product formulations support the growth of harmful microorganisms and, therefore, must be adequately preserved to insure quality over the shelf life and protect against contamination during consumer use. The efficacy of a preservation system is typically proven by means of microbiological challenge tests. Product test specimens are inoculated with test microorganisms (bacteria, mold and yeast) followed by periodic determination of viable microorganism counts, with clearly defined "pass and fail" criteria.

Stability

Chemical and physical stability testing of a product is an integral part of the development process. Its purpose is to ensure that the product meets the intended quality criteria, as well as functionality and aesthetics, when used and stored under normal or foreseeable conditions. Commonly used test conditions for physical and chemical stability are long-term storage at controlled room temperature, stress testing over several months at high and low temperatures, freeze–thaw cycles, as well as light exposure tests. Testing in the final package material is also performed to insure product/package compatibility.

Many stability-indicating parameters are monitored over time, such as viscosity, color, odor, texture, pH, particle size, and conductivity, as well as the analytical analysis of any active ingredients to predict product shelf life.

Product and packaging optimization

The final cosmeceutical formulation is subjected to various tests, including analytical testing of key ingredients, stability testing, and microbiological challenge testing. Once the formula has passed these tests, the package design, package engineering and product development teams determine the most appropriate package material (glass, plastic, metal) and container/ closure system. Product/package testing is conducted to insure the package not only dispenses the product, but also protects the product from adverse factors, and delivers the functionality, cost parameters, and package-specific marketing claims. Testing is conducted according to standardized procedures and the results confirm the integrity of the primary packaging and labeling, and insure the final quality of the product and package.

Consumer product-in-use testing

In-home usage testing is a necessary step to test the final product with consumers before launching a product. Consumers use the product as directed in their home environment and answer questions designed to capture the consumers' impressions and experiences. Product appeal and purchase intent are two key parameters that predict consumer accept-ability of the product. Overall satisfaction with the product and assessment of specific product attributes lead to further improvement to insure product acceptance.

Clinical testing, claims substantiation

Many well-established protocols are used by manufacturers to provide adequate and reasonable substantiation of the safety and effectiveness of various products prior to marketplace introduction. Efficacy testing of cos-metic products varies widely, depending on the claimed product benefits. Blind, double-blind, and open-label test designs may be used in controlled usage studies. They often incorporate both *expert clinical grading* of vari-ous skin parameters and objective instrumental *bioengineering methods* to evaluate skin status and facilitate statistical comparisons relative to vehi-cle controls or other comparative treatments, a pre-treatment state, an untreated control site, or comparisons among study timepoints. In the case of expert clinical grading, a variety of defined numeric scales are used to dimensionalize visual assessments: a specific skin parameter using a severity scale; the degree of improvement from the pre-treatment condition (e.g. worse, no change, improved, resolved); the presence or absence of a symptom; the surface area of involvement (e.g. eczema area and severity index), to rank the efficacy of various treatments or timepoints, or to characterize a specific progressive condition (e.g. xerosis) using specified, graduated descriptive scales.

Bioengineering methods use specialized instrumentation and procedures to make sensitive and reproducible measurements of numerous factors to assess skin condition and determine changes with product usage. There are dozens of bioinstrumental methods in use, such as electrical capacitance and/or resistance measurements of skin hydration, evaporimeters that assess transepidermal water loss, dermal torque meters, balistometers and cutometers that evaluate skin tensile properties such as elasticity and firmness, IR devices to assess skin temperature, and chromameters that evaluate skin redness or darkness. Skin oiliness and the presence of flakes are evaluated using specialized adhesive tapes that are applied to the skin. Features and properties of the skin below the stratum corneum can be assessed on live subjects using methods such as Confocal Microscopy, Optical Coherence Tomography, Far and Near Infra-red Spectroscopy, Nuclear Magnetic Resonance Spectroscopy, as well as other sophisticated optical and spectrographic methods.

Image analysis of visual information using computer algorithms facilitates the assessment of videomicroscopic images of the skin surface and digital clinical photographs taken under normal, polarized, fluorescent, and ultraviolet light conditions. Fringe or shadow projection techniques have been developed to assess skin topography (e.g. for wrinkle depth measurements or to quantify conditions such as cellulite intensity) of the live subject or skin replicas.

In addition to methods used to evaluate product effects on live subjects, biochemical, histological and biophysical assessments can be made using excised skin biopsies. All of these sophisticated methods strive for quantitative, sensitive and reproducible measurements to enhance testing options beyond what can be evaluated solely by clinical observation. However, robust demonstrations of product efficacy often employ clinical and instrumental evaluations, as well as subject self-perception parameters.

Subject self-assessment questionnaires can be used in a clinical study design (with product applications either in the clinic or at home in accordance with the study protocol) or in consumer home in-use tests (product use under real-life conditions). Clinical tests often query subjective irritation parameters (stinging, burning, itching, tightness, and tingling). These tests also often evaluate consumer perception of product aesthetics and functional benefits, one of the key aims of consumer home in-use testing.

The methods described above represent only a fraction of the test methods that are currently employed to evaluate the safety and efficacy of topically applied products. As the body of global scientific knowledge grows to unparalleled historical levels, so will the various protocols and methods that will be employed.

Manufacturing and quality control

The scale-up process begins with a series of lab batches, leading to mid-size pilot plant batches and successful full-scale production batches. Various product properties (e.g. viscosity, droplet distribution) are affected by changes in scale, and are dependent on many manufacturing variables or factors (e.g. mixing equipment and procedures, raw material quality, order of raw material addition, heating and cooling times, shear forces during manufacturing, etc.). Trial production batches are made prior to commercialization of the formula, and stability testing is critical to determine which actual processing conditions may have impacted the final product. Many intensive process reiterations are required to achieve a final, controlled process. The final production process is then validated according to cGMPs (current Good Manufacturing Practices) and quality control testing is conducted to insure a high quality product.

Conclusion

The complex development process of cosmeceuticals is both a science and an art involving multiple stages and many different disciplines. A number of key factors must be evaluated and considered to insure the final product is both efficacious and aesthetically pleasing to the end user. From the initial consumer insights to the final product launch, many steps are taken to deliver a safe, effective product that delivers the desired product benefits. The final product launch is the culmination of years of scientific research, numerous product optimizations, extensive stability, safety, clinical and consumer testing, various quality tests, legal/regulatory evaluations, and marketing claims substantiation. Cosmeceuticals are a fast-paced and continuously evolving area of research driven by the competitive marketplace, changing trends and high consumer expectations. New technologies, more effective formulations, and great advances in skin research will offer a bright future for this growing segment.

Further reading

Buell DS, Barclay KW, Block P, Crissian CA, Junker J, Melenkevitz DJ, Douglas J, Rotando JL, Van Ael RM, Victor BL, Yacko DP. The manufacture of cosmetics.

In: Rieger M (ed.) *Harry's Cosmeticology*, 8th edn. New York: Chemical Publishing, 2000, 787–874.

Draelos ZD. Formulation for special populations. In: Draelos ZD, Thaman LA (eds.) *Cosmetic Formulation of Skin Care Products*. New York: Taylor & Francis Group, 2006, 27–34.

Eccleston GM. Multiple-phase oil-in-water emulsions. *J Soc Cosmet Chem* 1990; **41**(1): 1–22.

Hyman PM, Rodriguez SN. Regulation of labeling and advertising claims. In: Estrin NF, Akerson JM (eds.) *Cosmetic Regulation in a Competitive Environment*. New York: Marcel Dekker, 2000, 43–53.

Jackson EM. Irritation and sensitization. In: Waggoner WC (ed.) *Clinical Safety and Efficacy Testing of Cosmetics*. New York: Marcel Dekker, 1990, 23–42.

Kligman AB. Cosmeceuticals: A broad-spectrum category between cosmetics and drugs. In: Elsner P, Maibach HI (eds.) *Cosmeceuticals and Active Cosmetics: Drugs vs. Cosmetics*, 2nd edn. Boca Raton, FL: Taylor & Francis Group, 2005, 1–8.

Orth DS. The keys to successful product preservation. In: *Insights into Cosmetic Microbiology*. Carol Stream, IL: Allured Publishing, 2010, **27–43**, 90–107.

Papakostas D, Rancan F, Sterry W, Blume-Peytavi U, Vogt A. Nanoparticles in dermatology. *Arch Dermatol Res* 2011; **303**(8): 533–550.

Taylor SC. Skin of color: Biology, structure, function, and implications for dermatologic disease. *J Am Acad Dermatol* 2002; **46**(2 Suppl.): S41–S62.

Wiechers JW, Souto EB. Delivering actives via solid lipid nanoparticles and nanostructured lipid carriers: Part III, Stability and efficacy. *Cosmetics & Toiletries* 2012; **127**(3): 164–173.

CHAPTER 3

Evaluating Cosmeceuticals

David H. McDaniel[1,2,3,4], Christina Steel[1,3], and Chris Mazur[1]

[1] McDaniel Institute of Anti-Aging Research/Laser & Cosmetic Center, Virginia Beach, VA, USA
[2] Eastern Virginia Medical School, Norfolk, VA, USA
[3] Old Dominion University, Norfolk, VA, USA
[4] Hampton University, Hampton, VA, USA

Introduction

Recent years have shown a dramatic increase in the number of cosmeceuticals being marketed, but no clear, industry standard protocol exists for safety and efficacy testing. Each company goes about demonstrating data to support claims in a different way resulting in the inability to do very few direct comparisons. This results in many examples of scientific and ethical questions that come from nonstandard test protocols and can cast doubt on cosmeceutical efficacy in general, which leads to a low acceptance rate in public opinion.

The very first use of the term "cosmeceutical" was coined by Dr. Albert Kligman who had a clear vision of three specific criteria that should be met in order to evaluate the proposed beneficial effect of a cosmeceutical product. Ironically, even though the originator had specific guidelines for product efficacy, upon review of the published results for some of the most popular products, very few fulfill all three criteria. The criteria proposed are not unreasonable, nor are they particularly difficult to fulfill. They are based on sound scientific principles similar to Koch's postulates for the identification of microbes. The three basic criteria to prove efficacy of a cosmeceutical compound, according to Dr. Kligman, are: (1) the active ingredient must penetrate the stratum corneum (SC) in sufficient concentrations to the intended target in a time frame consistent with the mechanism of action of the compound; (2) the ingredient should have a known specific biochemical mechanism of action in the target (skin, cell or tissue); and (3) statistically significant data from published, peer-reviewed, double-blind and placebo-controlled clinical trials sufficient to substantiate all the product's claims.

Briefly examining the three criteria, it is evident that these requirements for efficacy are logical and reasonable. The first criterion simply echoes the well-known facts about the stratum corneum serving as an efficient

Cosmeceuticals and Cosmetic Practice, First Edition. Edited by Patricia K. Farris.
© 2014 John Wiley & Sons, Ltd. Published 2014 by John Wiley & Sons, Ltd.

barrier mechanism for the skin which prevents proteins, sugars, peptides, nucleic acids and highly charged molecules with molecular weights over 1000 kDaltons from easily penetrating or being absorbed. Thus demonstrating the transport of the ingredient across such a barrier in the quantities needed to be biologically effective should be addressed. The second criterion addresses the need to demonstrate a known mechanism of action that allows for the physiological effect (activating/inhibiting gene expression, enzyme activity, cell cycle regulation, etc.). There are many popular ingredients that do not have clearly elucidated mechanisms of action or have incomplete mechanisms that require further study. Third, the clinical trials need to generate data with reproducible metrics that are statistically significant in both sample size and effect noted. Furthermore, the ideal study would be double-blind and vehicle-controlled so that there can be no bias introduced. Proper study design is one of the key factors missing in many of the published clinical trials for new ingredients (powders, cell extracts, cellular byproducts, etc.). Another common shortcoming is that the subject population is insufficient in size to make statistically valid conclusions.

As far as government regulatory agencies, the primary published guidelines speak not to efficacy, but to product safety and regulation of marketing claims. In both the published documents by the European SCCNFP (the Scientific Committee on Cosmetic Products and Non-Food Products Intended for Consumers in the EU and the FDA (the Food and Drug Administration) in the USA, there are detailed guidelines on how to test for various safety measures such as skin irritancy, and microbial content, but similar guidelines for efficacy are not to be found. In this chapter we will attempt to outline a procedure of testing from in vitro to human clinical trials (see Figure 3.1) that will demonstrate a variety of methods that both adhere to and expand on the scientific criteria for cosmeceutical effectiveness created by Dr. Kligman years ago.

In vitro evaluations

The initial testing of a cosmeceutical active ingredient ideally occurs in the laboratory and most often in cell cultures. Primarily human cells, of a type relative to the anticipated effects, for example, cultured human skin fibroblasts, serve as the basic cell for testing of most photoaging or skin care products. Other cell lines are used when the product has a more specific function, such as skin lightening (melanocytes) or hair growth stimulation (dermal papillae or whole hair follicles).

Using cultured human cells as the initial "test subject" is a cost-effective way to tie into later human testing. If a beneficial effect can be shown in a

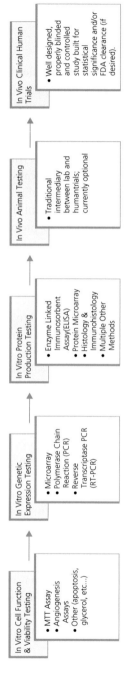

Figure 3.1 Outline of proposed testing protocol for evaluation of cosmeceuticals.

human cell (and also if a mechanism of action can be determined and meet the second criteria of cosmeceutical efficacy), it makes a more compelling, scientifically sound story when similar results are demonstrated in a human clinical trial.

Cell viability/function testing

The first series of tests that should be performed for any cosmeceutical active is to demonstrate there are no harmful effects when the compound is applied to the cells. This is most commonly done through cell viability testing. There are other tests involving measurement of a known product or marker related to cellular proliferation, angiogenesis, cell cycle/cellular proliferation and many other cellular processes. All of these tests will first help demonstrate that the compound is theoretically safe to use on humans (as evidenced by good results in the cell viability assays in cells related to the target tissue or application) and also will describe the effect(s) of the cosmeceutical on several cell functions or processes for relatively low cost. Briefly described below are some of the common testing methods that would aid in elucidating the mechanism of action and overall safety of a new cosmeceutical compound.

1 *The MTT assay:*   3-(4,5-Dimethylthiazol-2-yl)-2,5-diphenyltetrazolium bromide), is a tetrazolium salt that is reduced to a purple-colored formazan dye but only in living cells. This makes it an extremely useful tool for determining cytotoxicity in the cell cultures tested, as any decrease in quantity indicates a reduction in living cells and, when compared to untreated control samples, can be used to generate an approximate proportion of cell death. In contrast, an increase in formazan indicates a greater number of viable cells or increased proliferation.

2 *Angiogenesis assays:*   The process of angiogenesis is the generation of new capillary blood vessels. This is important in normal wound healing, as well as pathologies like diabetic retinopathy and tumor metastasis. Several in vitro tests exist, but most are based upon the principle of adding endothelial cells to an ECM-like matrix/gel in the presence of varying concentrations of the test compound and monitoring the rate and extent of the migration and tube formation of the added endothelial cells across the matrix. A recently developed in vitro test takes this one step further and allows for three-dimensional visualization of the full process of angiogenesis. By using embedded spheres of endothelial cells, the addition of an angiogenic compound will cause the spheres' tip cells to begin migrating and forming "sprouts" (equivalent to new blood vessels) which can then be measured for both number and length which can give an excellent measurement of the angiogenicity of the cosmeceutical.

3 *Other assays:* There are a large number of other assays that can be performed in vitro and can further help determine the mechanism of action of a particular cosmeceutical compound, but it is at this point that the assays must begin to be tailored to the specific tissue or desired effect that the compound is intended to have. Among the many additional tests which are readily available are: ATP production for cellular metabolism, metabolism of specific compounds like leptin, glycerol, etc., mitosis, DNA damage (useful for antioxidant compounds), mitochondrial membrane permeabilization states and many others.

Gene expression testing

The next step after determining any toxicity effects (as well as the maximum in vitro "safe" dosage) is to continue to examine the effects of the compound and look for any genetic expression or influence on signal transduction and related enzymes as a mechanism of action. The process would involve exposing target cells in the culture to concentrations of the active ingredient over a period of time and isolating DNA/RNA (depending upon the type of testing proposed) and comparing the results to untreated controls of the same duration. This generates a relative expression level for either: one gene, multiple genes, entire pathways of genes or the whole human genome (again, depending on the test). The results indicate if there is more or less mRNA (signal to the cell to create more of the protein(s) the gene encodes for) present in the treated cells, which would indicate either an upregulation (increased production) or downregulation (decreased production) of the genes studied. The availability of low cost genomic testing through multiple commercial labs or through in-house lab testing makes genetic expression studies both easy and vital to the evaluation of the efficacy of new cosmeceutical products.

The most effective method of genomic testing is the microarray, which can test a staggering number of genes (up to the entire human genome) all at once. These microarrays can be custom-designed (or are already commercially available) to focus on specific pathways relevant to the proposed mechanism of action for the compound. There are even microarrays that can be used to determine potential mechanisms of action by testing key markers of a variety of pathways for cellular processes, so that you can use the data to select a likely pathway (or pathways) that the compound may affect. Once that determination has been made, the specific mechanism of action or related genes can be studied and those results can confirm or refute the proposed mechanism of action as being valid for a cosmeceutical compound.

There are several overall types of microarray. In addition to the expression analysis arrays previously described, there are also CGH (Comparative

Genomic Hybridization) arrays which demonstrate the changes in the number of copies of a particular gene between samples; and the SNP (Single Nucleotide Polymorphism) arrays that determine if there are any mutations in the genetic sequence of a particular gene. This information is particularly useful in classifying disease states or pathologies and determining the potential for susceptibility to the same states. It is unlikely a cosmeceutical would directly alter anything these types of arrays measure, but they could be used to determine the genetic profile of the disease/pathology of the best responding subjects.

Alternatively, single gene PCR (or RT-PCR) can be performed, where only one gene is selected to be examined for genetic expression changes. While this can save time, it is only recommended that single gene PCR be used to confirm a specific hypothesis (such as, will treatment with this compound increase the gene expression of Collagen IA1?) or to be used as a sentinel marker for changes to concentration and formulation once both the mechanism of action and expected gene expression profile for a compound have been very well defined.

Protein production

Once testing for toxicity, cellular function and gene expression analysis has been completed, the next step in proving efficacy is to demonstrate that the observed changes in gene expression result in the actual production of the requisite protein. Gene expression simply determines the amount of mRNA the cell is receiving, post-translational modifications may occur and the protein is never actually created, so by verifying that both the gene signal is received and the protein itself is made, a strong scientific link can be made between the compound and efficacy.

One of the simplest methods for determining protein production is through the use of ELISA technology that detects protein content by binding the protein to a colorimetric or fluorescent reagent present in a 96-well dish and read using a spectrophotometer or fluorometer. The supernatant from the cell cultures treated with the compound is tested directly and concentrations of produced protein can be quantitated based on a standard curve run with the assay. This is perhaps the clearest evidence that the protein is being produced by the altered gene expression signals in the treated cells; in fact, the supernatant can be collected from the same experimental cells that yielded the microarray results.

Another method of determining protein production/deposition changes is through histochemical or immunohistochemical analysis of the protein. Commonly performed in ex vivo tissues, it is also possible to detect cellular proteins in in vitro cultures, as well as in cultured human tissue equivalents. Human tissue equivalents exist for a variety of tissue types and can be grown in a culture similar to cultured cells.

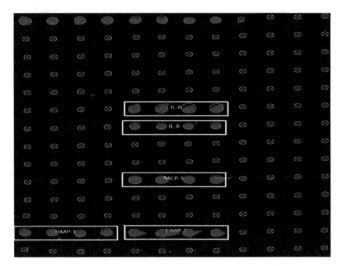

Figure 3.2 Image of protein array results showing several targeted proteins.

A relatively new method has been developed for testing protein production, and that is the protein microarray. Combining ELISA technology with the footprint and quantitation methods of microarrays, these new tests allow for the quantitation of large numbers of proteins to occur with one sample. (Sample image shown in Figure 3.2.) The arrays are also commonly pathway or disease-specific, for example, a set of inflammation proteins may comprise an Inflammatory Cytokine array and demonstrate a reduction in inflammatory markers following exposure to a cosmeceutical compound, further validating the mechanistic hypothesis of the tested compound.

There are many other methods of protein detection that can be used, such as gel zymography, flow cytometry, individual cell fluorescent imaging, etc. that are not discussed here. Indeed, the area of in vitro testing is expanding at a very rapid rate as the techniques become more advanced and less expensive. It is very possible that in vitro testing could become the dominant form of testing (evolving to the point of computer-modeled cellular responses to unknown compounds) of cosmeceutical compounds in the very near future.

In vivo evaluations

Once the in vitro testing is completed, the next steps are to design a study in vivo. The two main options for in vivo work are the animal model and a human clinical trial. While there are pros and cons to each method, both should be carefully designed, using the appropriate controls, safeguards and review committees to provide statistically valid data while protecting the human subjects and ensuring humane treatment of the animal subjects. Animal studies are usually an intermediate step between the lab and human trials and rarely (if ever) replace a solidly designed human clinical study of the near final cosmeceutical product.

By designing statistically valid studies, good scientific data can be generated in real-world application models that support the mechanistic claims and data discovered in vitro. In this way the action of the cosmeceutical can be traced at the cellular level, from gene expression to active protein production which is then verified with clinical results in human or animal subjects and creates solid evidence that the cosmeceutical is efficacious for a particular use.

Animal testing

Traditionally the testing phase between the lab and the human clinical trial was an animal model. In recent years the negative publicity involved in using animals to test cosmeceutical products has far outweighed any possible gains. In fact, many large cosmetic companies now have standard operating procedures that prohibit the use of animal testing of any kind in order to mitigate the bad publicity/protests and make the "No animal testing" claims for marketing purposes. It is mainly because of those reasons, as well as the expansion of the in vitro testing capabilities that many of the traditional animal testing models are superfluous for most common cosmeceutical items, and only in the case of a specialized form of testing are animal models the only testing methodology available.

Safety testing of final formulations

The formulation to be tested in human trials should be sufficiently tested before being used on humans. Unfortunately there is no universal set of tests to determine safety and, in many cases, stability. The FDA allows the use of previously established toxicology data of the individual components of a formulation as well as similar composition of formulations to be sufficient. For example, vitamin C has well-documented stability and toxicology testing so formulations using equivalent concentrations of vitamin C can tie safety to the previously established data. It is often the case that well-established, or GRAS (generally recognized as safe) compounds, have data already on file.

If the composition/formulation contains new compounds, it is up to the individual formulator to determine how best to prove, per the FDA guidelines, the safety and stability of the compound. The most common are RIPT (Repeat Insult Patch Test in 50–200 subjects), phototoxicity/photoallergy (typically for compositions containing a scent or UV-absorbing element), microbiological testing (to ensure there are no contaminants in

Figure 3.3 outline:

Safety
- Toxicology
- Repeat Insult Patch Test
- Microbiological testing
- Photoallergy
- Phototoxicity

Stability (all of these tests use the endpoints of pH, viscosity, odor and color as primary endpoints)
- 90 day stability test (at 45°C)
- Accelerated stability test (using higher temperatures and shorter durations)
- Cycle testing (from −10°C to 45°C)

Figure 3.3 Types of safety and stability testing.

the formulation), and various stability test models (to ensure the formula stays active and mixed throughout the shelf life of the product) (Figure 3.3).

Human clinical trials

Human clinical trials require IRB (Institutional Review Board) oversight and it is vital that all protections for human subjects are followed, as well as adhering to Good Clinical Practices (GCP) standards. Studies of these types are best handled by Certified Clinical Research Professionals and Coordinators to ensure that not only IRB requirements, human subject concerns, and in the case of products looking for FDA approval, all FDA requirements are met; including reporting of data and storage of the same.

Study design

Once the proper clinical staff have been established, the focus should be on proper study design. There are many clinical studies available in the literature on a variety of cosmeceutical products, but on further inspection many show poor study design that does not produce statistically significant results and read more like a collection of case studies or anecdotal evidence. The factors contributing to a well-designed study are (Figure 3.4):

1 Determination of sample size to generate statistically significant data sufficient to demonstrate efficacy of the product. The determination of the sample size can be quite difficult to accurately determine as it is based on the size of the overall population to be studied and requires an involved mathematical formula that has many factors, such as desired Confidence Interval of the statistics (e.g. a 95% Confidence Interval is basically an assurance that there is a 95% chance that the results did not occur randomly), degree of accuracy, and desired margin of error. In designing a study for FDA approval, the FDA may set the

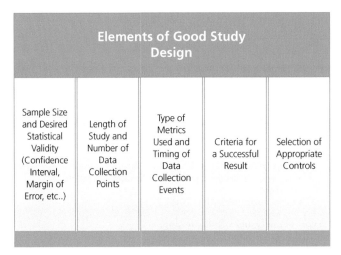

Figure 3.4 Elements of good clinical study design to ensure proper scientific validity in cosmeceutical trials.

required sample size; as a general rule of thumb, it is best to think about the expected level of change the cosmeceutical product is expected to produce (another reason extensive in vitro testing becomes vital). If the product is going to produce low level, subtle changes, than a larger sample size is required. Typically only relatively dramatic changes can be statistically proven with the small sample sizes common to many cosmeceutical studies.

2 After the sample size has been determined, the next critical decision is to determine the length of the study and how many data collection points will be used. In looking at the first of these variables, it becomes important to determine what will be the expected results of treatment with the cosmeceutical (again the extensive in vitro testing can be vital here). For instance, in studying a product designed to increase collagen, one must ensure that the study lasts long enough for the production of new collagen to occur and accumulate to clinically significant levels. Second, the study must include a follow-up period (a certain time span following treatment when the subject does not apply the product) to determine if the results can still be detected using the selected metrics. This period is sometimes termed a "washout period." This allows the product's results to be classified as temporary (3–12 weeks) or permanent (12 months or greater). Finally, the length of time the participant subjects will continue in the study without dropping out should also be a factor.

3 Another aspect of study design is determining which metrics will be used and the timing of those metrics. All good studies will have baseline and post-treatment measurements at a minimum. It is often useful to

collect data at points in the interim (commonly the midpoint of the study) or at selected milestones (for example, after each individual treatment, after the first wave of treatments, or after a certain number of weeks) and are unique to each study. Further information on metrics is discussed in the following section.

4 Another part of the study design is to determine what will be considered a "successful" treatment. This can be simple or complex depending on the nature of the results to be studied and the metrics used. It can be as easy as determining that a subject improving one grade on a grading scale for a particular characteristic is considered a success, or as complicated as using specific values on a measurement tool (for example, a reduction of 25% in the value of the post-treatment sebum meter score relative to the baseline measurement). These should be reasonable criteria to meet for a cosmetic product.

5 The final aspect, and possibly most crucial to study design, is the selection of appropriate controls. In the case of a cosmeceutical study it is always preferable to have the subjects and investigator blinded to which subjects are receiving the actual treatment to prevent bias. This requires the use of a placebo group, which typically will be handled in exactly the same fashion as the treatment group, except for the presence of the active ingredient. Deciding to use, for example, split face versus matched subjects can be complex.

Common metrics

1 In assessing cosmeceutical effectiveness, probably the single most important data capture tool is digital imaging. The minimum a good study design should include is baseline and post-treatment photos. The minimum criteria for good clinical photos are pictures that are taken in standardized lighting conditions, from the same camera angle and distance from the subject, using the same camera (as each digital chip can have slightly different resolution which may obfuscate subtle results), and against the same color background (or zoomed in close enough that the background is not visible in the image). A well-matched set of pictures is the greatest selling point a product can have to the general public as well as the scientific community. There are many imaging systems that are commercially available that consist of a high resolution camera and an immobilization device designed to ensure the proper positioning for sequential images. Some of these imaging systems are also equipped with sophisticated image analysis packages that allow for counting of features (pore size, hair counts, etc.), evaluations of skin tone through Red and Brown image composition analysis, and even 3D imaging/modeling of the imaged area, allowing for controlled analysis of volume and textural changes.

2 The "Gold Standard" of metrics in cosmeceutical studies is still the blinded expert grader. In this case, the well-matched images are randomized and placed before an expert, or panel of experts, in cosmeceutical use and testing, who then evaluate each individual image based on the decided upon characteristics and scale used. This method is still the preferred method of evaluation favored by the FDA. The scales can often be designed specifically for each study; or can be scales that have been well characterized and used for years in the scientific literature. Examples of widely used/accepted cosmetic scales are the Fitzpatrick wrinkle severity, the Glogau photoaging classification scale, and the Ascher scale for volume loss.

3 As previously mentioned, there are a large number of instruments that can be used to measure a variety of conditions useful to proving efficacy in a cosmeceutical product. There are elasticity meters that can measure the resilience of the skin (such as the BTC2000); chromameters that can detect changes in skin tone, sebum meters that record total levels produced, ultrasound images that show thickness of skin, skin profilometry, and others too numerous to list. These instruments are not always universally considered "valid" and also different brands of equipment may not produce the same data, so care should be taken when designing the study to ensure that the data will be acceptable for all end uses.

4 Finally there are subject assessments, exit questionnaires, and treatment logs/diaries. While these can generate some useful data, it is quite easy to inadvertently or intentionally skew the results by limiting the choices a respondent has, or by the phrasing of the question. It is significantly more difficult to skew the treatment log/diary since this is where the subject will record the use of the product to ensure compliance with the study protocol. These diaries can also be used to have the subject assess irritancy or other variables on a daily or weekly basis. While providing a variety of useful data, these should not be used as a substitute for expert grader data, and this data should not be used to determine the efficacy of a cosmeceutical product.

Conclusion

In conclusion, the evaluation of a cosmeceuticals efficacy should be a well-defined and linear process that can demonstrate all three of the criteria initially described by Dr. Kligman: (1) the active ingredient must penetrate the stratum corneum (SC) in sufficient concentrations to the intended target in a time frame consistent with the mechanism of action of the compound; (2) the ingredient should have a known specific biochemical mechanism of action in the target (skin, cell or tissue); (3) statistically significant data should be generated from published, peer-reviewed, double-blind and placebo-controlled clinical trials sufficient to substantiate all the product's claims. This data would be presented and published in peer-reviewed forums and journals. By using the steps of testing outlined in this chapter, these criteria can be met using good scientific principles and clinical practice. This will lend greater weight to any claims of efficacy and will set a standard for all other cosmeceutical compounds to be held to, which will remove much of the doubt surrounding the launch of a new product or application.

Further reading

Ascher B, et al. Full scope of effect of facial lipoatrophy: A framework of disease understanding. *Dermatologic Surgery* 2006; **32**(8): 1058–1069.

Auxenfans C, et al. Evolution of three-dimensional skin equivalent models reconstructed in vitro by tissue engineering. *Eur J Dermatol* 2009; **19**(2): 107–113.

Bhattacharyya TK, et al. Profilometric and morphometric response of murine skin to cosmeceutical agents. *Arch Facial Plast Surg* 2009; **11**(5): 332–337.

Christensen ML, Braunstein TH, Treiman M. Fluorescence assay for mitochondrial permeability transition in cardiomyocytes cultured in a microtiter plate. *Anal Biochem* 2008; **378**(1): 25–31.

Clinical Trials. [web page] June 12, 2012 [cited 2012 July 30]; Available from: http://www.fda.gov/ScienceResearch/SpecialTopics/RunningClinicalTrials/default.htm.

Defining Pathway-Specific Genes. [web page] [cited 2012 July 30]; Available from: http://www.sabiosciences.com/newsletter/pathwayAnalysis.html.

Gerlier D, Thomasset N. Use of MTT colorimetric assay to measure cell activation. *Journal of Immunological Methods* 1986; **94**(1–2): 57–63.

GmbH, P. PromoCell-3D-Angiogenesis Assay. [web page] 2012 July 9, 2012 [cited 2012 July 30]; Available from: http://www.promocell.com/products/cell-model-systems/angiogenesis-assays-and-kits/3d-angiogenesis-assay/.

Guidance for Industry Safety of Nanomaterials in Cosmetic Products [DRAFT GUIDANCE], U.S.D.o.H.a.H. Services, Editor. 2012, U.S. Food and Drug Administration.

Hall DA, Ptacek J, Snyder M. Protein microarray technology. *Mech Ageing Dev* 2007; **128**(1): 161–167.

Kimmich GA, Randles J, Brand JS. Assay of picomole amounts of ATP, ADP, and AMP using the luciferase enzyme system. *Anal. Biochem. (United States)* 1975; **69**(1): 187–206.

Lachenbruch PA, Rask C. *Thirteen Clinical Trial Design Questions and Answers.* Bethesda, MD: National Institute of Allergy and Infectious Disease, 2005.

Levin J, Momin SB, How much do we really know about our favorite cosmeceutical ingredients? *J Clin Aesthet Dermatol* 2010; **3**(2): 22–41.

Monheit GD, et al. Development and validation of a 6-point grading scale in patients undergoing correction of nasolabial folds with a collagen implant. *Dermatol Surg* 2010; **36** (Suppl. 3:1809–1816.

Office of Clinical Research: Education & Training. [web page] June 21, 2012 [cited 2012 July 30]; Available from: http://health.usf.edu/research/ocr/education.htm.

Participating in Clinical Trials. [web page] January 7, 2010 [cited 2012 July 30]. Available from: http://www.fda.gov/ForConsumers/ByAudience/ForPatientAdvocates/ParticipatinginClinicalTrials/default.htm.

Pinkel D, et al. High resolution analysis of DNA copy number variation using comparative genomic hybridization to microarrays. *Nature Genetics* 1998; **20**: 207–211.

Rode H-J, Eisel D, Frost I (eds.) *Apoptosis, Cell Death and Cell Proliferation*, 3rd edn. Roche Applied Science, 2004.

Shoshani D, et al. The Modified Fitzpatrick Wrinkle Scale: a clinical validated measurement tool for nasolabial wrinkle severity assessment. *Dermatologic Surgery* 2008; **34**: S85–S91.

Suga H, et al. Numerical measurement of viable and nonviable adipocytes and other cellular components in aspirated fat tissue. *Plast Reconstr Surg* 2008; **122**(1): 103–114.

Vijayananthan A, Nawawi O. The importance of Good Clinical Practice guidelines and its role in clinical trials. *Biomedical Imaging and Intervention Journal* 2008; **4**(1): e5.

Wang DG, et al. Large-scale identification, mapping, and genotyping of single-nucleotide polymorphisms in the human genome. *Science* 1998; **280**(5366): 1077–1082.

Yosipovitch G, et al. Time-dependent variations of the skin barrier function in humans: transepidermal water loss, stratum corneum hydration, skin surface pH, and skin temperature. *Journal of Investigative Dermatology* 1998; **110**(1): 20–24.

CHAPTER 4

Modalities for Increasing Penetration

Zoe Diana Draelos
Duke University School of Medicine, Durham, NC, USA

Introduction

Penetration of active ingredients into the skin is key for cosmeceutical efficacy. While there are some substances that belong on the stratum corneum to function properly, others must reach the viable epidermis or dermis to work. Moisturizers, for example, must coat the stratum corneum to inhibit transepidermal water loss and create an environment for barrier repair. Similarly, sunscreens must remain on the skin surface to either reflect UV radiation, as is the case with inorganic filters, or absorb the UV radiation, as is the case with organic filters. Antioxidants, on the other hand, must reach viable skin structures in order to prevent the effect of damaging oxygen radicals. Ideally, Vitamins C and E should penetrate to the dermis where viable DNA must be protected by donation of an electron to a reactive oxygen species.

Ingredient penetration is facilitated by penetration enhancers, which can be either physical or chemical in nature. This chapter examines penetration enhancement and cosmeceuticals. It begins with emulsions, the most basic of formulations, and then examines methods of barrier degradation. More specific penetration enhancement techniques, such as liposomes and nanodelivery, are also examined.

Emulsions

The most basic time-tested delivery system is the emulsion. An emulsion is formed from oil and water, which are mixed and held in solution by an emulsifier. The most common emulsions are oil-in-water, where the oil is dissolved in the water. This emulsion is the most popular delivery system because the water evaporates, leaving behind a thin film of oily ingredients. This is the basis for all moisturizers, the main method of transferring cosmeceuticals to the skin surface. If a large quantity of water is found in the emulsion, it is considered a lotion, while a thicker emulsion with less water is considered a cream.

Creams and lotions are the main cosmeceutical delivery systems because they are inexpensive to produce. They also impart moisturizing qualities to the skin surface, one of the main methods used by cosmeceuticals to improve skin texture and appearance. Thus, carefully constructed emulsions can accomplish moisturization and delivery of an active agent simultaneously. Moisturization accounts for approximately 50–75% of the consumer-perceived benefits of any cosmeceutical, with the active ingredients playing a secondary role.

Beyond the emulsion delivering the cosmeceutical to the skin, active ingredients can penetrate through defects in the stratum corneum. There are several methods of inducing barrier degradation that are discussed next to include physical and chemical modalities.

Barrier degradation

Damaging the barrier is the cheapest and simplest method for penetration enhancement. This can be achieved by encouraging loss of the corneocytes through physical removal or chemical degradation of the intercorneocyte bonds. Physical removal can occur with microdermabrasion or facial brushing. Microdermabrasion bombards the skin with small particles sprayed at the skin forcefully to remove the corneocytes, which are then removed with suction. Cosmeceuticals applied following microdermabrasion will penetrate more deeply. This same effect can be achieved with rotary or sonicating facial brushes that can also remove corneocytes.

Barrier degradation can also be accomplished chemically with substances that blow apart the stratum corneum. The most common penetration enhancer used in topical pharmaceuticals is propylene glycol. While propylene glycol can damage the stratum corneum and allow penetration, it also can cause barrier damage, leading to patient-perceived stinging, itching, and burning. This is why many lotions and creams cause noxious sensory stimuli when applied immediately after shaving to the legs, which is barrier-damaged skin.

Other chemicals that function as penetration enhancers include isopropyl myristate, glycolic acid, urea, and retinoids. Frequently, tretinoin is used as a penetration enhancer for other pharmaceuticals, such as 4% hydroquinone. The challenge with this type of penetration enhancement is the prevention of irritant contact dermatitis.

Liposomes

Newer delivery methods include liposomes, however, liposomes are usually suspended in emulsions for skin delivery. Liposomes are spherical vesicles with a diameter between 25 and 5000 nm, formed from membranes consisting of bilayer amphiphilic molecules, which possess both polar and nonpolar ends. The polar heads are directed toward the inside of the vesicle and toward its outer surface while the nonpolar, or lipophilic tails, are directed toward the middle of the bilayer.

Liposomes are based on the natural structure of the cell membrane, which has been highly conserved through evolutionary change. The name is derived from the Greek word "lipid" meaning fat and "soma" meaning body. Liposomes are primarily formed from phospholipids, such as phosphatidylcholine, but may also be composed of surfactants, such as dioleoylphosphatidylethanolamine. Their functionality may be influenced by chemical composition, vesicle size, shape, surface charge, lamellarity, and homogeneity.

The liposome is an extremely versatile structure. It can contain aqueous substances in its core, or nothing at all. Hydrophobic substances can dissolve in the phospholipid bilayer shell, which allows liposomes to deliver both oil-soluble and water-soluble substances. This characteristic is used in cosmeceutical delivery where an oil-soluble substance can be dissolved in water if placed in the phospholipid shell.

It is unlikely that traditional liposomes will diffuse across the stratum corneum barrier intact. The corneocytes are embedded in intercellular lipids, composed of ceramides, glycosylceramides, cholesterol, and fatty acids, which are structurally different from the phospholipids of the liposome. It is postulated that liposomes penetrate through the appendageal structures, but may also fuse with other bilayers, such as cell membranes, to release their ingredients. These penetration challenges are overcome with nanoliposomes that more readily traverse the stratum corneum due to their small size, which are discussed next.

Nanotechnology penetration enhancement

Nanotechnology penetration enhancement represents the next frontier in cosmeceutical delivery. This technology uses particles that are less than 100 nm in one dimension. These particles can be formulated as nanoemulsions, nanoliposomes, polymeric nanoparticle spheres, and quantum dots. Some of these nanocarriers will be discussed in the context of cosmeceutical delivery.

Nanoemulsions

Emulsions that are based on oil-in-water or water-in-oil formulations contain large droplets that do not penetrate the stratum corneum readily. Nanoemulsions possess the same formulation, except the droplets are on the nano scale of 20–100 nm. If the nano droplets are larger than 100 nm, the emulsion appears white, while nanoemulsions with droplets of 70 nm are transparent. Nanoemulsions offer the ability to deliver highly hydrophobic or lipophilic substances into the skin, which could not otherwise penetrate. This offers unique nanocarrier opportunities because the stratum corneum is an excellent barrier to lipophilic cosmeceuticals.

Cosmeceutical nanoemulsions of ubiquinone have been developed. Ubiquinone, also known as coenzyme Q10, is an important antioxidant manufactured by the body and found in all skin cells. Topical penetration had been challenging, however, Hoppe et al. were able to demonstrate coenzyme Q10 penetration into the viable epidermis and a reduction in oxidation with weak photon emission. Theoretically, higher concentrations of ubiquinone in the skin would enhance endogenous antioxidant capabilities, preventing oxidative damage to cellular structures.

Another cosmeceutical use for nanoemulsions is in the delivery of hyaluronic acid, a natural glycosaminoglycan found in the dermis that functions as a humectant. Nanoparticle hyaluronic acid can create an imperceptible film on and in the stratum corneum, attracting water and creating the illusion of smoothness by filling in fine lines and increasing skin water content. These examples highlight the utility of nanoemulsions as cosmeceutical penetration enhancers.

Nanoliposomes

Another utilization of liposome technology on a smaller scale is the formation of nanoliposomes for penetration enhancement. Nanoliposomes can be specially designed to release their internal contents under certain conditions. For example, nanoliposomes can be released when a desired pH or temperature is present in the stratum corneum. One of the main challenges with nanoliposomes is their inherent instability. They are readily deformed and possibly lysed when compressed. They are subject to fusion, aggregation, and precipitation. This means that nanoliposomes can fuse together and combine their contents and bilayer shells in suspension, possibly rending the newly created liposome larger than 100 nm, thus rendering it technically outside the liposome range. More commonly nanoliposomes can physically stick together, again creating liposome clumps outside the nano range. Finally, the nanoliposomes can fall to the bottom of the emulsion under the effect of gravity and leave their evenly distributed state. In many situations, it is likely that nanoliposomes possess the properties of traditional liposomes due to their instability.

Penetration-enhancing devices

The other mechanism for penetration enhancement is the use of physical devices that damage the stratum corneum. These devices can alter various attributes of the stratum corneum, such as the structure or electrical conductivity.

Poration

One method of changing the barrier capabilities of the stratum corneum is to literally poke holes in the barrier. Devices manufactured for this purpose are adapted from acupuncture equipment where tiny, tapered stainless steel, sterilized, solid core needles are placed around a roller. The roller is moved over the skin with pressure to push the needles into the skin, thus creating tiny pores. The needles are spaced to minimize pain and exquisitely sharpened to decrease skin crush injuries. The number of the times the poration roller is moved over the skin directly correlates with the number of pores created and the barrier damage.

There are two ways to physically increase the penetration of cosmeceuticals with poration, also known as microneedling. Either the cream can be applied prior to use of the roller or after the roller has created the pores. Most commonly, the cream is applied first and pushed into the skin with the porator needles. This strategy requires carefully formulated cosmeceuticals that do not contain irritants or cell toxic substances since the ability of the stratum corneum to block penetration is bypassed. Stinging and/or burning may ensue if low pH substances, such as lactic, glycolic, or ascorbic acid, are pushed into the skin. Also, preservatives designed to maintain cosmeceutical stability may not be the best ingredients to introduce into the dermis. Patients should not be encouraged to use standard skin care products with poration, but rather should use cosmeceuticals designed for this application.

Another goal of poration is to wound the skin in columns, much like the fractionated carbon dioxide lasers, encouraging tissue regeneration to occur. It is theorized that this controlled wounding increases collagen and glycosaminoglycan production, without producing visible scarring. Much of the success of poration is related to the expertise of the user and the design of the device. Many dermatologists in Europe use poration immediately following dermal hyaluronic acid injections to attempt to improve the result and longevity of the filler. No controlled studies on this technique have been published to date.

A variation on poration has been introduced onto the professional dermatology market. A device that looks like a hinged plastic spoon with pyramidal plastic spines on the back can be pressed into the skin. The plastic spines are so small that they theoretically can fit between nerve fibers, allowing poration of the skin painlessly. This application technique has been studied with little success for botulinum toxin and hyaluronic acid administration by the author. The major problem was the single use of the needles, which bent easily, and the concern that the needles might break off in the skin, producing a foreign body reaction. New material technology may solve this problem, but further research is required.

Electroporation

Poration as previously described can also be combined with electricity to augment the effect. The same solid needles placed on a metal roller can be electrified with high strength pulsed electric fields. If the field strength is small, with a transdermal voltage less than 100 volts, charged molecules can transport through the skin. If the field strength is large, greater than 100 volts, the lipid bilayers of the skin are disrupted and transbilayer transport occurs through the electropores within the lipid layers. A study by Vanbever et al. in 1997 demonstrated a two-fold increase in transdermal delivery of mannitol with electroporation.

Iontophoresis

Another related electrical penetration enhancement technique is iontophoresis, which also uses an electric current to allow substances to penetrate the skin. Iontophoresis applies a small voltage, using 10 volts or less, to the skin with a continuous constant current of 0.5 milliamps per centimeter square or less. This is much lower voltage than electroporation and is constant current instead of the pulsed current found in electroporation. Iontophoresis is under investigation for use with transdermal patches, discussed later, whereby a device to generate a constant electric current is affixed to the passive transdermal patch to facilitate cutaneous penetration. The advantage is that peptides and proteins, currently topically applied as cosmeceuticals, can be pushed across the stratum corneum by electromotive force. In addition, large charged molecules can be delivered, which is not possible passively.

Galvanic current

Galvanic current is different from electroporation in that it utilizes a constant very low voltage direct current. The principle is that the skin can be enhanced through an electrochemical process that either attracts or repels charged ions. The current is administered through electrodes that touch the skin. Galvanic devices have been used to cleanse the face, an esthetic procedure known as desincrustation, and for the treatment of cellulite on the body. It is thought that galvanism works on cellulite by increasing the vascular and lymphatic drainage by improving the functioning of the cellular membrane and allowing trapped fluid and lipids to be dispersed and eliminated. The galvanic current is used in conjunction with topical cosmeceuticals to enhance the effect and there are those who believe that the treatment alters electrical channels in the skin to enhance penetration of the topical agent. Little has been published in the medical literature regarding this technique.

Transdermal patches

Transdermal patches, also known as skin patches, were originally developed for pharmaceutical delivery and then adapted to cosmeceutical delivery of actives to a targeted area. The first commercialized patch was approved in 1979 for the delivery of scopolamine for motion sickness with the subsequent approval of nicotine, estrogen, and nitroglycerin patches. The patch contains four components: liner, active agent, adhesive, membrane, and backing materials. The liner protects the patch and is removed before application. Removal of the liner exposes the drug, which is fixed to the skin with an adhesive. The membrane controls the release of drug onto the skin surface and the backing protects the patch from anything that rubs the skin.

This same patch technology has been adapted to cosmeceutical delivery. Patches containing Vitamins C and E have been commercialized for application to wrinkles around the eyes, between the brows, and on the upper lip. These patches are an adaptation of an older product, known as frownies, which used adhesive to tape skin in place and minimize wrinkles overnight. The patch functions not only by immobilizing skin, but also by physically decreasing transepidermal water loss, delivering moisturizing ingredients, such as dimethicone to the skin surface, and placing vitamins or other cosmeceutical ingredients on the skin. The physical effect of the patch on the skin is just as important as the cosmeceutical delivered.

Transdermal patches are still a minor delivery method for cosmeceuticals. A variation of the transdermal patch is a film face mask. This delivery uses a polymer film to cover the face and deliver cosmeceutical moisturizers and other active ingredients without adhesive. The face is covered with the mask for 5 to 15 minutes, while reclining, delivering vitamins and botanicals to the skin surface.

Conclusion

This chapter has reviewed the various methods available for penetration enhancement. They can be divided in chemical penetration enhancement through the use of emulsions, barrier degradation, liposomes, and nanotechnology. Physical methods of penetration enhancement include poration, electroporation, iontophoresis, galvanic current, and transdermal patches. All of these techniques try to overcome the protective functions of the stratum corneum charged with keeping "out" what should stay "out" and keeping "in" what should stay "in." While penetration enhancement may be a way to enhance cosmeceutical functioning, it is also a way to introduce other challenges, including safety concerns and skin disease.

Further reading

Arora P, Mukherjee B. Design, development, physicochemical, an in vitro and in vivo evaluation of transdermal patches containing diclofenac diethylammonium salt. *Journal of Pharmaceutical Sciences* 2002; **91**(9): 2076–2089.

Banga AK, Bose S, Ghosh T. Iontophoresis and electroporation: Comparisons and contrasts. *Int J Pharm* 1999; **179**(1):1–19.

Blatt T, Mundt C, Mummert C, Maksiuk T, Wolber R, Keyhani R, Schreiner V, Hoppe U, Schachtschabel DO, Stab F. Modulation of oxidative stresses in human aging skin. *Z Gerontol Geriat*. 1999; **04**; 3f2(2): 83–88.

Edwards DA, Prausnitz MR, Langer R, Weaver JC. Analysis of enhanced transdermal transport by skin electroporation. *Journal of Controlled Release* 1995; **34**(3): 211–221.

Hoppe U, Bergemann J, Diembeck W, Ennen J, Gohla S, Harris I, Jacob J, Kielholz J, Mei W, Pollet D, Schachtschabel D, Saurermann G, Schreiner V, Stab F, Steckel F. Coenzyme Q10, a cutaneous antioxidant and energizer. *Biofactors* 1999; **9**(2–4): 371–378.

Hui SW. Low voltage electroporation of the skin, or is it iontophoresis? *Biophys J* 1998; **72**: 679–680.

Kaur IP, Agrawal R. Nanotechnology: A new paradigm in cosmeceuticals. *Recent Patents Drug Deliv Formulation* 2007; **1**: 171–182.

Nair V, Pillai O, Poduri R, Panchagnula R. Trandsdermal iontophoresis. *Methods Find Exp Clin Pharmacol* 1999; **21**(2): 139.

Rizwan M, Aqil M, Talegaonkar S, Azeem A, Sultana Y, Ali A. Enhanced transdermal drug delivery: An extensive review of patents. *Recent Patents on Drug Delivery and Formulation* 2009; **3**(2):105–124.

Solans C, Izquierdo P, Nolia J, Azemar N, Garcia-Celma MJ. Nanoemulsions. *Current Opinions in Colloid & Interface Science* 2005; **10**(3–4): 103–110.

Sonneville-Aubrun O, Simonnet JT, L'Alloret F. Nanoemulsions: A new vehicle for skincare products. *Advances in Colloid and Interface Science* 2004; **108–109**: 145–149.

Tadros T, Izqulerdo P, Esquena J, Solans C. Formation and stability of nano-emulsions. *Advances in Colloid and Interface Science* 2004; **108–109**, 303–318.

Vanbever R, Prausnitz MR, Preat V. Macromolecules as novel transdermal transport enhancers for skin electroporation. *Pharmaceutical Research* 1997; **14**(5): 638–644.

CHAPTER 5

Nanopharmaceuticals and Nanocosmeceuticals

Adnan Nasir
University of North Carolina at Chapel Hill, Chapel Hill, NC, USA

Introduction

Nanotechnology is the study of materials 1–100 nm in dimension. Disciplines embracing nanotechnology include biomedicine, optics, electronics, chemistry, engineering, consumer goods, foods and cosmetics. Nanomedicine and nanodermatology are dominated by nanoparticulate drug delivery systems.

Naturally occurring nanoparticles include viruses, lipid transport proteins, endosomes, and bacterial inclusion bodies. Synthetic nanomaterials (nanoparticles, carbon nanotubes, nanowires, fullerenes, quantum dots) may exhibit characteristics and unconventional behaviors (chemical, physical, biological, and electrical) which may depart from their bulk counterparts. Nanoparticles are able to cross biological barriers, selectively accumulate at sites of tumors or inflammation, and increase the solubility of drugs and other active ingredients. These have potential benefits as well as risks for manufacturers, transporters and consumers. Standards have been developed in the US, Europe, and Japan to assess these hazards and allow for proper handling and disposal procedures to minimize toxicity and environmental exposure in order to promote research and commercialization of nanotechnology.

Nanotechnology in dermatology

Dermatology requires new treatments. In the past few years the Food and Drug Administration in the US has approved very few new therapies for dermatologic disease. The future of dermatology requires either the creation of a novel arsenal of treatments, giving a new purpose to existing treatments with new indications, or enhanced formulation. With nanotechnology, all this is possible.

Nanoparticles used in cosmetics include nanoemulsions, nanocrystals, micelles, polymeric nanocapsules, niosomes, liposomes, nanostructured lipid carriers, solid lipid nanoparticles, dendrimers, fullerenes, and carbon nanotubes. Nanoparticulate ultraviolet light filters include mineral-based nanoparticles containing zinc, iron, or titanium. Carbon-based nanoparticles such as carbon nanotubes and fullerenes are being explored for their potent antioxidant properties.

Nanovehicles

One of the hallmarks of nanotechnology is the development of nanocarriers. The aim of nanocarriers is to safely and securely package and transport a payload from one part of the host (be it a tissue, a cell, or a subcellular structure) to another in a controlled fashion. Nanocarriers exist in nature. These include viruses, which protect and transport viral DNA, and RNA; nanoparticulate lipoproteins which package and transport hydrophobic lipids in the aqueous environment of plasma; and exosomes, which are nanoscale vesicles containing regulatory microRNAs that mediate cell–cell communication. The ideal nanocarrier should be safe, stable, and capable of transporting one or more active compounds. Examples of synthetic nanocarriers include liposomes, niosomes, ethosomes, and multifunctional nanoparticles (Figures 5.1, 5.2 and 5.3). By engineering the size, shape, and physicochemical properties of nanoparticles, it is possible to deliver active ingredients to a desired site in the epidermis or dermis with minimal toxicity. The depth of penetration and the permeation rate of drugs can be enhanced with nanoparticulate delivery.

Nanoparticle modification and functionalization

Engineering of nanoparticles to design specifications (such as desired dispersability, stability, bioavailability, tissue targeting, release kinetics)

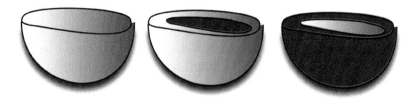

Figure 5.1 Nanoparticles: solid matrix (left), active core (middle), active shell (right).

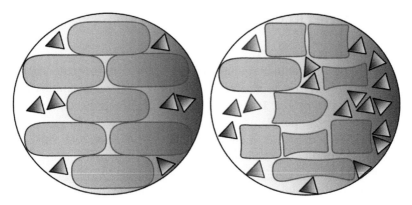

Figure 5.2 Solid lipid nanoparticles (left), nanostructured lipid carriers (right).

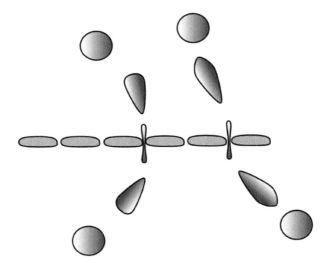

Figure 5.3 Elastic liposomes penetrating gaps between keratinocytes.

relies on careful functionalization. This is achieved through a variety of means. For example, covalent amide or ester bonding, avidin-biotin coupling, charge coupling, van der Waals, selective miscibility, or layered polymerization. Particles need to be designed to control their stability and aggregation characteristics. Coatings such as polyethylene glycol protect the nanoparticles from reticuloendothelial clearance. The particle charge can influence penetration. For example, cationic liposomes enter deeper into hair follicles than negatively charged liposomes. Cell membranes are negatively charged, and cationic nanoparticles are internalized more readily than anionic ones.

Nanoparticles in dermatology

Photoprotection

A number of longitudinal studies of large cohorts have demonstrated the importance of sun protection in the prevention of melanoma and nomelanoma skin cancer. Traditional methods of photoprotection include physical blockers, antioxidants, and DNA repair enhancers. Nanoparticles containing zinc oxide and titanium dioxide are effective at scattering, absorbing, and reflecting ultraviolet rays. There was initial concern over the safety of these particles, however, recent studies have shown that these nanoparticles do not enter viable epidermis or become absorbed systemically. Inorganic physical blocking sunscreens are coated with silicone or dimethicone, which reduces their ability to generate reactive oxygen species.

Nanoparticulate sunscreens distribute more evenly on the skin, and disperse with fewer gaps, which may enhance their sun protective efficacy. Nanoparticles also are more tightly adsorbed to the skin and remain on the surface longer and may require less frequent application. Sunscreens containing endonucleases which enhance DNA repair may be beneficial for immunocompromised patients or those who may have genodermatoses affecting DNA repair.

Sunscreens are more effective when in nanoparticulate form. Lipophilic sunscreens, such as 2-OH-methoxy-benzophenone (OMB) can be densely packed into solid lipid nanoparticles and chitosan polymeric nanoparticles. Nanoparticles disperse evenly on the skin. This denser packing and more even application allow for half the concentration of OMB in nanoparticulate preparations compared to standard emulsions. The use of less photoabsorber saves on manufacturing costs and reduces environmental and user exposure. When combined in nanostructured lipid carriers with TiO_2 OMB generates a higher SPF than either agent alone.

Rejuvenation

The use of retinoids for anti-aging has been well established. Retinoids bind nuclear receptors and elicit a cascade of events which leads to repair of ultraviolet-induced skin damage, epidermal differentiation and renewal, and increased dermal collagen. Topical retinol formulations can dry the skin, and cause an irritant dermatitis. Solid lipid nanoparticles containing retinol concentrate their payload in the upper portion of the stratum corneum. They also release retinol in a sustained fashion over six hours. These features may improve the overall tolerability and efficacy of retinol. Solid lipid nanoparticles containing tretinoin and isotretinoin show localization in the epidermis, no systemic absorption, and slow release kinetics which result in less irritation.

Botulinum toxin is typically injected into skeletal muscle, particularly in the face for rhytides. The pain and bruising associated with this therapy can be circumvented with topical application. Transdermal drug delivery is enhanced with nanoparticles. Topical nanoparticulate preparations of botulinum toxin have been studied in animal models and in pilot human trials shown to effectively paralyze skeletal muscle and efface dynamic rhytides. Side effects, such as ptosis, and diplopia preclude self-administration, and limit availability of this therapy to the clinic.

Fragrance

Perfumes typically contain organic compounds which readily disperse and evaporate. Their usefulness is dictated by their scent, and its release characteristics. Burst release results in a flood of perfume, and then none. If fragrance is bound too tightly to its carrier, it remains stable, however, so little is released that it loses its utility. Sustained release of perfume and shampoo scent has been successful with fragrance incorporated into solid lipid nanoparticles. The use of scent for repellance has also been explored. Lemon oil and N,N-diethyl-meta-toluamide (DEET) in liposomal preparations have shown sustained release kinetics.

Tanning

Nitric oxide is involved in a number of important skin activities including pathogen defense, wound healing, and inflammation (i.e., psoriasis). The role of nitric oxide in the promotion of cosmetic and photoprotective tanning has long been recognized. Nitric oxide is volatile and unstable. Nitric-oxide-stabilizing and releasing nanoencapsulated compounds have already been developed for wound healing. Adaptation in topical cosmetics may be useful for the creation of a new generation of sunscreens and tanning agents.

Nanofibers

Nanofibers are fibers with a diameter of $1\,\mu$m or less. This allows fibers to have an enormously large surface area to mass ratio, on the order of $100\,m^2/gm$. Nanofibers can be manufactured using a variety of techniques. Substrates can be natural (chitosan, collagen, gelatin, casein, hyaluronic acid, cellulose acetate, silk protein, chitin, fibrinogen) or synthetic polymers. It is possible to control a number of parameters for fiber synthesis including type of polymer, polymer solution (molecular weight, conductivity, viscosity, surface tension), and processing settings (electric potential, voltage, flow rate, capillary design). These allow for the precise fabrication of a variety of fibers with differing morphologies, molecular structures, and mechanical properties. Electrospun nanofibers have been used for microgels, tissue engineering, wound healing, and drug delivery (erythromycin, methylene blue, itraconazole, wound healing, tetracycline). Cosmetic nanofibers containing gold, or vitamin A and E are being used for masks.

Hair loss

Because nanoparticles preferentially accumulate in hair follicles, investigation of their use in the treatment of hair disorders has expanded. The encapsulation of pilotrophic agents in nanoparticles increased their permeability over aqueous controls. Nanoparticulate hinokitiol was superior to an aqueous solution in transitioning hair from the telogen to the angagen phase. Minoxidil nanoparticles made of block copolymers of poly (ϵ-caprolactone) and polyethylene glycol had enhanced follicular penetration. Finasteride has been incorporated into liposomes for topical delivery. Antiandrogens such as RU 58841 have been incorporated into solid lipid nanoparticles and have demonstrated enhanced permeation and penetration. Liposomal preparations of cyclosporine A induce hair regrowth in rat models of alopecia areata. Small siRNAs encapsulated in cationic microspheres are useful in the treatment of alopecia areata in a mouse model.

Hirsutism

Anti-androgens such as aldosterone and cyproterone acetate have been used for the treatment of hirsutism. Nanoparticulate delivery systems for topical cyproterone acetate have been developed and may be useful for the treatment of hirsutism. Anti-trypanosomal medications such as eflornithine have been used to manage hirsutism; nanoparticulate delivery systems may potentially increase efficacy and reduce toxicity.

Hair dying

Chitosan is a positively charged polyelectrolyte. It stabilizes zwitterionic phospholipid systems and can form nanoparticles, porous matrices, hydrogels, and films. It comes from natural marine sources, is biocompatible, biodegradable, and mucoadhesive. Hair dye containing chitosan carries less risk of side effects than traditional dyes.

Acne

Sebaceous glands are part of the pilosebaceous unit. Adapalene-loaded PLGA nanoparticles were shown to be more successful for the treatment of acne and rosacea. Dye studies have shown that PLA nanoparticles penetrate hair follicles and release dye within sebaceous glands. Retinoids, which are typically irritating, unstable, and can be systemically absorbed, are better tolerated in nanoformulations. Benzoyl peroxide formulations in nanoparticles show greater tolerability and efficacy than their nonencapsulated counterparts. Antiandrogens have also been shown to target sebaceous glands Solid lipid nanoparticles containing cyproterone acetate are preferentially localized to sebaceous glands. The result is diminished sebum production and acne. This accumulation does not extend to the surrounding dermis, resulting in less absorption and fewer systemic side effects.

Microneedles

Microneedles are manufactured to submicron tolerances. Microneedles can be coated or uncoated, and be solid or have a hollow core. They can be assembled on patches and on rollers. The length, diameter, and bore, if present, can be precisely engineered. Microneedles have been manufactured using a variety of techniques, some borrowed from the semiconductor industry. By controlling the dimensions and surfaces of the microneedles, it is possible to use them as cost-effective, and painless cosmetic, cosmeceutical, and drug delivery devices. Direct delivery enhances the efficacy of retinoids, hydroquinone, and hyaluronic acid, and reduces time to anesthesia for lidocaine. Wound healing with microneedle puncture can lead to collagen deposition comparable to intense pulsed light. Microneedles coupled with fractionated radiofrequency have been shown to reduce scarring associated with acne. Microneedles can work in conjunction with other therapies for multimodality facial rejuvenation.

Regulation and safety

The number of nanoparticulate preparations for the skin has exploded over the past decade, from a few dozen in 2005 to over a thousand in 2012. The growth of nanotechnology in the cosmeceutical marketplace and in dermatologic pharmaceuticals has led to cross-over in these two arenas. The distinction between cosmetics and drugs has to do with intended use. If a product is advertised and labeled to affect the skin's structure or function, it is regulated as a drug. If, however, it makes general statements about altering appearance, it is treated as a cosmetic. The importance of the claim is central, whether or not the product actually has a structural or functional impact on the skin. As more nanocosmeceuticals are developed, their potential for activity through altering skin structure and function increases, and the likelihood that they will be regulated as drugs increases. The regulatory process for drugs is typically much lengthier and costlier than the process for cosmetics. The FDA is working to develop regulations which address potential overlaps and possibly create a separate approval category for cosmeceuticals and nanocosmeceuticals.

Successfully penetrating this barrier is one of the chief goals of nanopharmaceuticals and nanocosmeceuticals. Yet penetration of harmful particles is not a desirable goal. Primary features of nanoparticles to consider include their shape, size, size range, surface reactive groups, coatings, charge, surface to volume ratio, pore density, porosity, water solubility, aggregability, size and phase of crystals (for example, rutile and anastase titanium dioxide crystals differ in their biologic reactivity), redox potential, ability to induce free radicals, water and oil solubility.

A good understanding of these properties may lead to engineered fail-safe mechanisms to mitigate toxicity, for example, coating of sunscreen nanoparticles with silicates or manganese to prevent the formation of reactive oxygen species; and engineering nanomaterials to minimize penetration. Toxicity studies need to be done on tissue cultures as well as animal models and should include an evaluation of the localization of nanoparticles (whether on the skin surface, or deeper penetration), absorption into the blood stream, and bioaccumulation, persistence or elimination of nanoparticles. Only nanoparticles selected for lack of toxicity, biocompatibility, biodegradability, and efficacy should be considered for consumer use.

Conclusion

Nanotechnology is the science of precise design on the nanoscale. The unique properties of matter on this scale allow for the creation of a whole new class of dermatologics termed nanocosmeceuticals and nanopharmaceuticals. Using nanocarriers for active ingredient stabilization and targeted delivery, nanomaterials are being used for the restoration of skin health and vigor and the alleviation of skin disease. Because of the potential overlap between cosmetics and drugs in the nanotechnology space and the widely different current approval and regulatory policies of the two, new regulatory frameworks to foster the safe and cost-effective introduction of nanomaterials in medicine and society will need to be developed. Nanotechnology heralds an era of renewed vigor and development in dermatology.

Further reading

Badran MM, Kuntsche J, Fahr A. Skin penetration enhancement by a microneedle device (Dermaroller) in vitro: Dependency on needle size and applied formulation. *Eur J Pharm Sci* 2009; **36**(4–5): 511–523.

Bikowski J, Del Rosso JQ. Benzoyl peroxide microsphere cream as monotherapy and combination treatment of acne. *J Drugs Dermatol* 2008; **7**(6): 590–595.

Cafardi JA, Elmets CA. T4 endonuclease V: Review and application to dermatology. *Expert Opin Biol Ther* 2008; **8**(6): 829–838.

Clementoni MT, B-Roscher M, Munavalli, GS. Photodynamic photorejuvenation of the face with a combination of microneedling, red light, and broadband pulsed light. *Lasers Surg Med* 2010; **42**(2): 150–159.

Collins A, Nasir A. Topical botulinum toxin. *J Clin Aesthet Dermatol* 2010; **3**(3): 35–39.

Friedman A, et al. Susceptibility of Gram-positive and -negative bacteria to novel nitric oxide-releasing nanoparticle technology. *Virulence* 2011; **2**(3): 217–221.

Gittard S, et al. Deposition of antimicrobial coatings on microstereolithography-fabricated microneedles. *JOM, Journal of the Minerals, Metals and Materials Society* 2011; **63**(6): 59–68.

Gordon LG, et al. Regular sunscreen use is a cost-effective approach to skin cancer prevention in subtropical settings. *J Invest Dermatol* 2009; **129**(12): 2766–2771.

Green AC, et al. Reduced melanoma after regular sunscreen use: Randomized trial follow-up. *J Clin Oncol* 2011; **29**(3): 257–263.

Jenning V, Gohla SH. Encapsulation of retinoids in solid lipid nanoparticles (SLN). *J Microencapsul* 2001; **18**(2): 149–158.

Kroubi M, Karembe H, Betbeder D. Drug delivery systems in the treatment of African trypanosomiasis infections. *Expert Opin Drug Deliv* 2011; **8**(6): 735–747.

Kumar R, et al. Development of liposomal systems of finasteride for topical applications: Design, characterization, and in vitro evaluation. *Pharm Dev Technol* 2007; **12**(6): 591–601.

Lademann J, et al. Influence of nonhomogeneous distribution of topically applied UV filters on sun protection factors. *J Biomed Opt* 2004; **9**(6): 1358–1362.

Lee HY, Jeong YI, Choi KC. Hair dye-incorporated poly-gamma-glutamic acid/glycol chitosan nanoparticles based on ion-complex formation. *Int J Nanomedicine* 2011; **6**: 2879–2888.

Munster U, et al. RU 58841-myristate--prodrug development for topical treatment of acne and androgenetic alopecia. *Pharmazie* 2005; **60**(1): 8–12.

Nakamura M, et al. Controlled delivery of T-box21 small interfering RNA ameliorates autoimmune alopecia (Alopecia Areata) in a C3H/HeJ mouse model. *Am J Pathol* 2008; **172**(3): 650–658.

Pardeike J, Hommoss A, Muller RH. Lipid nanoparticles (SLN, NLC) in cosmetic and pharmaceutical dermal products. *Int J Pharm* 2009; **366**(1–2): 170–184.

Pardeike J, et al. Nanostructured lipid carriers as delivery system for the phopholipase A2 inhibitors PX-18 and PX-13 for dermal application. *Pharmazie* 2011; **66**(5): 357–361.

Puglia C, et al. Evaluation of percutaneous absorption of the repellent diethyltoluamide and the sunscreen ethylhexyl p-methoxycinnamate-loaded solid lipid nanoparticles: An in-vitro study. *J Pharm Pharmacol* 2009; **61**(8): 1013–1019.

Rancan F, et al. Stability of polylactic acid particles and release of fluorochromes upon topical application on human skin explants. *Eur J Pharm Biopharm* 2012; **80**(1): 76–84.

Rastogi R, Anand S, Koul V. Electroporation of polymeric nanoparticles: An alternative technique for transdermal delivery of insulin. *Drug Dev Ind Pharm* 2010; **36**(11): 1303–1311.

Rolland A, et al. Site-specific drug delivery to pilosebaceous structures using polymeric microspheres. *Pharm Res* 1993; **10**(12): 1738–1744.

Romero-Graillet C, et al. Nitric oxide produced by ultraviolet-irradiated keratinocytes stimulates melanogenesis. *J Clin Invest* 1997; **99**(4): 635–642.

Shim J, et al. Transdermal delivery of mixnoxidil with block copolymer nanoparticles. *J Control Release* 2004; **97**(3): 477–484.

Siqueira NM, et al. Innovative sunscreen formulation based on benzophenone-3-loaded chitosan-coated polymeric nanocapsules. *Skin Pharmacol Physiol* 2011; **24**(3): 166–174.

Stecova J, et al. Cyproterone acetate loading to lipid nanoparticles for topical acne treatment: Particle characterisation and skin uptake. *Pharm Res* 2007; **24**(5): 991–1000.

Taepaiboon P, Rungsardthong U, Supaphol P, Vitamin-loaded electrospun cellulose acetate nanofiber mats as transdermal and dermal therapeutic agents of vitamin A acid and vitamin E. *Eur J Pharm Biopharm* 2007; **67**(2): 387–397.

Thery, C., Exosomes: Secreted vesicles and intercellular communications. *F1000 Biol Rep* 2011; **3**: 15.

Van Reeth, I., Beyond skin feel: Innovative methods for developing complex sensory profiles with silicones. *J Cosmet Dermatol* 2006; **5**(1): 61–67.

Verma DD, et al. Treatment of alopecia areata in the DEBR model using Cyclosporin A lipid vesicles. *Eur J Dermatol* 2004; **14**(5): 332–338.

Villaverde A, et al. Packaging protein drugs as bacterial inclusion bodies for therapeutic applications. *Microb Cell Fact* 2012; **11**(1): 76.

CHAPTER 6

Cutaneous Barrier Function, Moisturizer Effects and Formulation

Dee Anna Glaser and Adam R. Mattox
Saint Louis University School of Medicine, St Louis, MO, USA

Barrier function

Proper hydration is crucial for normal physiologic function of the skin. Hydration, in part, is regulated and maintained by the barrier function of the stratum corneum (SC). The SC is the biochemically active, self-regulated, superficial layer of the skin. This selectively permeable, heterogeneous, composite outer layer of the epidermis protects against desiccation and over-hydration. It must maintain adequate amounts of water to function in various environmental conditions. Disease states and extreme environmental conditions may compromise the barrier function, leading to excessively dry skin. Moisturizers are topical products of variable formulations designed to aid the SC in the task of regulating skin hydration. Specialty formulations may contain additives to assist the SC with the antimicrobial, antioxidant and UV protection necessary to repair and maintain a homeostatic barrier.

Stratum corneum structure and function

One common and over-simplified analogy to explain the anatomy of the SC is the brick and mortar model. Terminally differentiated corneocytes represent the bricks, while the intercellular lamellar lipids represent the mortar. While an easy concept to grasp, the image of a rigid, impermeable, non-restorative brick wall is in contrast to the functioning SC. Instead, the SC is pliable, semi-permeable, adaptable and capable of self-restoration.

No longer metabolically active, terminally differentiated keratinocytes become corneocytes. On most body sites, the SC consists of 12–16 layers of flattened corneocytes. Each layer is approximately $1\,\mu m$ thick. Within its protein shell, each corneocyte consists of a highly organized, insoluble,

Cosmeceuticals and Cosmetic Practice, First Edition. Edited by Patricia K. Farris.
© 2014 John Wiley & Sons, Ltd. Published 2014 by John Wiley & Sons, Ltd.

keratin macrofibrillar matrix. This protein matrix can bind substantial amounts of water, causing cellular swelling and changes in morphology. Furthermore, the physical packing of multiple corneocyte layers creates a tortuous path for water molecules to traverse during evaporation. Barrier function is improved as the diffusion length increases.

Aiding in selective water retention, terminally differentiated corneocytes contain high concentrations of a very efficient, natural, humectant referred to as Natural Moisturizing Factor (NMF). NMF consists of free amino acids and their derivatives such as pyrrolidone carboxylic acid, lactate and urea produced by the proteolysis of filaggrin. Filaggrin proteolysis is activated as corneocytes mature and dehydrate, a helpful homeostatic mechanism. By maintaining the delicate balance of free water in the SC, NMF optimizes the activity of enzymes responsible for its own synthesis. The amount of filaggrin produced increases in response to biochemical signals induced by barrier compromise from injury and harmful environmental conditions.

Though the majority of water in the SC originates from the viable epidermis and dermis, under the proper conditions, NMF may absorb atmospheric water. Corneocytes in the middle layers of the SC contain the highest concentration of biochemically functional NMF. They retain the most water, giving them a swollen appearance on microscopy.

Exogenous factors can reduce the concentration of NMF in the SC. NMF may be washed out by routine cleansing agents. There is a significant age-related decline in the level of NMF. Reduced synthesis of filaggrin is generally to blame, but the phenomenon is exacerbated by the concurrent age-related decline in general barrier function. Illustrating the benefit of sunscreen in moisturizer, UV light is sufficient to disrupt the enzymatic breakdown of filaggrin that produces NMF.

Lamellar granules in the stratum basale cells contain the biologic precursors of intercellular lipids. As maturation and upward migration occur, the intercellular lipids such as ceramides (50% by mass), cholesterol (25% by mass), and free fatty acids (10–20% by mass) are produced and discharged to the intercellular space. The intercellular lipid bilayer, also known as the intercellular lamellar lipid membrane, is the predominant structure directly functioning as the SC's permeability barrier. Experimentally, xerosis occurs proportionally to the amount of lipid removed by solvent extraction, indicating the integral contribution of lipids to barrier function. The permeability and barrier efficiency are determined by the relative ratio of SC lipids present in the intercellular lipid bilayer. Moisturizers can be formulated to mimic normal physiology and manipulate the balance of intercellular lipids to accelerate cutaneous barrier recovery.

In addition to the cohesive forces of the intercellular lipid bilayer, corneocytes are held together by direct intercellular protein structures called corneodesmosomes. Normal cell desquamation is only possible once proteolysis of the corneodesmosomes occurs. Maturing keratinocytes produce these proteolytic enzymes and package them with intercellular lipids in lamellar granules. The contents of the lamellar granules are subsequently secreted into the extracellular space. To describe the cleaving of corneodesmosomes, a model of precisely controlled protease-protease inhibitor interaction has been proposed. However, the coordinated manner of enzyme activation is still unknown. Ultimately, pH, water content and physical properties of the intercellular lipid layer are thought to greatly impact enzymatic activity.

Desquamation

Flaky skin is a cutaneous reaction pattern reflecting abnormal desquamation. Dryness may be the primary contributing factor causing this abnormality. Corneocytes are normally shed from the skin surface in groups too small to visualize. If desquamation is disturbed, larger collections form, visible as scales with rough texture.

In order to maintain tissue integrity, the complex process of normal physiologic exfoliation must be carefully regulated. The above mentioned corneodesmosomes (CD) provide the main cohesive force between corneocytes that must be degraded for release to occur. Hydrolytic proteases from the Kallikrein family are responsible for cleaving CD intercellular connections. Water is not only a substrate for hydrolysis, but it also regulates enzymatic activity. Desmosomal degradation is significantly reduced at low humidity, leading to suppressed desquamation and scale formation. Maintenance of SC hydration with moisturizers can help optimize enzymatic function. For increased efficacy, moisturizers may contain a special ingredient such as glycerin to promote dissociation of corneocytes.

Exogenous conditions effect barrier function

As terrestrial beings, human skin must adapt to a diverse range of environmental conditions. Relative humidity is perhaps the most significant environmental factor affecting barrier function and skin hydration. Low humidity is generally thought to induce or exacerbate disorders by reducing the capacity to produce NMF. Fortunately, compensatory mechanisms like exocytosis of lamellar bodies, SC thickening and increasing intercellular lipid content reduce transepidermal water loss (TEWL) and the effects of low humidity. Compensation mechanisms are remarkably efficient, evidenced by time spent in a dry environment leading to accelerated barrier recovery when compared to a humid environment.

Temperature also has a significant impact on barrier function. Barrier recovery is accelerated while the skin surface temperature is maintained between 36–40°C. Outside this range the rate of recovery is delayed. Despite robust mechanisms of compensation, the skin will require treatment in extreme or prolonged environmental conditions. Furthermore, compensatory mechanisms diminish with age and the presence of disease states.

In addition to thermal disruption, excessive bathing with soap leads to the depletion of NMF and SC lipids essential to maintaining the skin's permeability barrier. Without proper formulation, cleansers and moisturizing agents like humectants can lead to impaired barrier function. Other additives, including preservatives and fragrances can serve as irritants and allergens, triggering dermatitis exacerbations.

Water and its effect on the epidermis

In addition to affecting the activity of enzymatic processes described above, water is responsible for many of the physical properties of healthy skin. Giving plasticity to the superficial layers and allowing for their deformation and suppleness, water is one of the most important components. The viable epidermis has a remarkably high water content (70% or greater). Water content is sharply reduced beyond the corneo-epidermal junction, with a normal range of 15–30%. In the SC, water is associated with the hydrophilic portions of intercellular lipids, NMF and the intracellular keratin matrix of corneocytes.

The water gradient in the epidermis is maintained by endogenous glycerol and the distribution of aquaporins. Endogenous glycerol is derived from sebaceous glands and the systemic circulation and functions as a natural humectant. Aquaporins are membrane bound channels that increase the permeability of cell membranes to small uncharged molecules like glycerol. Aquaporin 3 (AQP3) is the most abundant aquaporin in the epidermis. AQP3 allows bidirectional osmotic diffusion of glycerol into cells, pulling water along with it. This explains the prolonged effect of glycerol on skin hydration referred to as the reservoir effect. The distribution of AQP3 mimics the epidermal water gradient as it is expressed more in the stratum basale than in the stratum granulosum (Figure 6.1). The expression of AQP3 channels is also reduced by chronic sun exposure and in aging, explaining the dryness seen in the elderly and photoaged skin. Studies are ongoing to identify compounds that can increase AQP3 levels and improve skin hydration.

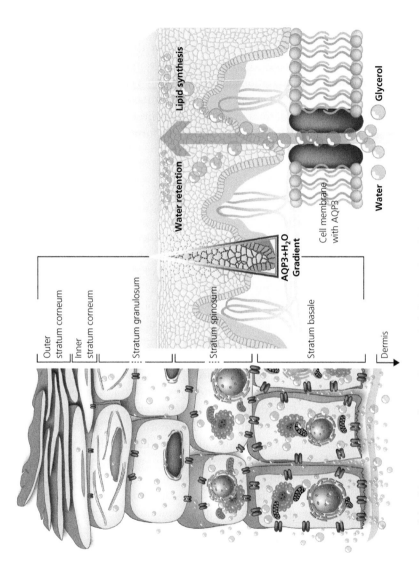

Figure 6.1 The structure of the skin. Source: Draelos, Z. *The Journal of Clinical and Aesthetic Dermatology* 2012; 5(7): 55. © Matrix Medical Communications, with permission.

Moisturizing basics

To the average consumer, the term moisturizer can be misleading. One might assume the term implies the product is actually putting moisture back into the skin. However, moisturizers put very little exogenous water back into the skin nor are they incorporated into the intercellular lipids. Moisturizers simply attempt to slow the rate of transepidermal water loss (TEWL) and create an optimal environment for the skin to restore the SC barrier. As mentioned above, the normal SC water content is between 15–30%. The four steps to remoisturization have been described as: (1) the initiation of barrier repair; (2) the reduction in cutaneous moisture evaporation; (3) the onset of dermal-epidermal moisture diffusion; and (4) the synthesis of intercellular lipids. Moisturizers are formulated to perform by one or more of these steps.

Emulsions

Most commercially available moisturizing products are emulsions. The most common type of skin care emulsion is an oil in water (O/W) emulsion. This type of emulsion consists of tiny droplets of oil finely dispersed in water. Oil in water emulsions can be used to deliver a variety of active ingredients including antioxidants, peptides and botanical extracts. Water in oil (W/O) emulsions consist of water droplets dispersed in an oil carrier and are used primarily for formulating sunscreen products. Water in silicone (W/Si) emulsions consist of water droplets dispersed in silicone and are used in color cosmetics, skin care products and sunscreens.

Creams and lotions can be differentiated by their physical properties and chemical composition. Creams are more occlusive and thicker than lotions. They contain less water than lotions and have a high oil phase made of heavier lipids such as waxes. Creams are preferred for night application and are favored for treating special areas like around the eyes and neck. Lotions contain more water and have lower oil content than creams. Lotions are less occlusive, absorb into the skin easily and are pourable. These properties make lotions an excellent choice for body applications.

Contents of a moisturizer

Table 6.1 shows the common ingredients found in a moisturizer.

Table 6.1 Common moisturizing ingredients.

Occlusives	Humectants	Emollients
Petrolatum	Glycerin	Dimethicone
Mineral oil	Honey	Cyclomethicone
Paraffin	Hyaluronic acd	Isopropyl myristate
Dimethicone, cyclomethicone	Panthenol	Sunflower oil
Vegetable and animal fats	Urea	Jojoba oil
Lanolin	Sorbital	Palm oil
Propylene glycol	Sodium pyrrolidine carboxylic acid	Castor oil
Stearyl stearate	Sodium lactate	Hexyldecanol
Beeswax	Glycolic acid	Oleyl alcohol
Vegetable waxes	Lactic acid	Octyldodecanol
Lecithin	Tartaric acid	Cetyl alcohol
Cholesterol	Propylene glycol	Stearyl alcohol

Water

With the exception of ointment-based products, the predominant component of moisturizers is water (65–95% by weight). Though dry skin lacks water content, the water in moisturizer does not directly contribute to re-moisturization. Even with generous application and repeated use, only a small amount of water is absorbed by the SC. Water serves as both the diluent to thin texture and the continuous phase containing colloids or emulsions. Once applied, the water evaporates to leave behind the lipids and active ingredients.

Occlusive ingredients

Occlusive ingredients physically prevent water loss from the stratum corneum by creating a hydrophobic barrier over the skin. Petrolatum is the most commonly used and most effective occlusive agent reducing TEWL by 99%. Petrolatum penetrates the SC, helping to restore the barrier function by stimulating intercellular lipid synthesis. The main drawback to petrolatum is its unaesthetic greasy appearance.

A silicone polymer, dimethicone is a less greasy alternative to petrolatum and the basis of all "oil-free" moisturizers. It is a hypoallergenic, noncomedogenic, and nonacnegenic ingredient that can be added to a formulation to reduce the petrolatum concentration. Lanolin is an effective occlusive agent although its use is limited by odor, expense and potential allergenicity. Mineral oil, paraffin wax, cetyl alcohol and stearyl alcohol are occlusive agents found in commercially available moisturizing formulations.

Humectant ingredients

In the SC, humectants attract and bind water originating from the lower layers of the skin, including the dermis and viable epidermis. If environmental humidity exceeds 70%, these hygroscopic molecules may be able to attract a small amount of exogenous water. Humectants used alone increase TEWL. Thus, in order to ensure effective moisturization, humectants must be combined with occlusives. Humectants are thought to alleviate the appearance of xerotic skin by inducing corneocyte swelling reducing the intercellular spaces and obscuring fine lines.

Glycerin is a highly effective humectant that can be applied topically to enhance skin hydration. As mentioned above, glycerin facilitates desmosome digestion and enhances skin hydration by creating a reservoir effect. Topical glycerol (but not topical sebaceous lipids) has been shown to correct hydration experimentally, providing the rationale for glycerol-containing moisturizers.

Other commonly used humectants include hyaluronic acid (HA), panthenol, sodium pyrrolidonic carboxyclic acid (PCA), propylene glycol, sodium lactate, sorbital and urea. The alpha hydroxy acids including lactic, glycolic and tartaric acid function as both humectants and exfoliators.

Emollient ingredients

Emollient ingredients contribute to the esthetics of a moisturizer by enhancing skin slip and smoothness. Emollients fill in the microscopic crevices between desquamating corneocytes and include a variety of compounds from esters to alcohols. Long chain fatty acids such as stearic, linoleic, linolenic, oleic and lauric are excellent emollients and are found in oils such as jojoba, castor, palm and sunflower seed. Emollient alcohols including cetyl, stearyl, octyldodecanol, hexyldecanol and oleyl alcohol have excellent skin-smoothing properties, without the drying effect traditionally associated with astringent alcohols like isopropyl. The choice of emollient may be limited by conflicting chemical interactions between ingredients. For example, monoester emollients hydrolyze in the presence of low pH, making them unsuitable for hydroxy acid additives.

Emulsifiers

Depending on the formulation, emulsions can be customized to have diverse physical traits. For this reason, most moisturizers are water-in-oil or oil-in-water emulsions. Additives known as emulsifiers serve to hold the aqueous and non-polar phases of a mixture together. Soap at a concentration of less than 0.5% is one of the more common emulsifying agents. At this low concentration, none of the soap directly contacts the skin; it is held at the interface of the water and oil in the product. Surfactants are the other main class of emulsifying agents.

Preservatives

The manufacture and distribution of moisturizers often require considerable distance and time. For this reason, it is not feasible to provide products free of preservative ingredients. Manufacturers are expected to provide the consumer a microbiologically preserved product while maintaining the lowest risk of toxic effects. A patient's preservative sensitivity profile is quite relevant when recommending a moisturizer, especially if allergic contact dermatitis is a contributing factor. Patch testing may be necessary to identify contributing allergens and provide clear avoidance guidelines. Parabens and formaldehyde-releasing compounds are common preservatives that also happen to be relatively common contact allergens.

Fragrance

Another additive with potential deleterious effects is fragrance. Complex fragrance mixes contain dozens of separate ingredients, including specific subsets known as fragrance keys. Though fragrance-free products are now more common than ever; fragrance is added to moisturizers to mask the often unpleasant odor of a lipid base. A pleasant scent may enhance patient compliance. Again, a patient's contact allergen sensitivity profile is relevant when providing recommendations. Fortunately, gentle, fragrance-free, moisturizers are prevalent and simplify the process.

Choosing a moisturizer

Facial moisturizers

More so than body products, facial moisturizers must provide consumers a highly aesthetic appearance. Facial moisturizers predominantly utilize lotion or cream vehicles. Facial products must be safe and free of stinging, burning or itching. Low residue formulations allow for the application of cosmetic products after moisturization.

Facial moisturizers only tend to affect wrinkles in direct and transient mechanisms. A plumping effect is achieved by increasing the water content of the periorbital skin. Moisturizers may fill in fine wrinkles by slightly smoothing the surface. Pigmented moisturizers even out facial skin tones by coloring over hyper- or hypopigmented areas. A facial moisturizer containing a broad spectrum sunscreen will be most effective preventing the effects of further photoaging.

Oily skin

Patients with oily skin are often troubled by their appearance, unpleasant feeling and sense of uncleanness. The origin of skin surface oil depends on the body area and density of sebaceous glands present. For example, on the forehead, oil is predominantly sebum generated by sebaceous glands with only minor contribution by intercellular lipids from keratinocytes (3–6%). However, on the palms, the majority of endogenous oil is from epidermal lipids. Sebum does not appear to directly contribute to the cutaneous barrier function of the SC. Harsh over-cleansing to remove excess sebum will remove epidermal lipids, resulting in barrier damage and excessive dry skin. It appears the skin content of sebum and water are separate characteristics.

Many moisturizers designed for oily skin types also claim to help control oil. This is typically accomplished by the addition of oil-absorbing substances such as talc, starch, or other synthetic polymers.

Aging skin
The distinct features of chronological aging and photoaging overlap to contribute to the overall changes. Chronologically aged skin tends to impact hydration and barrier function more significantly. Over time, keratinocytes lose the ability to terminally differentiate and form a stratum corneum with normal physiologic desquamation. The rate of formation of epidermal lipids contributing to barrier function slows as well. These factors, combined with the atrophy of the eccrine glands, precipitate dry skin in older adults. Though nothing can be done to reverse chronologic aging effects, the topics covered in this chapter regarding moisturizers and exfoliants play a significant role in optimizing the remaining physiologic function of aged skin.

Conclusion

Skin hydration and barrier function are essential to skin health and appearance. The use of moisturizers is an important part of any daily skin regimen and product selection should take into account any pre-existing skin conditions, age and personal preference. Our understanding of how skin maintains hydration and barrier function has evolved significantly in the past decade allowing for the development of more effective moisturizing products.

Further reading

Del Rosso JQ, Levin J: Clinical relevance of maintaining the structural and functional integrity of the stratum corneum: why is it important to you? *J Drugs Dermatol* 2011; **10**(10 Suppl):s5–12.

Del Rosso JQ, Levin J. The clinical relevance of maintaining the functional integrity of the stratum corneum in both healthy and disease-affected skin. *J Clin Aesthet Dermatol* 2011; **4**(9): 22–42.

Draelos Z. Aquaporins: An introduction to a key factor in the mechanism of skin hydration. *J Clin Aesth Derm* 2012; **5**(7): 53–56.

Lynde C. Moisturizers for the treatment of inflammatory skin conditions. *J Drugs Dermatol* 2008; **7**(11): 1038–1043.

Harding CR. The stratum corneum: Structure and function in health and disease. *Dermatol Ther* 2004; **17** Suppl. 1: 6–15.

Lee B, Warshaw E. Lanolin allergy: History, epidemiology, responsible allergens, and management. *Dermatitis* 2008; **19**(2): 63–72.

Levin J, Miller R. A guide to the ingredients and potential benefits of over-the-counter cleansers and moisturizers for rosacea patients. *J Clin Aesthet Dermatol* 2011; **4**(8): 31–49.

Man MM, Feingold KR, Thornfeldt CR, Elias PM. Optimization of physiological lipid mixtures for barrier repair. *J Invest Dermatol* 1996; **106**(5): 1096–1101.

Rawlings AV, Harding CR. Moisturization and skin barrier function. *Dermatol Ther* 2004; **17** Suppl 1: 43–48.

Rawlings A, Harding C, Watkinson A, Banks J, Ackerman C, Sabin R. The effect of glycerol and humidity on desmosome degradation in stratum corneum. *Arch Dermatol Res* 1995; **287**(5): 457–464.

Verdier-Sevrain S, Bonte F. Skin hydration: A review on its molecular mechanisms. *J Cosmet Dermatol* 2007; **6**(2): 75–82.

PART II
Cosmeceutical Ingredients

CHAPTER 7

Cosmeceutical Uses and Benefits of Alpha, Poly and Bionic Hydroxy Acids

Barbara A. Green
NeoStrata Company, Inc., Princeton, NJ, USA

Introduction

Van Scott and Yu discovered the benefits of a class of compounds they named the alpha-hydroxyacids (AHAs) nearly four decades ago (the mid-1970s) while researching a treatment for ichthyosiform disorders. Initially, AHAs were found to have a profound effect on keratinization and stratum corneum exfoliation. Subsequent research demonstrated that AHAs could also provide significant anti-aging effects through dermal matrix building. Together with the discovery of topical retinoids, anti-aging skincare was born. Today, AHAs remain important skincare ingredients. Discovery of next-generation hydroxyacid compounds such as the polyhydroxy acids (PHAs) and bionic acids (BAs) has enabled additional skin benefits and therapeutic uses.

Hydroxyacid classification: AHA, PHA, BA

Alpha-hydroxyacids (AHAs)

The AHAs are organic carboxylic acids having one hydroxyl group attached to the alpha position of the carboxyl group on an aliphatic or alicyclic molecule; the hydroxyl group is chemically neutral and the carboxyl group is the acidic substituent on the molecule. Many AHAs are present in foods and fruits and, thus, AHAs have been named fruit acids. The most commonly used AHAs include glycolic acid and lactic acid. Citric acid, an antioxidant AHA found in citrus fruits, is a unique hydroxyacid because it contains a single hydroxyl group relative to three carboxylic acid functional groups in both alpha and beta positions, making it an alpha and beta hydroxyacid. Citric acid is found naturally occurring in skin where it plays a prominent role in the human metabolic process known as the

Cosmeceuticals and Cosmetic Practice, First Edition. Edited by Patricia K. Farris.
© 2014 John Wiley & Sons, Ltd. Published 2014 by John Wiley & Sons, Ltd.

Kreb's (citric acid) cycle, which generates energy for the human body. Some AHAs contain a phenyl group as a side-chain substituent which changes the solubility profile of the AHA molecule providing increased lipophilicity over conventional water-soluble AHAs. These AHAs can be used to target oily and acne-prone skin. Examples include mandelic acid (phenyl glycolic acid) and benzilic acid (diphenyl glycolic acid) (Table 7.1).

Polyhydroxy acids (PHAs)

Polyhydroxy acids are second-generation AHAs. They are typically slightly larger sugar acids that are structurally similar to AHAs, however, they possess two or more (i.e. poly) hydroxyl groups in the molecule. In order to be a polyhydroxy AHA, one of the hydroxyl groups must be positioned alpha to the carboxylic acid group. Many PHAs are naturally occurring, endogenous metabolites of the human body. Gluconic acid and gluconolactone, for example, are important metabolites formed in the pentose phosphate pathway. Gluconolactone, a PHA used in cosmetic formulations, provides similar effects to glycolic acid, but offers the added benefit of gentleness, antioxidant/chelation effects, and increased hydrating capacity. Clinical studies have demonstrated compatibility with sensitive skin, including rosacea and atopic dermatitis, which may in part be due to inherent gentleness and a hydration effect, as well as its ability to strengthen skin barrier function. Repeated, twice-daily use of gluconolactone (8% cream, pH 3.8) over a one-month period significantly increases skin barrier function, making skin more resistant to chemical challenge.

The skin-conditioning benefits of PHAs make them ideal cosmetic options for clinically sensitive skin and for use as adjunctive care in combination with potentially irritating medications. Concomitant use of gluconolactone-containing products with prescription azelaic acid in the treatment of rosacea significantly improves therapeutic outcomes versus the medication alone, including erythema and appearance of telangiectasia, with improved tolerability of the prescription medication. Published research has demonstrated an anti-acne effect with gluconolactone versus benzoyl peroxide. Other studies have demonstrated that the PHA, gluconolactone, provides complementary exfoliation effects and reduces the irritation potential of benzoyl peroxide in the treatment of acne. PHAs are also proven compatible with topical retinoid therapy in the treatment of acne.

Bionic acids (BAs)

Bionic acids are third-generation AHAs. The molecular structure is comprised of two components: a polyhydroxy acid attached to a sugar molecule. Lactobionic acid, for example, is comprised of gluconic acid (a PHA) attached to galactose via an ether-like linkage, and maltobionic acid is comprised of gluconic acid attached to a glucose molecule. BAs are larger

Table 7.1 Evolution of the alpha-hydroxyacids.

Generation	Hydroxyacid class	Ingredients	Skin benefits	Skincare uses
First generation	Alpha-hydroxyacids (AHAs)	Glycolic acid, lactic acid, citric acid, mandelic acid	Anti-aging across all skin layers, superior exfoliation and cell turnover; stimulates dermal biosynthesis (GAGs, collagen)	Normal skin types (non-sensitive); exfoliation of hyperkeratotic skin; peels
Second generation	Polyhydroxy acids (PHAs)	Gluconolactone	Non-irritating anti-aging effects; builds skin barrier function; preserves skin's natural elasticity, free radical scavenger, light exfoliation	Sensitive skin; barrier-strengthening; rosacea-prone, acne-prone
Third generation	Bionic acids (BAs)	Lactobionic acid, maltobionic acid	Highly moisturizing, protects via MMP inhibition and antioxidant effects; reduces pigment production; helps build deep skin matrix for plumping and firming	All skin types, moisturization and gentle descaling (eczema), post-procedure skin conditioning

molecules than traditional AHAs; however, at approximately 358 daltons, they are small enough to penetrate skin. BAs are mild acids having pKa values that are similar to the smaller AHA molecules. For example, the pKa of lactobionic acid is 3.8, which matches that of glycolic acid.

One of the notable differences of BAs is their hygroscopic nature due to the multiple hydroxyl groups on the molecule. BAs readily attract and retain water, and can form a gel matrix when an aqueous solution evaporates at room temperature. BAs also possess antioxidant and chelation properties. Lactobionic acid, for example, is as an antioxidant chelator used in organ transplantation preservation solutions where it inhibits hydroxyl radical production via the complexation of oxidation-promoting iron found in blood. Additionally, lactobionic acid functions as an inhibitor of matrix metalloproteinase enzymes (MMPs), as described further below.

A distinguishing benefit of the PHAs and BAs is gentleness on skin. When compared with glycolic acid and lactic acid, PHAs and BAs are nonstinging and non-burning. They are also non-irritating. For example, a 12% PHA/BA cream at pH 3.8 scored equivalent to a normal saline control in an occlusive patch, 14-day cumulative irritation test. For this reason, PHAs and BAs are ideal for use on sensitive skin and post-procedurally.

Benefits of hydroxyacids by skin condition

Hyperkeratotic conditions

The AHA class of compounds influences hyperkeratosis by modulating corneocyte attachment at the base of the stratum corneum, resulting in a specific desquamation effect when compared with the nonspecific effect of traditional keratolytic agents. The effect is visually apparent on severely hyperkeratotic skin, such as lamellar ichthyosis, where topical application of high-strength AHAs can lead to marked desquamation and the appearance of normally textured skin in just a few days. AHAs can also be used to descale psoriatic plaques. A study of a 20% AHA/PHA blend cream demonstrated optimal descaling effects after one week of twice daily application, and the result was statistically superior to the prescription 6% salicylic acid control (Figure 7.1). AHAs may be preferred as descaling agents over salicylic acid due to their ability to increase dermal matrix components and counteract corticosteroid-induced dermal thinning. Conversely, salicylic acid has been shown to cause dermal thinning.

Application of AHAs to normal dry skin generally does not cause a visually obvious exfoliation effect. Dry skin conditions can be temporarily relieved with externally applied water, humectants and occlusive compounds, which, through hydration, enable skin enzymes to function properly and promote normal desquamation. However, the dry skin

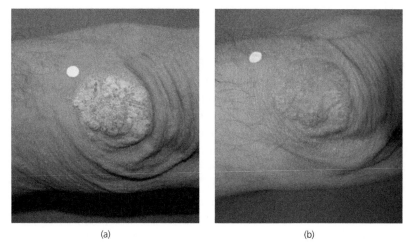

(a)   (b)

Figure 7.1 Psoriasis descaling effect of 20% AHA/PHA cream after twice daily application for 2 weeks. Statistically significant, clinically-graded improvement was observed after 1 week of use. Photos were taken at baseline (a) and after 2 weeks (b).

condition will persist if the stratum corneum and the barrier it provides are not formed properly. AHAs have been shown to increase ceramides within the stratum corneum, thus enhancing skin barrier function. PHAs and BAs are strong humectant compounds which have been shown to increase skin barrier function and can be used to treat eczema partly through gentle acidification of the stratum corneum.

Skin exfoliation can be evaluated using the dansyl chloride cell turnover model, which visually measures the disappearance of stained skin cells over time. Glycolic acid is considered the gold standard in this model. When the PHA, gluconolactone, and BAs, maltobionic acid and lactobionic acid, were tested using glycolic acid as a control, they were found to significantly increase exfoliation/cell turnover versus untreated controls. However, the magnitude of the effect was not as strong as what has been observed with glycolic acid, making the PHAs and BAs milder exfoliating agents. The light exfoliation effect of PHAs and BAs combined with increased barrier function, hydrating capacity and gentleness makes them ideal moisturizing agents for normal and sensitive dry skin conditions such as ichthyosis vulgaris and scaling associated with eczema.

Fine lines, wrinkles, loss of firmness

The AHAs are commonly considered to be exfoliating agents, however, the benefits of AHAs extend well beyond exfoliation. For example, AHAs have been shown to increase dermal biosynthesis of glycosaminoglycans and collagen, and improve the quality of elastic fibers. Notably, glycolic acid has been shown to increase the proliferation of fibroblast cells and to directly stimulate fibroblast cells in vivo and in vitro to produce collagen. In addition, indirect stimulation of collagen synthesis occurs following exposure of dermal fibroblast cells to factors that have been produced by epidermal keratinocytes in response to glycolic acid. This indicates a signaling effect that occurs between the epidermis and the dermis in response to glycolic acid which results in dermal matrix remodeling. Citric acid also significantly increases glycosaminoglycans including hyaluronic acid and the dermal proteoglycan, chondroitin sulfate in vivo. Maltobionic acid and lactobionic acid (BAs) have also been shown to increase hyaluronic acid synthesis in vivo. Stimulation of these cellular changes results in volume-building effects which help to improve symptoms of aging, including the appearance of fine lines, wrinkles and laxity.

Clinical studies with AHAs, PHAs and BAs demonstrate visual improvements in wrinkled skin, which have been supported by various objective measures including: image analysis of silicone replicas, skin thickness measurements utilizing digital calipers and dermal density assessments via ultrasound. Consistent use of these compounds results in a measurable and statistically significant increase in skin thickness versus untreated and vehicle controls. In as little as 12 weeks, significant plumping effects can be observed which provides the anti-wrinkle effect of these compounds (Figure 7.2).

Hyperpigmentation

Hyperpigmentation is a global aging concern spanning multiple races and ethnicities. The condition presents as hyperpigmented lesions that are

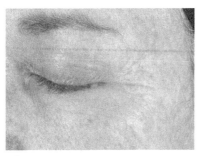 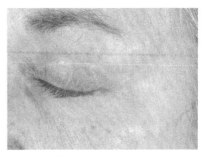

Before   After 16 weeks

Figure 7.2 Reduction in the appearance of crow's feet after 16 weeks use of a regimen including an eye cream containing 3% gluconolactone plus 3% maltobionic acid, pH 4.0 with other benefit ingredients including peptides, hyaluronic acid and antioxidant vitamins. Standardized light photography with facial positioning device; images are cropped and unretouched.

often hyperkeratotic including: lentigines, seborrheic keratoses and actinic keratoses. Other forms of hyperpigmentation, such as melasma, can be more expansive and are not typically hyperkeratotic in nature. Nearly all forms of hyperpigmentation involve sun exposure as a causative factor although some pigmentation is stimulated by other forms of inflammation (e.g. post-inflammatory hyperpigmentation).

Histologically, AHAs have been shown to reduce pigment clumping in the epidermis. These findings have been supported in clinical use studies where AHA containing formulations promote a more even complexion. The BAs, maltobionic acid and lactobionic acid, reduce melanin production in the presence of melanocyte stimulating hormone (αMSH) in the in vitro model utilizing B16 melanoma cells. In addition, the PHAs and BAs are efficient chelating agents, which may in part explain their pigment-evening effect on skin. Copper chelation is known to interfere with the production of the copper-containing enzyme tyrosinase, an essential enzyme in the production of melanin.

AHAs, PHAs and BAs can be formulated with hydroquinone or cosmetic skin brighteners to provide complementary pigment-evening effects as well as exfoliation of hyperkeratotic lesions. Moreover, the antioxidant properties of PHAs and BAs also help to stabilize hydroquinone.

Antioxidant effects

The PHA, gluconolactone, and the BAs, maltobionic acid and lactobionic acid, exhibit antioxidant properties. Gluconolactone was shown to inhibit free radical activation of the solar elastosis gene in an in vitro model of photoaging. This model was validated using other well-known antioxidants such as Vitamin C and Vitamin E, and gluconolactone provided comparable antioxidant effects. The experimental results were attributed to the chelation of oxidation-promoting metals and free radical scavenging. In addition, while glycolic acid can increase sunburn cell formation following UVB exposure in unprotected skin, topical application of gluconolactone does not cause an increase in sunburn cells following UVB irradiation, which may be due to its antioxidant effects. As described above, gluconolactone can also be formulated with oxidative drugs, for example, benzoyl peroxide, to help reduce irritation potential and erythema.

The BAs reduce UV-induced lipid peroxidation in the in vitro antioxidant model used to assess antioxidant capacity. UV-induced lipid peroxidation is an oxidative breakdown of polyunsaturated fatty acids, such as those found in cellular membranes, by free radicals generated during UV light exposure. Inhibitors of lipid peroxidation scavenge the hydroxyl radical, helping to maintain cellular membranes and healthy mitochondria.

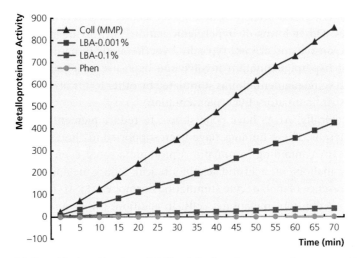

Figure 7.3 Lactobionic acid reduces MMP activity in a dose-responsive manner. Notes: Coll (MMP), Clostridum collagenase IV (collagen degrading MMP enzyme, negative control); LBA, lactobionic acid; Phen, phenantroline (a potent MMP inhibitor; positive control).

MMP inhibition

Matrix metalloproteinase enzymes (MMPs) are zinc-dependent endopeptidase enzymes that degrade collagen in skin as part of the natural process of collagen turnover. In youth, catabolism is balanced with neocollagenesis, resulting in a healthy dermal matrix and the appearance of youthful skin. With age and sun exposure, there is a shift in the balance in favor of collagen catabolism, resulting in dysfunctional collagen status and the formation of wrinkles, telangiectasia and loss of firmness. The BAs, lactobionic acid and maltobionic acid, function as MMP inhibitors, which may help to preserve youthful skin characteristics (Figure 7.3).

AHA peels

Alpha-hydroxy acid-based skin peels are topical procedures that, at high strength, are performed in physician's offices; medium-strength can be performed by aestheticians at spas and salons; and low-strength can be used by patients at home (Figure 7.4). Physician-strength, AHA peels are generally formulated at a low pH to deliver a high concentration of free acid quickly into skin. Concentrations of physician peels can reach or exceed 70% acid, with a pH of less than 1.0 when un-neutralized. Spa/salon peels, on the other hand, do not generally exceed 30%, and are adjusted to a minimum pH of 3.0. The pH of home peels is adjusted to a higher value to ensure safe use at home. Use of a sodium bicarbonate-based neutralizer solution terminates the activity of the AHA peel, generating

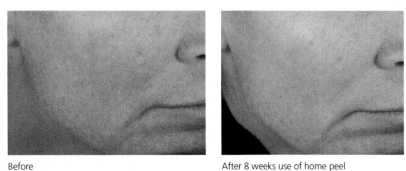

Before   After 8 weeks use of home peel

Figure 7.4 Reduced pigmentation after using a 20% (10% citric acid + 10% glycolic acid pH 3.6) home peel once weekly for 8 weeks with PHA home care products.

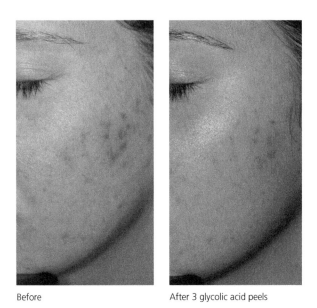

Before   After 3 glycolic acid peels

Figure 7.5 Reduced acne and post-inflammatory pigmentation following three free acid, glycolic acid peels: one 35% (pH 1.3), two 50% (pH 1.2) with adjunctive AHA/PHA home care products. No additional medications were administered.

visible carbon dioxide bubbles in the process, and ensuring completion of the procedure in a safe and predictable manner (Figures 7.4 and 7.5).

Physician-use AHA peels are classified as superficial peeling agents by the American Academy of Dermatology, meaning they primarily affect the epidermis. They have been coined "lunch time" peels due to the short length of the procedure and minimal-to-absent recovery time, with few potential side effects when performed carefully and superficially. At high strength and low pH, a deeper peel may occur, leading to an increase in the potential for side effects. Skin of color is prone to developing post-inflammatory hyperpigmentation, and caution is recommended in this population; it may be preferable to use lower strength AHA peels in order to prevent inflammation.

The most common AHA peeling agents are glycolic, lactic, mandelic and citric acids. Glycolic and lactic acids, as the smallest AHAs, are known to penetrate the skin rapidly in their free acid (un-neutralized) form. Mandelic acid, also known as phenyl glycolic acid, is a more lipophilic form of glycolic acid and is often used to target sebaceous skin; benefits with pigmentation have also been observed. Citric acid penetrates well and provides antioxidant benefits. Glycolic, lactic and citric acids cause stinging more readily than mandelic acid. All have been shown to have beneficial effects on skin in peeling application. Primary benefit areas include smoothing of wrinkles, pigmentation evening and adjunctive anti-acne and anti-rosacea effects (Figure 7.5). Many of these conditions are improved optimally when peels are combined with medications and/or other procedures with complementary mechanisms of action.

Formulating with AHAs

There are many factors to consider when formulating an effective AHA/PHA/BA product. Concentration and pH are two important factors because they impact the amount of acid delivered to the skin. As a general rule, AHA products that are formulated at the pH which matches the pKa of the acid will have approximately 50% of the AHA concentration present as free acid. This is important because the free acid form of an acid is un-ionized and can penetrate the skin more readily than the ionized, salt form which results upon neutralization. For example, a formulation containing 10% glycolic acid (pKa 3.8), which is adjusted to pH 3.8, will have approximately 5% of the glycolic acid bioavailable for rapid penetration in the free acid form. The remaining 5% will be converted to the neutralized salt form, which is significantly less bioavailable to skin. Since pH is a logarithmic scale, a change in pH by one unit impacts the concentration of free acid by a factor of ten.

Formulating technologies are available to help slow the penetration of free acid AHA molecules with the goal of reducing stinging and irritation potential. One such technology utilizes amphoteric amino acids as part of the pH adjustment process. Ingredients such as arginine, lysine or glycine, can function as bases and will raise the formulation pH. These ingredients can also form temporary bonds with the remaining free AHA molecules in formulations to provide a slow release effect. Studies show that use of amphoteric technology significantly reduces the sting and irritation potential of AHAs, while maintaining an effective pH and thus providing effective benefits to skin.

Conclusion

The hydroxyacids offer a selection of formulating and benefit options to meet the needs of varying patient populations, including those with clinically sensitive skin, dry skin, psoriasis and photoaging. First-generation AHAs such as glycolic acid offer significant anti-aging and exfoliation effects as a result of their stimulatory effects on stratum corneum desquamation and dermal biosynthesis, as well as pigment-evening benefits. AHAs continue to be used today due to their well-documented clinical benefits and proven safety profile. Second-generation polyhydroxy acids (PHAs) and third-generation bionic acids (BAs) provide similar anti-aging effects as AHAs, but offer additional benefits including enhanced moisturization and gentleness. In addition, these compounds provide protective benefits by functioning as antioxidants and MMP inhibitors, which may augment their anti-aging effects by helping to protect and preserve the skin's natural functions. AHAs, PHAs and BAs are highly adaptable anti-aging compounds that are likely to be used for years to come because they are effective in providing multiple benefits to skin from topical formulations.

Further reading

Berardesca E, Distante F, Vignoli GP, et al. Alpha hydroxyacids modulate stratum corneum barrier function. *Brit J of Dermatol* 1997; **137**: 934–938.

Bernstein EF, Brown DB, Schwartz MD, et al. The polyhydroxy acid gluconolactone protects against ultraviolet radiation in an *in vitro* model of cutaneous photoaging. *Dermatol Surg* 2004; **30**: 1–8.

Bernstein EF, Underhill CB, Lakkakorpi J, et al. Citric acid increases viable epidermal thickness and glycosaminoglycan content of sun-damaged skin. *Dermatol Surg* 1997; **23**: 689–694.

Ditre CM, Griffin TD, Murphy GF, et al. Effects of α-hydroxy acids on photoaged skin: A pilot clinical, histologic, and ultrastructural study. *J Am Acad Dermatol* 1996; **34**: 187–195.

Draelos ZD, Green BA, Edison BL. An evaluation of a polyhydroxy acid skin care regimen in combination with azelaic acid 15% gel in rosacea patients. *J Cosmet Dermatol* 2006; **5**: 23–29.

Hachem JP, Roelandt T, Schurer N, et al. Acute acidification of stratum corneum membrane domains using polyhydroxyl acids improves lipid processing and inhibits degradation of corneodesmosomes. *J Invest Dermatol* 2010; **130**(2): 500–510.

Kim SJ, Park JH, Kim DH, et al. Increased in vivo collagen synthesis and in vitro cell proliferative effect of glycolic acid. *Dermatol Surg* 1998; **24**: 1054–1058.

Okano Y, Abe Y, Masaki H, Santhanam U, Ichihashi M, Funasaka Y. Biological effects of glycolic acid on dermal matrix metabolism mediated by dermal fibroblasts and epidermal keratinocytes. *Exp Dermatol* 2003; **12** (Suppl. 2): 57–63.

Van Scott EJ, Yu RJ. Control of keratinization with α-hydroxy acids and related compounds. *Arch Dermatol* 1974; **110**: 586–590.

Yu, RJ, Van Scott, EJ. α-hydroxyacids, polyhydroxy acids, aldobionic acids and their topical actions. In: Baran, R, Maibach, HI (eds.) *Textbook of Cosmetic Dermatology*, 3rd edn. New York: Taylor & Francis, 2005: 77–93.

CHAPTER 8

Vitamin A: Retinoids and the Treatment of Aging Skin

Dana L. Sachs and John J. Voorhees
University of Michigan Medical Center, Ann Arbor, MI, USA

Introduction

Retinoids are Vitamin A-derived drugs that have been used to prevent and treat aging skin for decades. Patients applying topical retinoids as part of an anti-acne regimen were noted to have improved cosmesis following retinoid treatment. This observation led to an enormous body of research and literature on the application of topical retinoids for aging skin. In the US retinoids are available both by prescription and in over-the-counter cosmeceutical preparations. Natural and synthetic retinoids are available by prescription in various strengths and formulations and include the natural retinoid retinoic acid (tretinoin) and the synthetic retinoids adapalene, bexarotene, tazarotene, and alitretinoin. The natural retinoids retinol, retinaldehyde, and retinyl esters are available without a prescription and are formulated in innumerable over-the-counter preparations.

In this chapter, we address the natural retinoids specifically with the aims: first, to describe the nomenclature of these various compounds and the relationship of these compounds to each other; second, to discuss the signal transduction pathways in aged and photoaged skin; third, to discuss the biochemical mechanisms by which retinoids impact these aging pathways; and fourth, to discuss evidence-based medicine relevant to specific natural retinoids in their ability to improve aged skin.

Define the active ingredient

The term "retinoid" refers to a family of drugs that binds to and activates the retinoic acid receptors (RARs) eliciting transcriptional activation of retinoic acid responsive genes resulting in specific biologic responses. Retinoids are united in their ability to bind to intranuclear retinoid receptors and act as transcription factors. In skin, the retinoid target genes are cellular retinoic acid binding protein (CRABP) II, cellular retinol binding protein (CRBP),

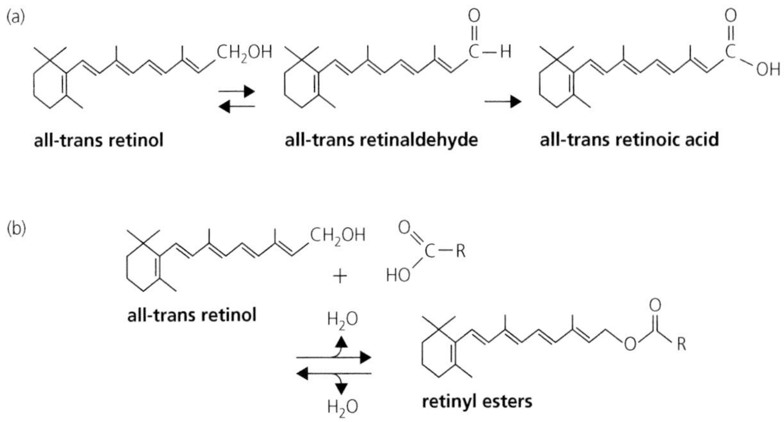

(a)

all-trans retinol   all-trans retinaldehyde   all-trans retinoic acid

(b)

all-trans retinol   retinyl esters

Figure 8.1 Structure of natural retinoids. (a) All-trans retinol is sequentially oxidized to all-trans retinoic acid in a two-step process. The first step of the reaction is a reversible one in which all-trans retinaldehyde can be reversibly converted back to all-trans retinol. The second step in which all-trans retinaldehyde is oxidized to all-trans retinoic acid is irreversible. (b) All-trans retinol undergoes esterification to retinyl esters. Some examples include retinyl linoleate, retinyl laurate, retinyl palmitate, and retinyl oleate.

retinoic acid 4-hydroxylase (CYP26) and keratin 6. RAR heterodimerizes with retinoid X receptors (RXR), and is critical for activating retinoic acid response elements in skin leading to retinoid signaling. There are various isoforms of both RAR and RXR; however, the RAR-γ/RXR-α heterodimer is the most important one in skin signaling.

Retinoids can be categorized as naturally occurring or synthetic (Figure 8.1). Naturally occurring retinoids include all-*trans*-retinol, all-*trans*-retinaldehyde and all-*trans*-retinoic acid. All-*trans* retinol is also known as retinol or Vitamin A; all-*trans*-retinaldehyde is referred to as retinal; and all-*trans*-retinoic acid is referred to as retinoic acid and tretinoin. For the purpose of clarity, all-*trans*-retinol, all-*trans*-retinaldehyde and all-*trans*-retinoic acid will be referred to as retinol, retinaldehyde and retinoic acid, respectively, throughout this chapter. Because the synthetic retinoids are not typically used in cosmeceutical preparations, they will not be discussed in this chapter.

The biology of aging skin

In order to understand the impact that topical retinoids have on improving the appearance of aging human skin, an understanding of skin aging biology specifically with a focus on the changes in dermal collagen is a prerequisite. Natural aging, or intrinsic skin aging, is optimally observed on sun-protected sites such as the upper inner arm or buttocks and is characterized by homogenous color, dryness and fine wrinkling. Photoaging, or extrinsic skin aging, is seen on sun-exposed sites such as the face, hands, and arms and displays fine and coarse wrinkling, dyspigmentation, erythema and predisposition to skin cancers. Though skin aging is apparent in both the epidermis and the dermis, the changes seen in the dermis likely make a much greater contribution to the overall appearance of skin aging.

Reactive oxygen species (ROS) are agents that drive complex signaling cascades in both natural and chronological aging, leading to both fragmentation of formed collagen and reduced new collagen synthesis. Ultraviolet (UV) light plays a significant role in photoaging and miniscule doses of UV lead to statistically significant ROS-mediated injury. Ultraviolet light is responsible for the generation of ROS specifically in the form of H_2O_2. Though ROS can cause direct cellular damage to cell walls, lipid membranes, mitochondria and DNA, H_2O_2 and other free oxygen radicals play an important role in cellular signaling pathways relevant to new collagen formation and breakdown of mature collagen. Through ROS signaling, transforming growth factor beta (TGF-β), a cytokine that promotes collagen production, is blocked and new collagen formation is decreased. Also regulated by ROS signaling is the epidermal growth factor receptor (EGF-R) pathway which signals activator protein (AP-1), a transcription factor responsible for increasing collagenase, a matrix metalloproteinase (MMP) important in collagen breakdown. This up-regulation of collagenase leads to an increase in collagen fragmentation which, in turn, leads to a decrease in the mechanical tension of the fibroblast. Loss of mechanical tension leads to the perpetuation of the cycle in which collagenase is increased, leading to further collagen fragmentation and ultimately permanent collagen loss clinically manifested as photoaging. Fragmented collagen accumulates in the dermis, yet it interacts poorly with integrins or collagen receptors. Each ultraviolet insult results in "micro" solar scars which ultimately coalesce to manifest clinically as "macro" scars or wrinkles.

In the case of natural aging, time leads to the generation of reactive oxygen species. Analogous to photoaging, ROS signaling leads to a blockade in TGF-β resulting in a decrease in new collagen formation. However, in contrast to extrinsic aging, AP-1 mediated breakdown of collagen by MMPs is signaled through the JNK pathway instead of through the EGF-R pathway.

Mechanisms of action

Retinoic acid is the retinoid which exerts an effect on tissues. In the first step of retinoid metabolism, retinol, a functionally inactive retinoid, is oxidized to retinaldehyde by the enzyme retinol dehydrogenase. This reaction is rate limiting for the formation of retinoic acid. In addition, retinaldehyde can be hydrolyzed back to retinol. In the second step, retinaldehyde is oxidized to retinoic acid by retinol dehydrogenase. Retinol and retinaldehyde serve as the ligands for CRBP. Retinoic acid and its metabolites are the ligands for CRABP-II. The ratio of ligand to binding protein is heavily skewed in the direction of binding protein such that receptors are never saturated by ligand. The activity of the p450 enzyme, retinoic acid 4-hydroxylase, also known as CYP 26, catalyzes the conversion of retinoic acid to 4-hydroxyretinoic acid (4-OH RA), the major retinoic acid metabolite.

Retinyl esters are the predominant metabolites of retinol and are important in the molecular storage of retinol in the skin. Two enzymes catalyze the conversion of retinol to retinyl esters: lecithin retinol acyltransferase (LRAT) and Acyl CoA;retinol acytransferase (ARAT). The substrates for LRAT are both retinol and retinol-CRBP complex whereas ARAT has just one substrate, retinol. LRAT is the predominant enzyme regulating retinol esterification in skin, and it is regulated by retinoic acid. Retinoic acid regulation of LRAT provides a mechanism by which RA is auto-regulated by controlling the levels of retinol available for conversion to retinoic acid. In basal keratinocytes, retinol which is supplied to the skin through dermal capillaries is esterified to retinyl esters by LRAT. These retinyl esters can be hydrolyzed back to retinol in basal keratinocytes as the cells differentiate and migrate to the stratum corneum. Topically applied or exogenous retinol can be esterified to retinyl esters by ARAT in suprabasal keratinocytes as well as by LRAT. This auto-regulatory loop in which retinoic acid regulates its own biosynthesis from retinol through regulation of retinol esterification has been well studied. This mechanism assures a lack of toxicity from topical ROL applied in excess for over-zealous patients.

Retinol is esterified with various fatty acids such as palmitic acid, stearic acid, and oleic acid to form retinyl palmitate, retinyl stearate, and retinyl oleate, respectively (Figure 8.2). Hydrolysis of retinyl esters reconstitutes retinol. In skin, approximately 99% of retinoids are retinol and retinyl ester whereas less than 1% of skin retinoids are retinaldehyde and retinoic acid. Application of retinol to skin results mainly in retinyl esters in skin cell membranes. Very little retinol is oxidized to retinoic acid, thus preventing side effects of excess retinoic acid. Application of retinoic acid to skin gives a vast excess of retinoic acid over that needed to load the RARs; this excess may produce some of the irritating side effects known to occur after RA application.

Once retinoic acid enters the nucleus of keratinocytes, it binds to RAR which forms a heterodimer with RXR. RAR/RXR activates various retinoic acid response elements (RAREs) which regulates the transcription of target genes and are responsible for retinoid actions in various tissues (Figure 8.3).

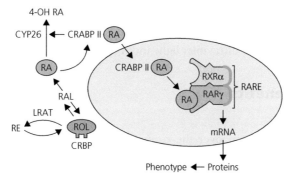

Figure 8.2 Mechanism of action of retinoids in skin. Retinol (ROL) binds to cellular retinol binding protein (CRBP) and undergoes sequential oxidation reactions to form retinoic acid (RA), or it is esterified by lecithin:retinol acyltransferase (LRAT) to retinyl esters (RE). RA binds to cellular retinoic acid binding protein II (CRABP II), and this protein-ligand complex enters the nucleus. In the nucleus, retinoic acid binds to the retinoic acid receptor-γ (RAR-γ) which heterodimerizes with retinoid X receptor-α (RXR-α) to activate retinoic acid response elements (RARE). Activation of RARE leads to transcription of mRNA and subsequent encoding of proteins that play a role in the signal transduction pathways leading to the improved clinical phenotype of retinoid treated aged skin. In the cytoplasm, RA is also hydrolyzed by CYP 26 to 4-hydroxyl retinoic acid (4-OH-RA), the major metabolite of RA which possesses just a fraction of the biologic activity of RA.

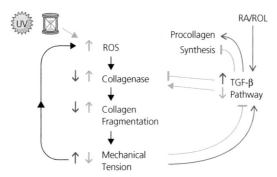

Figure 8.3 Site of action of retinoids in signal transduction pathways in aging skin. Whether due to ultraviolet light damage or the passage of time, reactive oxygen species are generated leading to an increase in collagenase. Collagenase is the major matrix metalloproteinase responsible for leading to the degradation and fragmentation of dermal collagen. Collagen fragmentation results in decreased mechanical tension of the fibroblast which in turn leads to a decrease in the activity of TGF-β signaling resulting in the blockade of new procollagen formation. Blockade of TGF-β also leads to a resulting increase in collagenase thus perpetuating the cycle of collagen fragmentation. Retinoids, specifically retinoic acid and retinol, improve the appearance of aging skin by increasing TGF-β leading to both an increase in procollagen synthesis and a decrease in collagenase.

In skin, retinoic acid is known to work through the TGF-β pathway and has been specifically demonstrated to inhibit the ultraviolet-induced matrix metalloproteinase mediated breakdown of collagen. In addition, retinoic acid protects against ultraviolet light-induced decreases of procollagen.

Clinical benefits

Retinol

Retinol is available in over-the-counter cosmeceutical preparations but labeling is often elusive with respect to determining the precise concentration of the compound. In general, cosmeceutical preparations seem to have retinol concentrations ranging from 0.1% to 1%, but this information is often vague and unclear. Compared to retinoic acid, retinol is fairly non-irritating at low concentrations. This fact, coupled with what is known about its metabolism to retinoic acid, and easy availability, would seemingly render retinol the ideal retinoid. Though there are numerous clinical trials of various concentrations of retinol demonstrating clinical improvement, studies establishing collagen enhancement accompanying the clinical improvement are lacking. In fact, it is unclear whether retinol at commercially available doses has collagen-enhancing properties. Other issues that further complicate the matter are those of drug degradation and improper release from vehicle (partition coefficient issues).

In an in vivo study of retinol, tretinoin, and vehicle applied to human skin, retinol 1.6% was found to significantly increase epidermal thickening comparable to tretinoin 0.025% but without the erythema associated with tretinoin. Other studies have demonstrated that retinol inhibits UV induction of collagen degrading enzymes and stimulates collagen production in photoaged skin. Low dose retinol 0.1% was found to improve clinical photoaging of fine lines and skin tone of the lateral periorbital regions with minimal irritation.

In a study of intrinsically aged skin, retinol 0.04% applied to the sun-protected skin of the arms in an elderly population was demonstrated to significantly increase glycosaminoglycan expression and procollagen I immunostaining compared with vehicle, and only mild irritation was noted in subjects. The improvement following retinol therapy seen in intrinsically aged skin is notable because the degree of collagen damage tends to be much less compared with photoaged skin.

Concentrations of retinol greater than 1% are desirable in cosmeceuticals to achieve the results seen in lab studies, but this information is rarely available on labels. Additionally, "consumer-friendly" dosing (likely exceptionally low retinol concentrations) is often used by companies to mitigate retinoid irritation, yet it is irritation that is a true biomarker of efficacy. Until studies are performed determining that dosing regimens and concentrations that do not cause irritation lead to collagen enhancement, it is unclear whether retinol is clinically effective in commercially available doses.

Retinaldehyde (retinal)

There are very few studies examining the effects of retinal for photoaging. An internet search for cosmeceuticals containing retinal as the main ingredient yielded one product produced by Avene/Pierre Fabre (Ystheal containing retinaldehyde 0.05%).

In a study of photodamaged human facial skin, retinal 0.05% was compared with retinoic acid 0.05% and vehicle. Silicone replicas of skin were performed at baseline, 18 and 44 weeks in the crow's feet region and optical profilometry was employed to study wrinkles and roughness as well as tolerance. At week 18, there was a statistically significant reduction in wrinkles and roughness in both the retinaldehyde and retinoic acid groups; no improvements were noted in the vehicle group. Retinal was well tolerated throughout the duration of the study compared with retinoic acid which was associated with local irritation leading to issues with subject compliance. The study design intentionally avoided the bias of sun exposure by starting all subjects at the same time such that week 18 evaluations were performed during the summertime and week 44 evaluations were performed during the winter.

Retinoic acid (tretinoin)

Retinoic acid is considered to be the penultimate retinoid and has been the most extensively investigated topical retinoid for its ability to improve aging skin. Its safety profile is well established. Retinoic acid binds to and activates the nuclear retinoic acid receptor RAR-γ and is derived from sequential oxidation of retinol and retinaldehyde as discussed earlier. In the US, retinoic acid is available by prescription and exists in cream, gel, microsphere gel, and emollient base formulations as branded names and generic drugs. Though there are multiple commercially available strengths including 0.025%, 0.05%, and 0.1% formulations, the optimal concentration of retinoic acid needed to improve aging skin has not been established. What is clear though is that higher concentrations of retinoic acid are associated with increased irritation. It is important to note, however, that the irritation effects are not responsible for improvement in aged skin.

Retinoic acid improves several characteristics of photoaged skin: surface roughness, dyspigmentation and fine wrinkles. Within the first week of therapy, tactile smoothening is noted, which corresponds with the histologic changes of compactness of the stratum corneum and spongiosis in the epidermis. Wrinkle improvement, however, is not observed until after two to four months of therapy. Importantly, with continued treatment with retinoic acid, the epidermis reverts to its pretreatment state and therefore wrinkle improvement is attributed to dermal changes instead of epidermal ones. Clinical and histological endpoints demonstrated significant improvement of photodamaged skin after four months in a double-blind, vehicle-controlled study of 30 subjects with photoaged forearms and facial skin. Type I collagen formation has been established to be significantly less in sun-damaged sites compared with sun-protected sites and following retinoic acid therapy of sun-damaged skin, an 80% increase in extracellular type I collagen was observed compared with only 14% increase in vehicle-treated skin. When retinoic acid 0.05% cream was applied to facial skin for a minimum of six months, the collagen band in the papillary dermis was demonstrably thickened.

Retinyl esters

As discussed earlier, retinyl esters are the main storage form of retinol in the epidermis. When natural stores of retinol are low, retinyl esters are hydrolyzed to retinol. The composition of retinyl esters in stripped human skin has been studied in vivo and found to be composed of retinyl linoleate, retinyl laurate, retinyl palmitate and retinyl oleate. Retinyl linoleate accounted for the majority of retinyl esters at up to 96 hours following retinol application. The other retinyl esters (oleate, palmitate, laurate, and stearate) each comprised less than 10% of the total.

The clinical benefits of retinyl esters have not been studied to any great extent. Though they are widely present in over-the-counter anti-aging treatments, little data exists supporting their use over retinol. They are often found on ingredient lists alongside retinol but given the superb autoregulatory functions of retinol, it is not clear whether these compounds have any true additive value in aging skin therapy. Table 8.1 is far from comprehensive but illustrates the variety of retinoid containing topical products available around the world. Examples of drugs and cosmeceuticals that contain natural retinoids are listed. Strengths are listed for all of the retinoic acid containing drugs. Strengths and dosages for retinol, retinaldehyde and retinyl esters are rarely easily accessed or listed. The auto-regulatory nature of natural retinoids suggests that there is really no need to look at pricey retinyl esters when formulating cosmeceuticals as retinol will be formed as needed and therefore subsequent retinoic acid will be available. In addition, the penetration of retinol through the stratum corneum is known to be much more optimal than that of retinyl esters or even retinoic acid.

Indications and contraindications

Retinoic acid has FDA approval for the treatment of fine wrinkles, mottled hyperpigmentation and tactile roughness of facial skin. Retinoic acid has

Table 8.1 Select commercially available topical retinoids.

	Over the counter		Prescription
		Tretinoin	Retin-A (0.025%, 0.05%, 0.1% cream; 0.01%, 0.025% gel)
			Renova (0.02% cream
			Atralin (0.05% gel)
			Avita (0.025% cream, gel)
			Refissa (0.05% cream)
			Retin A micro (0.04%, 0.1% microsphere gel)
			Tri-Luma cream (0.05%)
Retinol	Peter Thomas Roth Retinol PM Fusion (1.5%) Replainx		
	Retinol Plus Smoothing Serum 5x (1%, 0.5%, 0.3%, 0.2%)		
	La Roche Posay Biomedic Retinol 60 (0.06%, 0.03%, 0.15%)		
	Neova Retinol ME (0.3%, 0.15%)		
	Roc (?)		
	Avon (?)		
	Txsystems Afirm 3x (0.6%, 0.3%, 0.15%)		
	Skinceuticals (1%, 0.5%)		
	Ysthéal® Pierre Fabre (0.05%, 0.015%)		
	Eluage Pierre Fabre (0.05%, 0.015%)		
Retinal	Glytone (0.05%)		
	Osmosis Serum (0.1%, 0.05%)		
	Sircuit® (?)		
	Derma E®: Vitamin A		
Retinyl Esters	Palmitate	Equate--Anti Wrinkle Cream	
	Linoleate	Garnier Nutritioniste Ultra Lift Anti-Wrinkle Firming Eye Cream	
		Elizabeth Arden Crème Hydratante Continue 24H	

a pregnancy Category C rating, meaning that there are no adequate or well-controlled clinical trials in pregnant women. Oral retinoic acid is, however, a known teratogen so most practitioners advocate withholding topical retinoic acid therapy during pregnancy.

The other natural retinoids – retinol, retinaldehyde and retinyl esters – are used in innumerable cosmeceutical preoparations for the treatment of photoaged skin and because these compounds are not regulated as drugs, indication and contraindication data is not available.

In general, topical retinoids are applied nightly for the treatment of aging skin. Clinical efficacy can be gauged based on irritation; however, the degree of irritation, if any, needed for a biologic effect is unknown at this time. Therefore, it is unclear if once weekly dosing (or even less) is comparable with nightly dosing in terms of clinical efficacy. It is fairly well established, however, that increased frequency of use is associated with increased irritation.

Side effects

Photosensitivity

Topical retinoids have been considered to be phototoxins, but this concern is likely overstated. In fact, retinoids are photo-labile which is why they are packaged in materials that do not allow ultraviolet penetration. Due to the double bonds in their structures, retinoids are susceptible to photochemical reactions and are therefore considered to be photoreactive agents. Photoreactivity does not, however, imply that these agents cause phototoxicity or photoallergenicity. It is interesting that FDA labeling of retinoids continues to warn patients of these risks. Studies have demonstrated that tretinoin is neither phototoxic nor photoallergic in vivo.

In one series of four separate trials to investigate the photoxicity and photosensitizing properties of retinoic acid 0.05% gel (Atralin), no appreciable erythema compared with vehicle or white petrolatum was observed.

In skin pretreated with tretinoin and irradiated with ultraviolet light, no effect on the minimal erythema dose is seen, indicating that tretinoin has no phototoxic activity; retinoic acid lacks sunscreen properties as well. It is interesting that retinoids have been formulated into certain sunscreens given their photo-labile nature.

Retinoid dermatitis/irritation

Retinoid dermatitis results when topical retinoids are applied activating the RAR/RXR heterodimers in subrabasal keratinocytes (Figure 8.4). These heterodimers activate unknown transcription factors which activate the two main EGF-R ligands, heparin binding EGF (HB-EGF) and

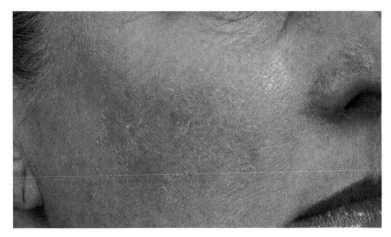

Figure 8.4 Retinoid dermatitis. Retinoid dermatitis is one of the major barriers to topical retinoid application. It is characterized by erythema and desquamation within days to weeks after initiation of therapy and often leads to cessation of treatment. On the molecular level, the RAR-RXR heterodimer is activated in suprabasal keratinocytes resulting in increased HB-EGF and amphiregulin expression. These two ligands are the main EGF-R ligands in human skin. EGF-R activation leads to proliferation of basal keratinocytes and resulting stratum corneum desquamation. This undesirable side effect may be partially mitigated by newer vehicle formulations and certain agents such as genistein.

amphiregulin. Binding of HB-EGF and amphiregulin to the EGF-R leads to proliferation of basal keratinocytes leading to epidermal hyperplasia and resulting in stratum corneum desquamation. As a result, there is disruption of the stratum corneum barrier, leading to cytokine release, causing erythema in the skin. The resulting scaling and erythema comprise the clinical findings of retinoid dermatitis. It is predictable and reproducible and has been heralded as a true indicator of efficacy and penetration. However, this is the side effect that patients most frequently report leading to poor compliance when using this drug class.

Newer formulations with emollient bases and microsphere technology have been created to mitigate these side effects. Various dosing regimens are used but without clear evidence of their efficacy. Dosing retinoic acid just once or twice per week can be an effective way to introduce patients to retinoic acid. Titration to the point of tolerable irritation by one additional weekly application every month can also be a useful way to build up a patient's tolerance to this agent. Some patients, however, do not tolerate much more than once or twice weekly dosing schedules. It is interesting that there has been so little data regarding the proper dosing of retinoic acid or even retinol in terms of achieving maximal increases in procollagen. It may, indeed, be that once weekly (or possibly less frequently) is adequate for procollagen enhancement. The biology of retinoids is predictable and well understood with many years of studies backing biologic activities of this class of agents. But it still has not been established that dermatitis is necessary for retinoid efficacy. It is quite possible that dermatitis is not a prerequisite for biologic activity. Identifying non-irritating retinoid regimens is an area for great potential growth in cosmeceuticals.

Genistein is the major isoflavone in soy extracts and has been shown to inhibit epidermal hyperplasia in organ culture. Daidzein and glycetin, two other soy isoflavones, were also shown to inhibit epidermal hyperplasia in organ cultures but to a lesser extent than genistein. Interestingly, soy extract was observed to stimulate both proliferation and synthesis of type I procollagen. Together, these data make a good case for the use of soy extract, genistein in particular, to mitigate the undesirable retinoid hyperplasia that accompanies retinoic acid use. In addition to mitigating the scaling and erythema, the increase in type I procollagen makes for a potential effect to the anti-aging effect of retinoic acid. It should be noted, however, that the use of genistein in combination with retinoic acid has not been rigorously studied in randomized controlled clinical trials. It would also be interesting to study the timing of genistein application in conjunction with retinoid use. Application of genistein pre-retinoid, with retinoid or post-retinoid would be reasonable regimens to consider in a study.

A recent publication studied the effects of the tree *Alstonia Scholaris* found in Southeast Asia with known anti-inflammatory effects. In the in vitro studies, *Alstonia Scholaris* was demonstrated to have anti-inflammatory effects mainly thought to be due to the major components echitamine and loganin. Specifically *Alstonia Scholaris* down-regulated MCP-1 and IL-8 from human keratinocytes, thereby alleviating symptoms of retinoid dermatitis in a cumulative irritation patch test with retinol. In addition, *Alstonia Scholaris* enhanced the ability of retinoids to inhibit MMP-1 expression, suggesting that it could potentiate the anti-aging effect of retinoids. Further investigation into agents that can mitigate retinoid dermatitis and enhance procollagen expression such as genistein and *Alstonia Scholaris* is exciting as new cosmeceuticals are developed and tested.

Conclusion

Topical retinoids are the mainstay of anti-aging therapy and their use is supported by scores of studies in vivo human skin studies. Retinoic acid is the key player in this arena as it is the compound that interacts directly with intranuclear retinoid receptors leading to transcription of proteins that impact aging pathways. Application of natural retinoids to aged human skin likely leads to adequate amounts of retinoic acid binding to retinoid receptors, given the highly regulated biology of these compounds. More detailed studies of retinyl esters and retinaldehyde with supporting clinical and biochemical data in human skin in vivo would be interesting. Studies of adequate dosing regimens to mitigate retinoid dermatitis would likely yield greater patient compliance with these agents. Identification and further studies of compounds such as genistein in conjunction with retinoids to reduce irritation is highly desirable.

Further reading

Chien AL, Voorhees JJ, Kang S. Topical retinoids. In: Goldsmith LA, Katz SI, Gilchrest B, Paller AS, Leffell DJ, Wolff K (eds.) *Fitzpatrick's Dermatology in General Medicine.* New York: McGraw-Hill Medical, 2012, pp. 2665–2273.

Duell EA, Kang S, Voorhees JJ. Unoccluded retinol penetrates human skin in vivo more effectively than unoccluded retinyl palmitate or retinoic acid. *J Invest Dermatol* 1997; **109**(3): 301–305.

Ellis CN, Weiss JS, Hamilton TA, Headington JT, Zelickson AS, Voorhees JJ. Sustained improvement with prolonged topical tretinoin (retinoic acid) for photoaged skin. *J Am Acad Dermatol* 1990; **23**(4 Pt 1): 629–637.

Fisher GJ, Kang S, Varani J, Bata-Csorgo Z, Wan Y, Datta S, et al. Mechanisms of photoaging and chronological skin aging. *Arch Dermatol* 2002; **138**(11): 1462–1470.

Kang S, Chung JH, Lee JH, Fisher GJ, Wan YS, Duell EA, et al. Topical N-acetyl cysteine and genistein prevent ultraviolet-light-induced signaling that leads to photoaging in human skin in vivo. *J Invest Dermatol* 2003; **120**(5): 835–841.

Kang S, Duell EA, Fisher GJ, Datta SC, Wang ZQ, Reddy AP, et al. Application of retinol to human skin in vivo induces epidermal hyperplasia and cellular retinoid binding proteins characteristic of retinoic acid but without measurable retinoic acid levels or irritation. *J Invest Dermatol* 1995; **105**(4): 549–556.

Kurlandsky SB, Duell EA, Kang S, Voorhees JJ, Fisher GJ. Auto-regulation of retinoic acid biosynthesis through regulation of retinol esterification in human keratinocytes. *J Biol Chem* 1996; **271**(26): 15346–15352.

Napoli JL. Retinoic acid biosynthesis and metabolism. *FASEB J* 1996; **10**(9): 993–1001.

Varani J, Fisher GJ, Kang S, Voorhees JJ. Molecular mechanisms of intrinsic skin aging and retinoid-induced repair and reversal. *J Investig Dermatol Symp Proc* 1998; **3**(1): 57–60.

Weiss JS, Ellis CN, Headington JT, Voorhees JJ. Topical tretinoin in the treatment of aging skin. *J Am Acad Dermatol* 1988; **19**(1 Pt 2): 169–175.

CHAPTER 9

Vitamin C Cosmeceuticals

Marianne N. O'Donoghue[1] and Patricia K. Farris[2]

[1]Rush University Medical Center, Chicago, IL, USA
[2]Tulane University School of Medicine, New Orleans, LA, USA

Introduction

Cosmeceuticals, as defined by Albert Kligman, M.D., are skin care products that have a favorable impact on the condition of the skin. They have revolutionized topical skin care by their ability to improve the skin's appearance without procedures. Vitamin C (L-ascorbic acid) is a water-soluble vitamin that is an essential naturally occurring antioxidant. As a systemic medicine, it prevents scurvy, a syndrome characterized by alterations in bones, mucous membranes, and the skin. Although most plants and animals can synthesize vitamin C, humans must rely on dietary sources since we lack the enzyme L-gulono-gamma-lactone oxidase that is necessary for its synthesis. Vitamin C is plentiful in citrus fruits and dark green, leafy vegetables. It is well absorbed by the intestines in physiologic doses. Interestingly, oral supplementation with high doses of vitamin C does not increase the amount absorbed and also does little to increase skin levels. Thus topical application of this vitamin is considered the best way to afford skin benefits.

Vitamin C: stability and derivatives

Cosmeceuticals containing vitamin C were among the first to enter the marketplace. Most early cosmeceutical formulations contained the active form of vitamin C, L-ascorbic acid (AA). Although these products were highly sought after by consumers, they were quickly found to be problematic in that exposure to air quickly oxidized L-ascorbic acid to dehydroascorbic acid and turned the products yellow. More recent formulations have produced chemically modified forms of ascorbic acid produced by esterification of the hydroxyl group. Such derivatives include magnesium ascorbyl phosphate (MAP), sodium ascorbyl phosphate, ascorbyl-6-palmitate and ascorbyl tetraisopalmitate (ATIP). These derivatives are more stable than L-ascorbic acid (AA), and are favored by cosmetic chemists for this reason.

Pinnell et al. have demonstrated that topical L-ascorbic acid can be formulated in a manner that ensures both stability and skin penetration. In their studies, daily application of 15% L-ascorbic acid at a pH of 3.2 saturated skin levels 20-fold over control after three days. After saturating the skin reservoir, the AA remained in the tissue with a half-life of four days. In contrast, topical 1M dehydroascorbic acid, 13%MAP and 10% ascorbyl-6-palmitate failed to increase levels of ascorbic acid when applied to porcine skin. Many current formulations stabilize and deliver L-ascorbic acid to the skin using delivery systems such as nanosuspensions and microemulsions.

Vitamin C: an important antioxidant

The skin uses antioxidants to protect itself from damaging free radicals. These reactive oxygen species (ROS) are produced most notably by sun exposure but also accumulate as part of the natural or intrinsic aging process. ROS exert damaging effects on proteins, DNA and cell membranes and affect cellular function by influencing transcription factors. In the skin, transcription factor activator protein 1 (AP-1) is up-regulated by ROS triggering the production of matrix-degrading metalloproteinases and reducing pro-collagen production. In addition, ROS up-regulate transcription factor nuclear factor kappa beta (NF-kB), resulting in the synthesis of variety of pro-inflammatory cytokines including tumor necrosis factor-α, interleukin-1 (IL-1), IL-6 and IL-8. Through cell surface receptors these inflammatory mediators further activate AP-l and contribute to skin aging. ROS are also known to increase elastin mRNA in dermal fibroblasts which may explain the elastotic changes that characterize actinically damaged skin.

The skin is armed with a set of naturally occurring antioxidants that help neutralize free radicals. Vitamin C is the most plentiful antioxidant in human skin and functions in the aqueous compartment of the cell. Vitamin C works in combination with other skin antioxidants including vitamin E, ubiquinone, alpha lipoic acid, glutathione. The skin is also armed with a set of enzyme antioxidants including superoxide dismutase, glutathione peroxidase, glucose-6-phosphate dehydrogenase and catalase. Together these two groups of antioxidants function to help control free radicals and protect cells from damage.

Vitamin C helps neutralize free radicals by donating an electron, generating the more stable ascorbate free radical and then by donating a second electron resulting in dehydroascorbic acid. Dehydroascorbic acid can either be broken down by dehydroascorbic acid reductase or be converted back to L-ascorbic acid. L-ascorbic acid is an efficient antioxidant capable of neutralizing the hydroxyl radical, superoxide anion, singlet oxygen and peroxynitrite. In in vitro studies comparing AA with its derivatives, AA was found to be the most effective antioxidant in an aqueous environment followed by MAP and ATIP. In contrast, ATIP was a more effective an antioxidant than MAP when tested in a lipid system.

It is important to remember that at the same time UV light is generating ROS, it is also impairing the skin's ability to neutralize them. Studies have shown that UV exposure depletes the skin of antioxidants in a dose-dependent manner. Ubiquinol and vitamin E are the most photosensitive, while L-ascorbic acid is somewhat more resistant. This is important since vitamin C helps regenerate ubiquinol and vitamin E after they are oxidized, and glutathione helps to regenerate vitamin C.

Vitamin C and photoprotection

While sunscreens remain the cornerstone for protecting the skin from UV light, the use of topical antioxidants in conjunction with sunscreen is gaining favor. Studies have shown that sunscreens do little to prevent oxidative stress although they are effective for reducing UV-induced erythema and thymine dimer formation. Studies have demonstrated that following UVA exposure, sunscreen prevents only 55% of UVA-induced free radicals. Cosmeceutical formulations containing antioxidants are now considered complementary to sunscreens by providing additional protection against free radical formation. While L-ascorbic acid is known to have photoprotective effects, it does not act as a sunscreen and does not absorb light above 295 nm.

In studies designed to evaluate the photoprotective effects of vitamin C, topical L-ascorbic acid (10% solution) was applied twice daily to porcine skin three days prior to UV exposure. Pre-treatment with L-ascorbic acid induced a 40% reduction in sunburn cells and a 52% reduction in UVB-induced erythema compared to vehicle treated skin. Additionally, 10% L-ascorbic acid solution has been shown to reduce UVB-induced immunosuppression and increase systemic tolerance to contact allergens in animal models. Studies in human skin confirm the benefits of topically applied vitamin C for photoprotection. A 10% L-ascorbic acid solution applied to human volunteers daily for five days prior to UVB irradiation significantly reduced minimal erythema dose (MED), while the same protocol using a 5% solution did not have an effect.

Studies have demonstrated that synergistic photoprotection can be achieved by combining topical antioxidants. A combination of 15% L-ascorbic acid and 1% α-tocopherol applied to pig skin four days prior to irradiation with a solar simulator (295 nm) offered superior photoprotection to either agent used alone. The vitamin C and E combination reduced sunburn cell formation, erythema and thymine dimer formation. The combination provided a four-fold increase in protection when compared to vehicle control. More recently, a stable formulation containing vitamins C, E and ferulic acid was tested for photoprotective effects. Ferulic acid is a potent plant antioxidant that stabilizes the vitamin C and E formulation. In a comparative study, 0.5% ferulic, 15% L-ascorbic acid and 1% vitamin E offered an eightfold increase in photoprotection compared to a four-fold increase with vitamin C and E alone. This ferulic acid-stabilized vitamin formulation reduced erythema, sunburn cell and thymine dimer formation and inhibited apoptosis. Additional studies demonstrated that the same ferulic acid-stabilized vitamin C and E formulation provided significant protection against sunburn and thymine dimer formation while 1% idebenone, 1% ubiquinone and 1% kinetin were ineffective. Finally, a combination antioxidant solution containing vitamin C with ferulic acid and phloretin was evaluated for photoprotective effects in ten subjects with Fitzpatrick skin types II and III. Subjects were pre-treated with the antioxidant product four days prior to receiving solar simulated light. Pre-treatment conferred photoprotective effects including prevention of sunburn cell production, thymine dimer formation, matrix metalloproteinases-9 expression and P53 expression. Thus it appears that the use of cosmeceutical formulations containing a combination of vitamin C and other antioxidants may be useful for mitigating both the acute and chronic effects of UV damage.

It is important to note that studies have suggested that topical antioxidants must be applied prior to UV exposure in order to confer photoprotective effects. In a double-blind placebo-controlled human study the short-term effects of antioxidants applied to skin after UV exposure showed no effects. In this study, melantonin, vitamin C and vitamin E were applied 30, 60 and 120 minutes after UV irradiation and all were found to be ineffective.

Vitamin C, collagen synthesis and wrinkles

In addition to being a skin antioxidant, vitamin C has other essential functions. It serves as a co-factor for both prolyl and lysyl hydroxylases. These enzymes are essential for collagen synthesis as the hydroxylated forms of proline and lysine facilitate excretion of procollagen from fibroblasts. Studies have demonstrated that vitamin C is also important for preserving dermal collagen in that it increases stability and decreases the heat sensitivity of collagen. In vitro studies suggest that ascorbic acid may increase the proliferative capacity of elderly dermal fibroblasts. Comparing newborn fibroblasts (3–8 days) with aging fibroblasts (80–95 years old), younger cells were more proliferative. When vitamin C was added, both sets of fibroblasts proliferated faster and reached higher densities than controls. Vitamin C also increased collagen production in both sets of fibroblasts. Subsequently, in vivo studies have confirmed the benefit of vitamin C on collagen production. Skin biopsies from 10 post-menopausal women who applied 5% L-ascorbic acid for 6 months to one forearm and vehicle to the other showed an increase in mRNA levels of collagen. Levels of tissue inhibitor of MMP-1 were also increased in the vitamin C-treated side. Thus vitamin C improves the dermal matrix by increasing collagen production and reducing collagen degradation.

Clinical studies: treating photoaging

While there are relatively few studies in the literature, there is an extensive amount of clinical experience confirming the benefits of topical vitamin C for treating sun damaged skin (Figures 9.1 and 9.2). In a 3-month, double-blind, randomized split-face study, 19 subjects applied 10% L-ascorbic acid or vehicle serum to half the face for 3 months. The vitamin C-treated side showed a significant improvement in optical profilometry image analysis compared to the vehicle-treated side in 14 patients. Clinical assessment showed significant improvement in fine wrinkles, tactile roughness, coarse rhytides, skin laxity/tone, sallowness/yellowing and overall skin appearance on the treated side in 16 of 19 patients.

In a 6-month, double-blind, vehicle-controlled study of patients with moderate photoaging, subjects applied 5% vitamin C cream to the neck and forearms. Improvement in global score was noted by investigators and subjects after three months and included skin hydration, roughness, laxity, suppleness, fine and coarse wrinkles. Clinical improvement was further increased after six months. Silicon replicas confirmed the improvement in fine and coarse wrinkles. Histologic examination of the vitamin C-treated side showed evidence of elastic tissue repair. The authors conclude that vitamin C may be helpful for improving the clinical stigmata of photoaged skin.

Fitzpatrick and Rostan conducted a split-face double-blind study where 10 patients were treated with 10% L-ascorbic acid and 7% tetrahexyldecyl ascorbate in an anhydrous polysilicone gel base. The gel base without active served as a control. At 12 weeks there was statistically significant improvement overall on the vitamin C-treated side. Skin biopsies

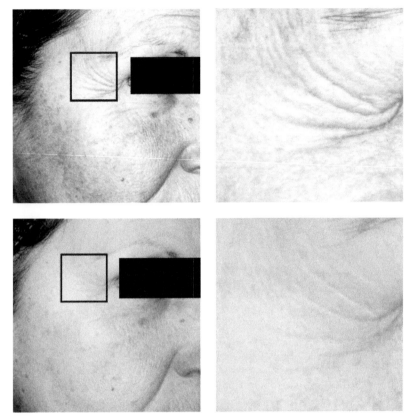

Figure 9.1 Patient before and after one-year treatment with 15% L-ascorbic acid serum and daily sunscreen SPF 20 with zinc oxide and octinoxate. Note improvement of fine lines and wrinkles in the periorbital area. Source: Draelos, Z. (Ed.) Procedures in Dermatology. Cosmeceuticals, 2nd Edn. 2009: Sauders. Reproduced with permission of Elsevier.

performed showed an increase in grenz zone collagen and increased staining for mRNA for type I collagen.

Vitamin C: an important skin lightener

Skin lightening is a desired cosmetic effect in patients with photoaging and with conditions like melasma. Although hydroquinone remains a mainstay of treatment for these conditions, consumer and regulatory concerns about the safety of hydroquinone have promoted interest in alternatives for skin lightening. Regulation of pigment production can be controlled at many levels. Vitamin C is known to inhibit tyrosinase, the enzyme that is the rate-limiting step in melanogenesis, and acts as a reducing agent for melanin

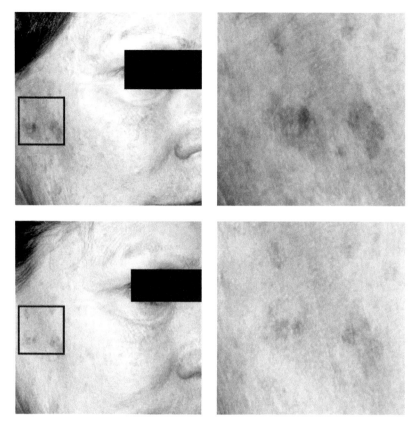

Figure 9.2 Patient before and after one year with 15% L-ascorbic acid serum and
SPF 20 sunscreen containing zinc oxide and octinoxate. Note marked improvement in
photodamage and lightening of mottled pigmentation. Source: Draelos, Z. (Ed.)
Procedures in Dermatology. Cosmeceuticals, 2nd Edn. 2009: Sauders. Reproduced with
permission of Elsevier.

and melanin intermediates. Thus, vitamin C has been considered as an
alternative for treating a variety of pigmentary disorders.

In a clinical study, patients were instructed to apply 10% magnesium-L-
ascorbyl-phosphate cream to treat either melasma or lentigines. Significant
lightening was seen in 19 out of 34 patients. A split-face, randomized,
double-blind study compared 5% L-ascorbic acid cream and 4% hydroquinone cream in 16 patients with melasma. Patients were evaluated
by colorimetry, digital photography, regular color slides and subjective
evaluations. Subjective improvement was seen in 93% of hydroquinone
users who reported good to excellent improvement compared to 62.5%
on the L-ascorbic acid side. It is of interest that the objective measure
colorimetry showed no statistical difference between the treatment modalities. Not surprisingly, the vitamin C-treated side experienced far fewer

side effects (6.2%) compared to the hydroquinone-treated side (68%). Hydroquinone produced a more rapid response at one month compared to the vitamin C-treated side at 3 months. Vitamin C has also been shown to improve melasma when delivered with iontophoresis. In a split-face study comparing weekly 70% glycolic acid peels with a nanosome L-ascorbic acid solution delivered with iontophoresis, both sides showed improvement after 6 weeks. The vitamin C-treated side outperformed the glycolic acid peels with greater improvement in melasma area and severity score. Thus the use of penetration-enhancing techniques may afford greater skin lightening benefits for topical vitamin C.

Vitamin C: A potent anti-inflammatory

Vitamin C is known to have anti-inflammatory activity. Cultured human cells loaded with vitamin C show a reduction in the activity of transcription factor NF-kB. It is believed that this down-regulation occurs by blocking TNF-α induced activation of NF-kB. In view of its anti-inflammatory activity, it has been suggested that topical vitamin C may be helpful for treating patients with inflammatory conditions such as acne. In addition, it has been noted that antioxidants may prevent the oxidation of sebum that contributes to comedogenicity.

In a randomized, double-blind, vehicle-controlled study, patients with acne applied 5% sodium-L-ascorbyl-2-phosphate lotion (APS) or vehicle for 12 weeks. Patients were evaluated by investigator and patient global assessment scores, inflammatory and non-inflammatory lesion counts, and cutaneous adverse events. Thirty-seven patients completed the study and a statistically significant improvement was seen in all parameters measured, including inflammatory and non-inflammatory lesion counts in the patients treated with 5% APS. The APS lotion was well tolerated; only four patients reported minor irritation in both the active and vehicle group.

Conclusion

Topical vitamin C continues to be a valuable and sought-after cosmeceutical ingredient. Consumers view vitamin-based skin care products as safe, natural and effective, making them among the most widely used. Topical vitamin C products include serums, lotions and creams and many current formulations contain vitamin C in combination with other antioxidant compounds. Currently available data suggests that cosmeceuticals containing vitamin C may be useful to enhance photoprotection, reduce the visible

Table 9.1 Effects of vitamin C.

Vitamin C feature	Effect
Antioxidant and photoprotection	Neutralizes free radicals.
	Reduces UV-induced erythema
	Reduces sunburn cell formation
	Reduces thymine dimer formation
	Reduces UV-induced immunosuppression
Preserves collagen	Acts as a co-factor for lysyl and prolyl hydroxylase
	Increases stability and decreases heat sensitivity of collagen
Lightens hyperpigmentation	Inhibits tyrosinase
	Reducing agent for melanin and melanin intermediates
Acts as anti-inflammatory	Down-regulates NF-kB
	Blocks TNF-α induced activation of
	NF-kB

signs of photoaging, improve hyperpigmentation, and treat inflammatory conditions like acne (Table 9.1).

Further reading

Darr D, Combs S, Durston S, et al. Topical Vitamin C protects porcine skin from ultraviolet radiation-induced damage. *Br J Dermatol* 1992; **127**: 247–253.

Espinal-Perez LE, Moncada B, Castanedo-Cazares JP. A double-blind, randomized trial of 5% ascorbic acid vs. 4% hydroquinone in melasma. *Int J Dermatol* 2004; **43** :604–607.

Humbert PG, Haftek M, Credid P et al. Topical ascorbic acid on photoaged skin: Clinical, topographical and ultrastructural evaluations: double-blind study vs placebo. *Exp Dermatol* 2003; **12**: 237–244.

Murray JC, Burch JA, Streilein RD, et al. A topical antioxidant solution containing vitamins C and E stabilized by ferulic acid provides protection for human skin against damage caused by ultraviolet irradiation. *J Am Acad Dermatol* 2008; **59**: 418–425

Phillips CL, Combs SB, Pinnell SR. Effects of ascorbic acid on proliferation and collagen synthesis in relation to donor age of human dermal fibroblasts. *J Invest Dermatology* 1994; **103**: 228–232.

Pinnell SR, Yang HS, Omar M, et al. Topical L-ascorbic acid: percutaneous absorption studies. *Dermatol Surg* 2001; **27**: 127–142.

Ronchetti IP, Quaglino D, Bergamini G. Ascorbic acid and connective tissue. In: Harris JR, ed. *Biochemistry and* Biomedical Cell Biology, New York: Plenum Press, 1996.

Traikovich SS, Use of topical ascorbic acid and its effects on photodamaged skin topography. *Arch Otolaryngol Head Neck Surg* 1999: **125**: 1091–1998.

Woolery-Lloyd J, Baumann L, Ideno H. sodium L-ascorbyl-2-phosphate 5% lotion for the treatment of acne vulgaris: A randomized, double-blind, controlled trial. *J Cosmet Dermatol* 2010; **9**(1): 22–27.

Zussman J, Ahdouf J, Kim J. Vitamins and photoaging: Do scientific data support their use? *Jour Am Acad Dermatol* 2010; **63**(3): 507–527.

CHAPTER 10

Niacinamide: A Topical Vitamin with Wide-Ranging Skin Appearance Benefits

Diane S. Berson[1], Rosemarie Osborne[2], John E. Oblong[2], Tomohiro Hakozaki[2], Mary B. Johnson[2], and Donald L. Bissett[2]

[1]Weill Medical College of Cornell University, New York-Presbyterian Hospital, New York, NY, USA
[2]The Procter & Gamble Company, Cincinnati, OH, USA

Introduction

Niacinamide is vitamin B3, an essential nutrient. In the body, it is converted to the co-factors NADH and NADPH that are involved in many biochemical reactions. Dietary deficiency of this water-soluble member of the vitamin B family causes pellagra, a disease which includes dermatitis and red lesions. Pellagra caused thousands of deaths in the United States in the first half of the twentieth century, until simple dietary supplementation with this absorbable vitamin was found to cure the disorder.

NAD+ and NADPH levels in skin cells decline with age. Thus, supplementing skin with the precursor to these vital co-factors has the potential to provide appearance benefits to aging skin. Since niacinamide penetrates the skin's surface readily, it is bioavailable from topical application for targeted delivery to specific skin sites. Clinical evaluations of topical formulations containing this vitamin have identified a wide range of skin care benefits. Among the many cosmetic effects for skin are reductions in the appearance of hyperpigmented spots, redness, yellowing (sallowness), surface sebum, pore size, surface texture, and fine lines and wrinkles. Additionally, there are improvements in moisturization, stratum corneum barrier integrity and elasticity. Further clinical evaluations have found that specific combinations of niacianamide with other cosmetic skin care ingredients can provide an even greater magnitude of appearance benefits.

Dermatological effects of topical niacinamide have also been observed in human testing, such as improvements in acne and bullous pemphigoid. A more recent evaluation demonstrated that topical niacinamide can provide appearance benefits in rosacea patients by improving skin barrier properties. The effect on the skin barrier also underlines the ability of

Cosmeceuticals and Cosmetic Practice, First Edition. Edited by Patricia K. Farris.
© 2014 John Wiley & Sons, Ltd. Published 2014 by John Wiley & Sons, Ltd.

this vitamin, when applied topically prior to, or with, topical retinoids to increase the skin's tolerability to retinoid treatment and enhance the visible improvement of photodamaged skin.

This brief review chapter will focus on only a few of these skin appearance effects: surface sebum, pore size, surface texture, hyperpigmentation, and fine lines and wrinkles. In particular, new mechanistic insights underlying niacinamide's effects on skin's appearance and enhanced visible improvements when combined with other ingredients will be highlighted.

Active ingredient

Vitamin B3 is present in many food sources (e.g., meat, nuts, wholegrains, legumes, yeast, to name a few). There are, of course, several commercial sources of the pure vitamin.

Three primary forms of vitamin B3 have been used in topical skin care products: niacinamide (aka nicotinamide), nicotinic acid, and nicotinate esters (e.g. benzyl nicotinate, myristoyl nicotinate). The bulk of the published in vitro and clinical studies revealing skin effects have been done with topical niacinamide (see below). Due to skin irritation concerns (see discussion on possible side effects below), clinical skin benefit studies with nicotinic acid and most nicotinate esters have not been done. There is some published clinical work with myristoyl nicotinate revealing effects on aging skin.

Mechanisms of action

Since niacinamide is a precursor to the co-factors NAD(H) and NADP(H), which are involved in many biochemical reactions in the skin, it has the potential to impact a wide variety of metabolic pathways and thus impact skin functions that rely on those pathways. As a result of the complex interactions, several mechanisms for the actions of niacinamide in vitro have been described. For example, NADPH is a cofactor in the synthesis of fatty acids and more complex lipids such as ceramides. Also, NADH has been observed to inhibit some of the enzymes involved in the synthesis of glycosaminoglycans (GAGs) in vitro. Thus, niacinamide's precursor role appears to be important in connection with the observed increase in stratum corneum ceramides in vitro and subsequent improvement in skin barrier function, and with the observed reduction in excess dermal GAGs in vitro and the improved appearance of wrinkles. For other effects observed in vitro such as the increase in production of proteins (barrier layer proteins and collagen) and the inhibition of melanosome transfer,

Table 10.1 Mechanistic effects of niacinamide and the postulated skin appearance benefits.

Niacinamide effect (ex vivo, in vitro)	Postulated skin appearance benefits
Inhibition of sebum production, specifically reducing the content of diglycerides, triglycerides, and fatty acids	Reduced acne Reduced pore size Improved texture
Stimulation of epidermal skin barrier lipids (ceramides) and proteins (keratin, involucrin, filaggrin)	Improved skin barrier and moisturization Reduced skin redness Rosacea appearance benefits
Anti-inflammatory (inhibition of inflammatory cytokines)	Anti-aging Reduced skin redness Rosacea appearance benefits
Increased production of collagen	Anti-wrinkle
Inhibition of production of excess dermal GAGs (glycosaminoglycans)	Anti-wrinkle
Inhibition of melanosome transfer from melanocytes to keratinocytes	Reduced hyperpigmentation
Inhibition of protein glycation via anti-oxidant effects (niacinamide, as precursor, increases levels of the redox co-factors NADH and NADPH)	Inhibit skin yellowing Sun protection

the specific mechanisms have not been elucidated to make connections to the skin benefits observed. However, it is possible that these effects also are a consequence of niacinamide's precursor role, the specifics of which have not been investigated in detail to define the processes involved. While all the mechanistic details have not been fully elucidated, Table 10.1 briefly presents an overview based on in vitro research and their potential connection to skin appearance benefits (discussed in more detail under Clinical Benefits).

More recent in vitro mechanistic studies have greatly expanded the number of potential skin targets affected by niacinamide in vitro. These new discoveries are summarized briefly in Table 10.2, and include a range of biomarkers related to skin structure, elasticity, wound healing and pigmentation. A relatively recent finding is the ability of niacinamide to impact UV-induced changes in skin. For example, in vitro testing showed that niacinamide can reduce production of PGE_2 from keratinocytes when stressed with non-lethal fluencies of UVB. Observations of cellular morphology also suggest an ability to protect overall integrity of the cellular structure from UV-induced changes in vitro. This supports published data showing the ability of both topical and oral niacinamide to prevent UV-induced immunosuppression. It has been hypothesized that, mechanistically, niacinamide protects cellular energy metabolism in vitro. The

Table 10.2 Newly discovered mechanistic effects of niacinamide and the postulated skin appearance benefits.

Niacinamide effect (ex vivo, in vitro)	Postulated skin appearance benefits
Stimulation of keratinocyte proliferation via potentiation of KGF-mediated effects	Wound healing
Stimulate production of collagen and mRNA transcripts of several matrix components, associated enzymes, and cytokines: fibulin-1, fibronectin-1, elastin, lysyl oxidase (1 and 2), procollagen, collagen (I and III), TGF-beta (1, 2, and 3), actin, CTGF, tenascin XB)	Anti-wrinkle (anti-aging)
Down regulation of MITF, tyrosinase, TRP1, TRP2, and PMEL17	Reduce hyperpigmentation
Reducing UV-induced PGE_2 synthesis from keratinocytes	Inflammation
Preventing UV-induced immunosuppression	Actinic keratosis
Metabolic oscillator for circadian rhythm regulation	Skin barrier

concept of niacinamide impacting cellular metabolism is based on its rapid incorporation into both the NADH and NADPH cellular pools. However, newer research on regulation of circadian rhythms suggests that niacinamide plays an even more critical role in connecting cellular metabolism with regulator processes in vitro.

Clinical benefits

In vehicle-controlled, randomized, double-blind, statistically powered human clinical testing (of duration up to six months), a wide range of skin care benefits have been observed with topical niacinamide.

Reduction in surface sebum, pore size, and texture appearance

These effects are discussed as a group since reduction in facial surface sebum has been observed to be associated with reductions in pore size and count and in the appearance of skin surface texture. Niacinamide significantly reduces surface sebum in human skin biopsy specimens and in facial testing (after four weeks of topical treatment on Caucasian skin), with decreases specifically in the glyceride and fatty acid components of skin surface sebum. These surface sebum component changes are accompanied by significant reductions in the appearance of pore size and rough skin texture.

More recent testing has confirmed this effect on Caucasian facial skin, showing significant reductions in surface sebum, sebum spots, pore size, and pore count (based on Sebutape® and quantitative image analyses). This testing also extended the observation to Japanese facial skin, revealing significant reductions in surface sebum and pore size after two and four weeks of treatment.

In the search for additional ingredients, screening in an in vitro sebocyte assay confirmed the effectiveness of niacinamide and identified another potent surface sebum-reducing ingredient, dehydroacetic acid or its salt sodium dehydroacetate (SDA), which has previously been used in the cosmetic industry as a preservative. In facial skin testing, the topical combination of niacinamide and SDA was significantly more effective than topical niacinamide alone, the combination more than doubling the reductions in skin surface sebum and bumpy facial texture appearance.

In other testing, a regimen of products containing niacinamide (N) and salicylic acid (SA) versus an OTC benzoyl peroxide (BP) product regimen were evaluated in women with Skin Types I–V. The N-SA regimen provided a significantly better skin hydration effect than the BP regimen and comparable acne lesion benefits. The former was also significantly more effective in improving visible skin surface texture, pore size, and pore count (Figure 10.1). Additionally, significant correlations among these skin parameters were found, indicating a connection between pore parameters and texture appearance, establishing that reduction of surface sebum, and thus visible pore size, is a valid target for improving skin texture appearance. The surface sebum and pore effects are also relevant to acne treatment.

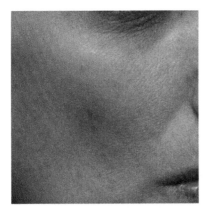 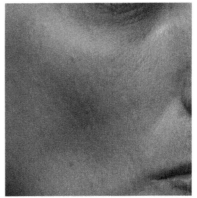

Figure 10.1 Topical regimen of niacinamide and salicylic acid significantly reduces the appearance of facial skin texture and pore size (baseline vs. week 12).

Reduction in fine lines and wrinkle appearance

Previous studies have shown a decrease in the appearance of facial fine lines and wrinkles following topical application of a niacinamide-containing moisturizer. Results from the clinical study showed significant reductions in these parameters after 8 and 12 weeks of treatment.

In recent clinical facial testing, a cosmetic moisturizing product regimen containing the combination of niacinamide (N), peptide (pal-KTTKS, which affects the dermal matrix in vitro), and retinyl propionate (RP) was evaluated versus a regimen that included a prescription 0.02% tretinoin product. While both regimens improved the appearance of facial fine lines and wrinkles significantly and to the same extent by the end of the study (24 weeks), the N/peptide/RP regimen was significantly more effective early in the study (after 8 weeks) and better tolerated by the test subjects, based on measures of skin barrier, erythema, and skin dryness (Figure 10.2).

Reduction in hyperpigmentation appearance

Topical niacinamide has been shown in several clinical studies to significantly reduce facial hyperpigmentation appearance, in particular, hyperpigmented spots. The effect is significant after four weeks of treatment.

More recent clinical testing has revealed the greater effectiveness of niacinamide in reducing the appearance of facial hyperpigmentation when combined with ingredients that inhibit different points in the pigmentation pathway in vitro. For example, N-acetyl glucosamine (which inhibits activation of tyrosinase in vitro) and N-undecyl-10-enoyl-L-phenylalanine (which blocks alpha-MSH in vitro) both significantly increase the skin appearance benefits of topical formulations containing niacinamide (Figure 10.3).

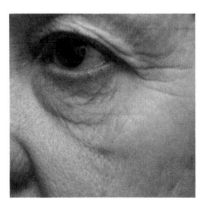 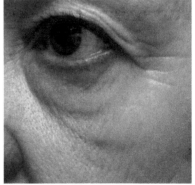

Figure 10.2 Topical regimen of niacinamide, peptide (pal-KTTKS), and retinyl propionate significantly reduces the appearance of facial fine lines and wrinkles (baseline vs. week 8).

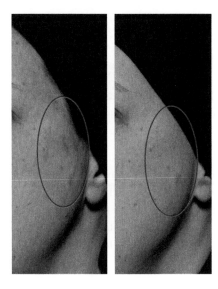

Figure 10.3 Topical niacinamide in combination with N-undecyl-10-enoyl-L-phenylalanine significantly reduces the appearance of facial hyperpigmented spots (baseline vs. week 8).

UV-induced immunosuppression and actinic keratosis

Continued research assessing the impact of both topical and oral niacinamide on preventing UV-induced immunosuppression establishes the ability of this vitamin to block this critical pathway in cancer onset, as exemplified through the reduction in the onset of actinic keratosis. While the effect appears to be more notable in the male population, this is an important finding for both genders.

Uses

Niacinamide is used topically in cosmetic skin care products for the facial appearance benefit effects discussed above. Topical niacinamide has also been used dermatologically for the treatment of acne in some countries and more recently to provide appearance benefits in rosacea patients and as an adjunct skin care with topical retinoids. Facial appearance benefits in a rosacea patient after four weeks of topical niacinamide are shown in Figure 10.4.

Possible side effects

Niacinamide can be used at high doses topically (at least up to 5%, the dose used in several commercial cosmetic products) and is generally well tolerated; however, in some rare cases mild skin irritation has been observed. The nicotinic acid form of Vitamin B3 can be problematic for topical use due to a skin reddening (vasodilation) response that can occur

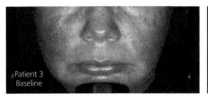 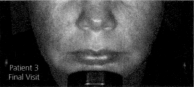

Figure 10.4 Topical niacinamide provides facial appearance benefits in rosacea patients (baseline vs. week 4).

at doses less than 1%. Often irritation and itching can accompany this response. Some nicotinic acid esters, even at doses much lower than 1%, can be difficult to use in cosmetic skin care products due to skin hydrolysis to free nicotinic acid, resulting in the reddening and irritation/itch effects. One ester (myristoyl nicotinate) has been reported to lack these effects, while still providing chronic skin benefits.

Conclusion

This chapter illustrates the myriad dermatological and topical uses of niacinamide in cosmetic formulas, from simple moisturization to providing appearance benefits in patients with dermatological skin disorders such as rosacea via improvement in skin barrier integrity. Since many of the skin appearance issues improved with this vitamin are encountered by dermatologists in their daily practices, having a cost-effective, skin-friendly material such as niacinamide is a welcome addition to the skin care options available for dermatologists to recommend to their patients.

While in vitro-based mechanistic understanding is a critically important component of selecting ingredients for cosmetic formulations, the importance of clinical proof of effectiveness cannot be over-emphasized to demonstrate real-world utility. Clinical studies demonstrating ingredient effectiveness must involve the following key design elements: statistically powered, double-blinded, vehicle-controlled, randomized, utilizing state-of-the-art objective measures (e.g. computer image analysis), and peer review of the study design and its results. These clinical efforts, which support the studies reported here for topical niacinamide, should provide the basis for recommending ingredients, and the products that contain those ingredients, to improve skin appearance in a noticeable and patient-relevant manner.

As laboratory and clinical research continues, additional skin care benefits of niacinamide and its combinations with other ingredients are likely to be found for this versatile, yet potent, water-soluble vitamin. Those new discoveries are expected to broaden even further the clinical utility of topical niacinamide.

Further reading

Bissett DL. Anti-aging skin care formulations. In: Draelos ZD, Thaman LA (eds.) *Cosmetic Formulation of Skin Care Products*. New York: Taylor & Francis Group, 2006, 167–186.

Bissett DL, Miyamoto K, Sun P, et al. Topical niacinamide reduces yellowing, wrinkling, red blotchiness, and hyperpigmented spots in aging facial skin. *Int J Cosmet Sci* 2004; **26**: 231–238.

Bissett DL, Oblong JE, Saud A, et al. Topical niacinamide provides skin aging appearance benefits while enhancing barrier function. In: Elsner P, Maibach HI (eds.) *Cosmeceuticals and Active Cosmetics*, 2nd edn. New York: Taylor & Francis Group, 2005, 421–440.

Bissett DL, Robinson LR, Raleigh PS, et al. Reduction in the appearance of facial hyper-pigmentation by topical N-undecyl-10-enoyl-L-phenylalanine and its ombination with niacinamide. *J Cosmet Dermatol* 2009; **8**: 260–266.

Damian DL, Patterson CR, Stapelberg M, et al. UV radiation-induced immunosuppression is greater in men and prevented by topical nicotinamide. *J Invest Dermatol* 2008; **128**: 447–454.

Draelos ZD, Ertel KD, Berge CA. Niacinamide-containing facial moisturizer improves skin barrier and benefits subjects with rosacea. *Cutis* 2005; **76**: 135–141.

Draelos ZD, Ertel KD, Berge CA. Facilitating facial retinization through barrier improve-ment. *Cutis* 2006; **78**: 275–281.

Final report on the safety assessment of sodium dehydroacetate and dehydroacetic acid. *J Am Coll Toxicol* 1985; **4**: 123–159.

Fu JJJ, Hillebrand GG, Raleigh P, et al. A randomized, controlled comparative study of the wrinkle reduction benefits of a cosmetic niacinamide/peptide/retinyl propionate product regimen vs. a prescription 0.02% tretinoin product regimen. *Br J Dermatol* 2010; **162**: 647–654.

Hakozaki T, Minwalla L, Zhuang J, et al. The effect of niacinamide on reducing cutaneous pigmentation and suppression of melanosome transfer. *Br J Dermatol* 2002; **147**: 20–31.

Imai S. Clocks in the NAD world: NAD as a metabolic oscillator for the regulation of metabolism and aging. *Biochim Biophys Acta* **2010**; 1804: 1584–1590.

Kaczvinsky JR, Li JX, Mack CE, et al. Effectiveness of a salicylic acid-niacinamide regimen for improvement in the appearance of facial skin texture and pores in post-adolescent women. In manuscript.

Kimball AB, Kaczvinsky JR, Li J, et al. Reduction in the appearance of facial hyperpig-mentation after use of moisturizers with a combination of topical niacinamide and N-acetyl glucosamine: Results of a randomized, double-blind, vehicle-controlled trial. *Br J Dermatol* 2010; **162**: 435–441.

Lammers K, Bushnell D, Laughlin T, et al. Niacinamide inhibits melanogenesis related gene expression in melanocytes when co-cultured with keratinocytes. *J Am Acad Dermatol Sup* 2010; **62**: AB118.

Matts PJ, Oblong JE, Bissett DL. A review of the range of effects of niacinamide in human skin. *Int Fed Soc Cosmet Chem Mag* 2002; **5**: 285–289.

Osborne RO, Rose-Mansfield R, Matsubara A, Swanson C. Reduction in skin sur-face sebum with cosmetic ingredients. Oral presentation, 22nd World Congress of Dermatology 2012, Seoul, Korea (poster number FC 02-06).

Park J, Halliday GM, Surjana D, et al. Nicotinamide prevents ultraviolet radiation-induced cellular energy loss. *Photochem Photobiol* 2010; **86**: 942–948.

Robinson MK, Mills KJ, Trejo AV, et al. Reduction in gene expression related to inflammation by skin barrier improving agent, niacinamide. *J Am Acad Dermatol Sup* 2009; **60**: AB83.

Sivapirabu G, Yiasemides E, Halliday GM, et al. Topical nicotinamide modulates cellular energy metabolism and provides broad-spectrum protection against ultraviolet radiation-induced immunosuppression in humans. *Br J Dermatol* 2009; **161**: 1357–1364.

Surjana D, Halliday GM, Martin AJ, et al. Oral nicotinamide reduces actinic keratoses in phase II double-blinded randomized controlled trials. *J Invest Dermatol* 2012; **132**: 1497–1500.

CHAPTER 11

Innovative Botanicals

Jennifer David[1], Candrice R. Heath[2], and Susan Taylor[1,3]

[1] Society Hill Dermatology, Philadelphia, PA, USA
[2] St Luke's-Roosevelt Hospital Center, New York, NY, USA
[3] University of Pennsylvania, Philadelphia, PA, USA

Introduction

Significant innovations have occurred in the past several years in the development of botanical agents. Botanical agents are now included in a wide array of skin care and personal care products. These innovative botanicals are also utilized to complement medical therapy for disorders such as acne, melasma, and rosacea. As an increasing number of botanicals are at the center of basic science and clinical research studies, we now have evidence-based medicine to support therapeutic claims and understand potential adverse events. In this chapter, we will define the active ingredients, outline the mechanisms of action, clinical benefits, uses and potential adverse events of five innovative botanicals: pine bark extract (PBE), Coffea arabica, pomegranate, tea tree oil, and grape seed extract.

Pine bark extract (PBE)

Pine bark extract (PBE) is obtained from the bark of the French maritime pine tree, *Pinus maritime*. It is commonly marketed under the trade name Pycnogenol®. The active ingredients in PBE are phenolic acids, vanillin, and condensed flavonoids (procyanidins and proanthocyanidins). With its complex composition, PBE exhibits anti-inflammatory, antioxidant, vasomotor and anti-allergic effects through a variety of mechanisms (Table 11.1).

The use of pine bark for medicinal purposes can be traced back to the "Father of Medicine", Hippocrates, in 400 BC. Currently, PBE has been reported to treat wide-ranging skin disorders from hyperpigmentation, to systemic lupus erythematosus, photoaging, and venous insufficiency.

The anti-allergic and anti-inflammatory properties of PBE have been evaluated by Choi and Yan. Through both in vitro and in vivo models, PBE was demonstrated to inhibit liberation of histamine and other

---

Cosmeceuticals and Cosmetic Practice, First Edition. Edited by Patricia K. Farris.
© 2014 John Wiley & Sons, Ltd. Published 2014 by John Wiley & Sons, Ltd.

Table 11.1 Active ingredients and mechanism of action for PBE.

Active ingredient	Mechanism of action
Pine bark extract (PBE)	*Anti-inflammatory*: Blocks nuclear factor kappa-light-chain-enhancer of activated B cells Inhibits production of the adhesion proteins: vascular cell adhesion molecule-1 (VCAM-1) and intercellular adhesion molecule-1 (ICAM-1) Blocks gene expression of 5-lipoxygenase (5-LOX) and cyclooxygenase-2 (COX-2) and activity of phospholipids A2 (PLA2) *Anti-oxidant*: Protects against the degradation of endogenous antioxidant substances. (tocopherol and glutathione) *Vasodilatation*: Increases nitric oxide production *Anti-allergic* Inhibits the release of histamine from mast cells

inflammatory cytokines when stimulated through IgE-mediated immune responses.

PBE has also been investigated for its effect in protecting human skin against solar UV-simulated light-induced erythema. A study conducted by Saliou et al. demonstrated that a higher minimal erythema dose (MED) was required to elicit an erythematous response when human subjects were taking oral PBE supplements versus not taking them.

PBE, in the form of Pycnogenol, has been declared GRAS (generally regarded as safe) by an independent panel of toxicology experts. Although not demonstrated through research studies, it has been speculated that the potent antioxidant effects of PBE may interfere with the action of certain chemotherapeutic drugs and radiation therapy.

Coffea arabica

Coffea arabica (*C. arabica*), also known as green coffee, is a species of Coffea originally indigenous to the mountains of Yemen, in the Arabian Peninsula, as well as the highlands of Ethiopia. Bioactive metabolites such as phenolic diterpenes, tocopherols, and fatty acids have been isolated from Coffea arabica. Coffea arabica extract (CAE) and green coffee seed oil extract (GCO) have anti-aging and anti-inflammatory effects, the mechanism of which have been studied (Table 11.2).

Table 11.2 Active ingredients and mechanism of action for Coffea arabica.

Active ingredient	Mechanism of action
Green Coffee seed oil extract (GCO)	*Anti-aging*: Increases synthesis of collagen, elastin and glycosaminoglycans by direct release of TGF-β and GM-CSF Increases Aquaphorin-3 mRNA expression in human cultured keratinocytes
Coffea arabica leaves extract (CAE)	*Anti-aging*: Stimulates type I procollagen expression *Anti-inflammatory*: Inhibits MMP-1, -3, -9 expression and inhibits the phosphorylation of JNK, ERK and p38

Coffea arabica metabolites are commonly used in anti-aging products to address fine lines, wrinkles, hyperpigmentation, skin firmness, and erythema.

A double-blind, randomized, controlled clinical usage study *C. arabica*, evaluated the efficacy and tolerability of a novel topical, multi-ingredient (key component being *C. arabica*) skin care system (face wash, day lotion, night cream and eye serum) in reducing the appearance of the signs of photoaging. Forty Caucasian female participants were randomly assigned to apply either the *C. arabica* enriched regimen or an unspecified anti-oxidant free skin care regimen. Statistically significant improvement in the appearance of wrinkles, firmness, hyperpigmentation, redness, tactile roughness and clarity in phototdamaged skin was noted as compared to controls (Figure 11.1). *C. arabica* was well tolerated with no adverse effects.

Pomegranate

Pomegranate is a fruit grown on the tree, *Punica granatum*, of the Punicaceae family. Many forms of pomegranate are currently available including pomegranate juice, cold-pressed seed oil, peel extract, fruit extract, hydroalcoholic and gel-based pomegranate extract which may be included in various products. Pomegranate has antioxidant, anti-inflammatory, and anti-carcinogenic properties (Table 11.3). Therapeutic efficacy is derived from ellagic acid and flavonoid (anthocyanidins and anthocyanins) components of pomegranate.

Pomegranate and its derivatives have been used to treat bacterial and fungal infections, sunburns, photoaging, and for photochemoprevention by ameliorating the adverse effects of UV-B radiation.

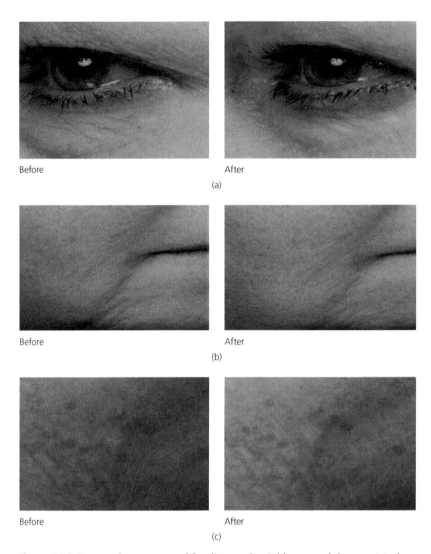

Before   After

(a)

Before   After

(b)

Before   After

(c)

Figure 11.1 Improved appearance of fine lines and wrinkles around the eyes (a), the mouth (b) and hyperpigmentation (c) after using a novel, topical multi-ingredient skin care system with (c). Arabica as the key component.

Many in vitro assays have proven the anti-bacterial properties of pomegranate. One study evaluated the actions of pomegrante methanolic extract (PGME) combined with antibiotics against 30 clinical isolates of methicillin-resistant *Staphylococcus aureus* (MRSA) and methicillin-sensitive *Staphylococcus aureus* (MSSA). Susceptibility testing of the isolates to PGME and antibiotics was performed by the broth dilution method. Synergic activity was detected between PGME and the five antibiotics tested, chloramphenicol, gentamicin, ampicillin, tetracycline, and oxacillin, ranging from 38% to 73%.

Table 11.3 Active ingredients and mechanism for action for pomegranate.

Active ingredient	Mechanism of action
Pomegranate by-product (PBP)	*Antioxidant*: Decreases cellular lipid peroxide content and increases the level of reduced glutathione
Cold pressed pomegranate seed oil	*Anti-inflammatory*: Inhibits cyclooxygenase and lipoxygenase *Anti-carcinogenic*: Inhibits skin edema, hyperplasia, and epidermal ornithine decarboxylase activity
Pomegranate fruit extract (PFE)	*Anti- tumorgenesis*: Inhibits TPA-induced phosphorlyation of ERK1/2, p38, and JNK1/2, along with activation of NF-κ B

A double-blind, placebo-controlled trial evaluated the protective effects of ellagic acid-rich pomegranate extract and showed when ingested orally, pomegranate extract has an inhibitory effect on pigmentation in the human skin caused by UV irradiation.

The safety profile of oral pomegranate supplement has been evaluated in numerous studies with no adverse effects noted.

Tea tree oil

Tea tree oil, an essential oil, is produced from the tree, *Melaleuca alternifolia*, which is native to Australia. The active ingredients in tea tree oil include terpinen-4-ol, α-terpineol, α-pinene, 1-8-cineole, sesquiterenoid and terinolene. Tea tree oil has broad-spectrum antimicrobial and antiseptic properties, as well as anti-inflammatory, and antioxidant, properties (Table 11.4).

Tea tree oil has been used for bacterial, fungal, insect and viral infections, as well as acne, psoriasis, cuts and burns.

The clinical benefits of tea tree oil have been reviewed through a few research studies. A randomized, controlled trial compared standard MRSA decolonization treatment regime of 2% nasal mupirocin ointment and 4% chlorhexidine topical wash versus a topical tea tree oil regime, which included 10% tea tree oil nasal cream and 5% tea tree oil body wash. The results demonstrated similar decolonization rates for both the standard decolonization methods and the tea tree oil techniques. When data was analyzed for decolonization of superficial skin surfaces, the tea tree oil decolonization was deemed superior.

Table 11.4 Active ingredient and mechanism of action for tea tree oil.

Active ingredient	Mechanism of action
α-terpineol	*Antioxidant:* Rapidly autoxidizes free radicals *Antimicrobial:* Damages bacteria cell wall membrane

terpinen-4-ol	*Anti-inflammatory:*
	Inhibits the production of the inflammatory mediators, tumor necrosis
	    factor alpha (TNF-α), interleukin-1β (IL-1β), and IL-10
	Antimicrobial:
	Loss of nucleic acids through cytoplasmic membrane damage in S. aureus
	    (260-nm absorbing material lost)

1,8-cineole	*Antifungal:* Inhibits the formation of germ tubes, or mycelial conversion, in C. albicans

A randomized, control trial of 123 subjects with head lice demonstrated that a treatment regime that combined tea tree oil, lavender oil and a lice suffocation product was an effective alternative to the traditional pyrethrin-based lice treatment.

Additionally, in a randomized double-blind trial of 60 patients with mild-to-moderate acne, half were treated with 5% tea tree oil gel and the other half treated with placebo (gel vehicle with no anti-acne activities). The tea tree oil was found to be 3.55 more effective than placebo for total acne lesion count and 5.75 times more effective than placebo for acne severity index.

Tea tree oil's anti-fungal properties have also been proven effective against *Pityrosporum ovale*, the causative agent of dandruff. A randomized, single-blind, parallel-group study to investigate the efficacy and tolerability of 5% tea tree oil and placebo in patients with mild to moderate dandruff was conducted. The 5% tea tree oil shampoo group showed a 41% improvement in the quadrant-area-severity score compared with 11% in the placebo group ($p < .001$). Statistically significant improvements were also observed in the total area of involvement score, the total severity score, and the itchiness and greasiness components of the patients' self-assessments.

Anecdotal evidence from almost 80 years of use suggests that the topical use of the oil is relatively safe, and that adverse events are minor, self-limiting and occasional. Published data indicate that tea tree oil is toxic if ingested in higher doses and can also cause skin irritation at higher concentrations. Allergic contact or irritant dermatitis are possible side effects of tea tree oil.

Table 11.5 Active ingredients and mechanism of action for grape seed extract.

Active ingredient	Mechanism of action
Grape Seed Proanthocyanidin Extract (GSP)	*Antioxidant*: Free radical scavenger *Anti-inflammatory*: Inhibits the effect of inflammatory markers produced by TNF-alpha *Anti-carcinogenic*: Inhibits ornithine decarboxylase and myeloperoxidase activities Prevents UVB-induced tumor initiation and promotion *Wound healing*: Promotes vascular endothelial growth factor expression in keratinocytes

Grape seed extract

Grape seed extract, derived from whole grape seeds of the plant *Vitis vinifera*, has significant concentrations of vitamin E, linoleic acid, resveratrol, and flavonoids (anthocyanins and proanthocyanidins). It has potent antioxidant, anti-inflammatory, anti-carcinogenic and wound-healing properties (Table 11.5).

Grape seed extract is used in treating hyperpigmentation, photoaging and wound healing. A multi-dimensional study by Cornacchoine et al. evaluated the antioxidant properties of *Vitis vinifera* shoot extract (Samartine) along with a biotechnological extract (Ronacare® Hydroine) through in vitro and in vivo studies. Ronacare Hydroine is a patented topical agent composed of organic molecular compounds ectoine and hydroxyectoine that are isolated from halophilic microorganisms living in extreme environments. These compounds prevent protein denaturing by reducing water loss. In vitro, *V. vinifera* shoot extract appeared to have stronger antioxidant capacity than vitamin C or vitamin E on keratinocytes after H_2O_2 exposure. In vivo evaluation showed that a four-week, twice-daily application of Sarmentine (1%) serum showed significant improvement in all skin characteristics (firmness, radiance, texture, fine lines and wrinkles). However, improvements in skin texture, smoothness, evenness, hydration and softness were significantly higher in the Samartine plus Ronacare Hydroine group.

Grape seed extract has been shown to inhibit the cytochrome P450 system and can affect the intracellular concentration of drugs metabolized by this enzyme.

Conclusion

Innovative botanical agents have been demonstrated to have a variety of useful applications in medicine including anti-inflammatory, anti-oxidant, anti-aging, anti-microbial and anti-carcinogenic properties. A thorough understanding of the value and application of these agents remains incomplete. However, as additional clinical studies are performed, the efficacy and safety profile of botanicals will continue to shift from anecdotal to evidence-based medicine.

Further reading

Barker SC, Altman PM. A randomized assessor blind, parallel group comparative efficacy trial of three products for the treatment of head lice in children – melaleuca oil and lavender oil, pyrethrins and piperonyl butoxide, and a "suffocation" product. *BMC Dermatol* 2010; **10**(1): 6.

Carson CF, Mee BJ, Riley TV, et al. Mechanism of action of *Melaleuca alternifolia* (tea tree) oil on *Staphylococcus aureus* determined by time-kill, lysis, leakage, and salt tolerance assays and electron microscopy. *J Antimicrob Chemother* 2002; **46**(6): 1914–1920.

Chiang H, Lin T, Chiu C, Chang C, Hsu K, Wen K, et al. Coffea arabica extract and its constituents prevent photoaging by suppressing MMPs expression and MAP kinase pathway. *Food Chem Toxicol* 2011; **49**(1): 309–318.

Choi Y, Yan G. Pycnogenol inhibits immunoglobulin E-mediated allergic response in mast cells. *Phytother Res* 2009; **23**(12): 1691–1695.

Cornacchione S, Sadick N, Neveu M, Talbourdet S, Lazou K, Perrier E, et al. In vivo skin antioxidant effect of a new combination based on a specific *Vitis vinifera* shoot extract and a biotechnological extract. *J Drugs Dermatol* 2007; **6**(6 Suppl.): s8–s13.

Del Carmen Velazquez-Vereda M, Dieamant G, Eberlin S, Nogueira C, Colombi D, Queiroz M, et al. Effect of green Coffea arabica L. seed oil on extracellular matrix components and water-channel expression in in vitro and ex vivo human skin models. *J Cosmetic Dermatol* 2009; **8**(1): 56–62.

Dryden M, Dailly S, Crouch M. A randomized, controlled trial of tea tree topical preparations versus a standard topical regimen for the clearance of MRSA colonization. *J Hosp Infect* 2004; **56**(4): 283–286.

Enshaieh S, Jooya A, Siadat AH, Iraji F. The efficacy of 5% topical tea tree oil gel in mild to moderate acne vulgaris: A randomized, double-blind placebo-controlled study. *Indian J Dermatol Venereol Leprol* 2007; **73**(1): 22–25.

Jurenka J. Therapeutic applications of pomegranate (*punic granatum l.*): A review. *Altern Med Rev* 2008: **13**(2): 128–144.

Maimoona A, Jameel K, Saddiqe Z, Naeem I. A review on biological, nutraceutical and clinical aspects of French maritime pine bark extract. *J Ethnopharmacol* 2011; **133**(2): 261–277.

Mittal A, Elmets CA, Katiyar SK. Dietary feeding of proanthocyanidins from grape seeds prevents photocarcinogenesis in SKH-1 hairless mice: Relationship to decreased fat and lipid peroxidation. *Carcinogenesis* 2003; **24**: 1379–1388.

Palmer D, Kitchin J. A double-blind, randomized, controlled clinical trial evaluating the efficacy and tolerance of a novel phenolic antioxidant skin care system containing Coffea arabica and concentrated fruit and vegetable extracts. *J Drugs Dermatol* 2010; **9**(12): 1480–1487.

Pazyar N, Yaghoobi R. Tea tree oil as a novel antipsoriasis weapon. *Skin Pharmacol Physiol* 2012; **25**(3): 162–163.

Saliou C, Rimbach G, Moini H, McLaughlin L, Hosseini S, Packer L, et al. Solar ultraviolet-induced erythema in human skin and nuclear factor-kappa-B-dependent gene expression in keratinocytes are modulated by a French maritime pine bark extract. *Free Radic Biol Med* 2001; **30**(2): 154–160.

Santosh, K. Grape seed proanthocyanidines and skin cancer prevention: Inhibition of oxidative stress and protection of immune system. *Mol Nutr Food Res* 2008; **52**(1): S71–S76.

Satchell A, Saurajen A, Bell C, Barnetson R. Treatment of dandruff with 5% tea tree oil shampoo. *J Amer Acad Dermatol* 2002; **47**(6): 852–855.

CHAPTER 12

Green Tea Extract

Neil Houston[1] and Alexa Boer Kimball[1,2]

[1]Clinical Unit for Research Trials and Outcomes in Skin (CURTIS), Massachusetts General Hospital, Boston, MA, USA
[2]Harvard Medical School, Boston, MA, USA

Introduction

Tea is the second most consumed beverage after water and has been enjoyed around the world for centuries. Very few substances are thought to be as widely beneficial to a person's health with as few side effects as green tea. Green tea is a commonly used botanical cosmeceutical due to the antioxidant and anti-inflammatory properties found in refined tea leaves. Even though green tea is commonly consumed as a beverage, green tea extract (GTE) can be applied topically or taken in pill form to utilize the beneficial health effects of the tea plant. In this chapter, we will review the major studies and findings on GTE, as well as discuss the potential health benefits that have yet to be substantiated.

Active ingredient

The tea plant, *Camellia sinensis*, is most commonly known in three forms: (1) fully fermented black tea; (2) partially fermented oolong tea; and (3) unfermented green tea (Figure 12.1). After harvesting, black and oolong tea leaves are dried and begin to oxidize. To produce black tea, the tea leaves are completely dried and crushed to encourage further oxidation and give the tea its distinctive dark-brown color. Oolong tea is partially oxidized. Green tea, on the other hand, is immediately steamed or heated after harvesting in order to prevent oxidation (Figure 12.2). Many of the beneficial ingredients that are lost through the processing of black and oolong tea are retained in green tea, resulting in a cosmeceutical botanical with superior health benefits. Although black tea contains many of the same ingredients as green tea, a comparative in vitro study by Chatterjee et al. has shown black tea to have less antioxidant and anti-inflammatory potential than green tea.

Cosmeceuticals and Cosmetic Practice, First Edition. Edited by Patricia K. Farris.

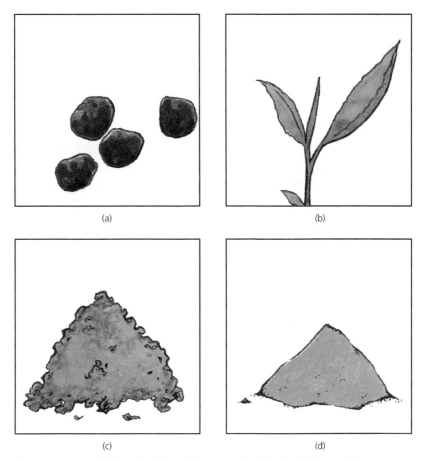

(a)   (b)

(c)   (d)

Figure 12.1 *Camellia sinensis*: (a) Seeds from the *Camellia sinensis* plant; (b) Green tea leaves; (c) Dried and processed green tea leaves; (d) Finely ground green tea leaves, commonly known as matcha. Source: Artwork by Ryan Denman.

Green tea's antioxidant properties are attributed to polyphenolic catechins, also known as flavan-3-ols. Catechins are a form of flavonoid, and although green tea contains a variety of catechins, three in particular – epicatechin, epicatechin-3-gallate (ECG) and epigallocatechin-3-gallate (EGCG) – account for the known health benefits of GTE. Catechins make up about 30–35% of the dry weight of the green tea leaf, and 90% of all polyphenols in green tea. In black tea, the catechins are oxidized during processing so the final product contains only 4% catechins, compared to 30% in green tea.

EGCG is the most potent of the catechins and the active ingredient in green tea and GTE (Figure 12.3). To date, EGCG is the most studied

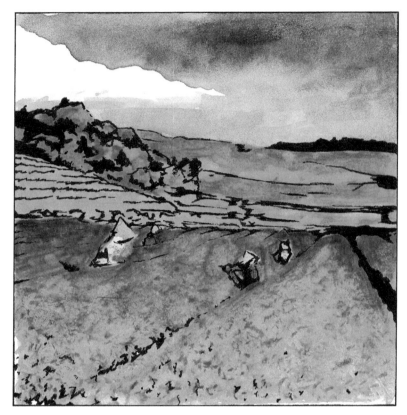

Figure 12.2 Fields of green tea planted for harvesting. Source: Artwork by Ryan Denman.

polyphenol in green tea. While other catechins have an antioxidant effect, EGCG is the largest and most plentiful catechin in green tea and is the most active antioxidant in any tea available. After processing, green tea retains the highest concentration of EGCG, which makes it a desirable botanical for use in cosmeceutical products.

The catechins in GTE positively affect the human body through three related mechanisms of action: (1) as an antioxidant; (2) as an anti-inflammatory agent; and (3) by protecting against ultraviolet (UV) radiation. All three of these properties will be outlined below. Green tea has been used in many forms and is commonly taken orally as a nutritional supplement. GTE has more recently been utilized in cosmeceutical products to take advantage of potential anti-aging properties and, to a lesser degree, UV protection. There is also evidence supporting GTE action in lessening collagen breakdown in the skin and combating the natural decomposition that occurs with aging.

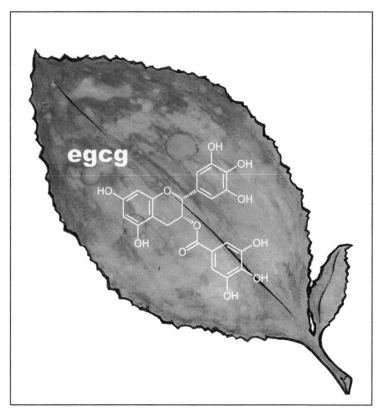

Figure 12.3 Epigallocatechin-3-gallate (EGCG) is the active ingredient in green tea extract, accounting for the extract's potent antioxidant properties. Source: Artwork by Ryan Denman.

Mechanisms of action

Skin aging has been largely attributed to free radical damage and inflammation. Green tea's anti-aging properties are thought to be due to the ample supply of antioxidants available to scavenge free radicals. EGCG, EGC, and epicatechin collectively quench the following reactive oxygen species: singlet oxygen, hydrogen peroxide, superoxide radical, hydroxyl radical, and peroxyl radical. According to a study by Kim et al., these polyphenols limit UV-induced lipid peroxidation in skin. In addition, Nakagawa et al. found that these polyphenols reduce the oxidation of proteins in free radical-generating systems in vitro.

The antioxidant properties of GTE have a downstream effect that provides anti-inflammatory and UV protective qualities to skin, further contributing to GTE's anti-aging properties. Free radicals up-regulate certain transcription factors, such as activator protein 1 (AP-1) and nuclear transcription factor-kappa B (NF-kB), which, in turn, up-regulate pro-inflammatory mediators. AP-1 contributes to the production of metallo-proteinases that break down collagen in the skin. NF-kB up-regulates transcription of interleukin (IL)-1, IL-6, IL-8, and tumor necrosis factor alpha. These cytokines further activate NF-kB and AP-1, which continues the cycle and results in inflammatory damage and collagen breakdown that both lead to skin aging. By reducing free radicals, EGCG thereby down-regulates AP-1 and NF-kB expression and reduces inflammatory and UV damage to the skin (Figure 12.4).

Green tea's photoprotective properties were studied by Elmets et al. in a trial to determine the effect of EGCG and ECG on UV-induced erythema. In this study, topical GTE was shown to provide photoprotection from 24 to 72 hours. Topical green tea reduced the number of sunburned cells by 66% when applied 30 minutes prior to UVB exposure. In addition to UVB protection, GTE prevented psoralen-UVA photodamage with both pre- and post-treatment application, reducing erythema, hyperplasia, and hyperkeratosis. They concluded that GTE can reduce DNA damage after UV radiation as well as reduce photoaging. The UV protective properties of GTE were also demonstrated in a study by Katiyar et al., in which topical EGCG reduced UVB-induced inflammatory responses and infiltration of leukocytes in human skin (Table 12.1).

Some limitations of topical formulations of EGCG are caused by the hydrophilic nature of polyphenolic catechins. The outermost layer of the epidermis, the stratum corneum, is hydrophobic, making it challenging for EGCG to penetrate to the required depths necessary to exert its full antioxidant and anti-inflammatory effects. In order to increase the likelihood of proper skin penetration, the recommended concentration of polyphenols in GTE is 90% or more. This concentration can be difficult to discern from products currently on the market since there is little standardization regarding GTE potency in cosmeceuticals. GTE can be processed in a variety of ways, providing different amounts of EGCG. Products may detail the concentration of GTE without mentioning the concentration of polyphenols within the extract, which may misrepresent the effectiveness of the product and be misleading to the consumer (Figure 12.5).

Catechins in green tea are typically unstable and easily oxidized, further limiting the effectiveness of a substance that cannot readily permeate the epidermis. This amplifies the importance of a high concentration of catechins in topical products, in order to increase the likelihood of skin penetration before the product becomes oxidized and is rendered ineffective as an antioxidant. Even though high concentrations of catechins are important for efficacy, higher concentrations of GTE are not cosmetically elegant and have a green brown color that may temporarily stain the skin.

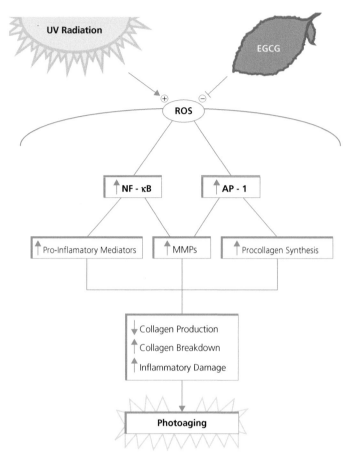

Figure 12.4 UV radiation induces reactive oxygen species (ROS) in the skin, which can lead to up-regulation of nuclear transcription factor-kappa B (NF-kB) and activator protein 1 (AP-1). NF-kB signals an increase in pro-inflammatory cytokines. AP-1 leads to activation of matrix metalloproteinases (MMP), as well as a decrease in procollagen synthesis. Collectively, this results in an increase in collagen breakdown, decreased collagen production, and increased inflammatory damage, resulting in photoaging. EGCG quenches various ROS, which down-regulates NF-kB and AP-1. Source: Artwork by Ryan Denman. Adapted from: Chen L, Hu JY, Wang SQ. The role of antioxidants in photoprotection: a critical review. *J Am Acad Dermatol*. 2012; **67** (5): 1013–1024.

Clinical benefits

Treatment of photoaging

GTE's photoprotective properties, similar to its antioxidant and anti-inflammatory properties, are attributed to green tea's potent concentration of EGCG and other catechins. GTE can be applied topically or taken orally as a supplement. Green tea supplements allow the body to utilize the antioxidant properties of GTE differently from topical application, but many of

Table 12.1 Various health benefits of green tea extract and the primary mechanism of action.

Health benefit	Active ingredient	Route of administration	Mechanism
Antioxidant	EGCG	Topical, Oral	Catechins scavenge the following ROS: singlet oxygen, hydrogen peroxide, superoxide radical, hydroxyl radical, and peroxyl radical.
Anti-inflammatory	EGCG	Topical, Oral	Anti-inflammatory benefits result from antioxidant properties of catechins. Free radicals up-regulate certain transcription factors, such as activator protein 1 (AP-1) and nuclear transcription factor-kappa B (NF-kB), which, in turn, up-regulate pro-inflammatory mediators such as interleukin (IL)-1, IL-6, IL-8, and tumor necrosis factor alpha. By reducing free radicals, EGCG thereby down-regulates AP-1 and NF-kB expression and reduces inflammatory damage to the skin.
UV protection	EGCG	Primarily Topical, Oral	UV protection results from antioxidant properties of catechins. EGCG quenches free radicals, which down-regulates AP-1 and NF-kB expression, thereby reducing UV damage to the skin.
Decrease in collagen breakdown	EGCG	Primarily Topical, Oral	AP-1 contributes to the production of matrix metalloproteinases (MMP) that break down collagen in the skin. By reducing free radicals, EGCG down-regulates AP-1, which has the downstream effect of reducing MMPs that break down collagen

the same health benefits still apply. Both topical and oral administration provide UV protection and reduce inflammation, providing encouraging support for regular GTE supplement use in conjunction with topical use to lessen UV damage and signs of skin aging.

The largest double-blind, placebo-controlled, randomized clinical trial examining oral green tea polyphenol supplements and their effect on sun damage was conducted by Janjua et al. in 2009. The study followed 56 women, with the treatment group receiving 250 mg of green tea polyphenols twice daily over a 2-year period. The results suggested that

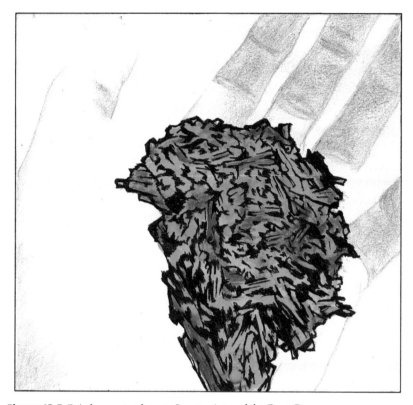

Figure 12.5 Dried green tea leaves. Source: Artwork by Ryan Denman.

green tea polyphenols may improve sun damage at 12 months, yet no clinical differences were seen at 24 months.

To date, only one double-blind, placebo-controlled, randomized clinical trial has been conducted regarding GTE's anti-aging properties from topical application. This study by Chiu et al. examined 24 women over an 8-week period. The treatment group received 10% GTE cream and 300 mg GTE supplements twice a day, while the other group received placebo. After 8 weeks, no significant clinical difference could be seen; however, there was improvement in elastic tissue content of the treatment group, suggesting a longer time period may be needed for clinically visible effects. Further clinical trials must be undertaken to determine the most effective and practical way to deliver the antioxidant and anti-inflammatory potential of GTE.

Collagen is thought to maintain skin thickness and elasticity. With age, collagen production decreases and existing collagen degrades. GTE may delay collagen breakdown with age, reducing wrinkles and keeping the skin looking healthier and more youthful. More studies will need to be conducted in human subjects in order to substantiate these claims, although the existing evidence shows some validation of GTE's effect on collagen and provides a good reason to pursue future studies. An in vitro study showed that green tea polyphenols inhibit the activity of collagenase and increase the collagen biosynthesis rate of human fibroblasts. Other studies have demonstrated that topical GTE suppresses metalloproteinase and age-related collagen cross-linking in mice.

Treatment of warts

Sinecatechins 15% ointment, known under the trade name Veregen®, is derived from green tea leaves and is the first botanical product that the U.S. Food and Drug Administration (FDA) has approved for the treatment of external genital and perianal warts. Sinecatechins ointment is a mixture of catechins and other green tea components. The ointment is 85–95% catechins by weight, and 55% of these catechins are comprised of EGCG. Although the ointment's efficacy has been demonstrated, the mechanism of action is not yet known. The ointment is applied three times daily and causes complete clearance of warts in 53–58% of patients after 16 weeks of treatment, compared with a 33–37% clearance rate with placebo.

Chemoprevention

In addition to the benefits of polyphenolic catechins listed above, GTE has been shown to have anti-carcinogenic properties and has been studied extensively both in vitro and in vivo. EGCG has shown tumor-suppressive effects on an animal carcinogenesis model, a mouse xenograft model, and on various cancer cell lines. EGCG has also displayed anti-UV carcinogenic potential through topical and oral administration in mice. When put in the drinking water of mice, the polyphenolic components of green tea significantly protected against UV-induced skin carcinogenesis in terms of tumor incidence, size, and multiplicity, compared to a control group.

Possible side effects

Green tea has been used in a variety of ways throughout the development of modern medicine and no serious conditions are linked to its use. The main side effects of oral GTE are directly related to the caffeine content, although decaffeinated options of the extract are available. Caffeine can lead to insomnia, nausea, and frequent urination. Pregnant women and people with high caffeine sensitivity should avoid taking caffeinated GTE supplements. Topical application has not been shown to cause side effects from the caffeine content of GTE.

Two studies by Chow et al. examined the consumption of up to 1200 mg of EGCG per day taken as a supplement for 1–4 weeks by healthy adults. Reported adverse effects included intestinal gas, nausea, stomach ache, heartburn, abdominal pain, dizziness, headache, and muscle pain. These effects were all rated as mild events and no lasting conditions or serious adverse events were reported. Chow et al. also determined that 800 mg EGCG supplements are well tolerated and optimize the biological effects of tea catechins.

Contraindications

There are few known contraindications for GTE. According to a study at the University of Southern California, various catechins in green tea can bind with the anticancer drug bortezomib, reducing its efficacy. The interaction between EGCG and bortexomib is highly specific and can render the drug practically useless for cancer treatment. Green tea products containing EGCG should be avoided by patients undergoing bortexomib treatment.

Conclusion

GTE is a promising addition to the cosmeceutical market, with potent antioxidant and anti-inflammatory properties that can help combat free radical damage and skin aging. Over centuries, people have used green tea to sharpen their minds and rejuvenate their bodies, and more studies are needed to reveal the best way to utilize GTE's beneficial effects. GTE can be found in moisturizing creams, sunscreen, anti-aging cream, make-up, moisturizing lotion and hand soap, and the prices of these products can vary considerably. Consumers have many GTE products available to them with no clear standards outlining which products effectively utilize GTE's health benefits. The optimal concentration, dosage, and route of administration must be determined and substantiated through future studies in order for GTE to reach its full potential as a botanical cosmeceutical.

Further reading

Chatterjee P, Chandra S, Dey P, Bhattacharya S. Evaluation of anti-inflammatory effects of green tea and black tea: A comparative *in vitro* study. *J Adv Pharm Tech Res* 2012; **3**: 136–138.

Chow HH, Cai Y, Hakim IA, et al. Pharmacokinetics and safety of green tea polyphenols after multiple-dose administration of epigallocatechin gallate and polyphenon E in healthy individuals. *Clin Cancer Res* 2003; **9**(9): 3312–3319.

Elmets C, Singh D, Tubesing K, et al. Cutaneous photoprotection from ultraviolet injury by green tea polyphenols. *J Am Acad Dermatol* 2001; **44**: 425–432.

Farris P. Idebenone, green tea, and coffeeberry extract: New and innovative antioxidants. *Dermatol Ther* 2007; **20**: 322–329.

Janjua R, Munoz C, Gorell E, Rehmus W, Egbert B, Kern D, Chang AL. A two-year, double-blind, randomized placebo-controlled trial of oral green tea polyphenols on the long-term clinical and histologic appearance of photoaging skin. *Dermatol Surg* 2009; **35**(7): 1057–1065.

Katiyar S, Elmets CA, Katiyar SK. Green tea and skin cancer: Photoimmunology, antiogenesis, and DNA repair. *J Nutr Biochem* 2007; **18**: 287–296.

Katiyar SK, Matsui MS, Elmets CA, Mukhtar H. Polyphenolic antioxidant (−)-epigallocatechin-3-gallate from green tea reduces UVB-induced inflammatory responses and infiltration of leukocytes in human skin. *Photochem Photobiol* 1999; **69**: 148–153.

Kim J, Hwang JS, Cho YK, et al. Protective effects of epigallocatechin-3-gallate on UVA and UVB induced skin damage. *Skin Pharmacol Appl Skin Physiol* 2001; **14**: 11–19.

Levine J, Momin SB. How much do we really know about our favorite cosmeceutical ingredients? *J Clin Aesthet Dermatol* 2010; **3**(2): 22–41.

Ueda JI, Saito N, Shimazu Y, Ozawa T. A comparison of scavenging abilities of antioxidants against hydroxyl radicals. *Arch Biochem Biophys* 1996; **333**: 377–384.

CHAPTER 13

Soy and Oatmeal-Based Cosmeceuticals

Jason Emer[1] and Heidi A. Waldorf[1,2]
[1]Icahn School of Medicine at Mount Sinai, New York, NY, USA
[2]Waldorf Dermatology & Laser Associates, PC, Nanuet, NY, USA

Introduction

The desire to protect, maintain and improve skin quality and appearance combined with fears of long-term effects of synthetic chemicals has sparked interest in alternative, "natural" topical therapies. Oatmeal and soy are two of the most widely used and efficacious botanicals in dermatology. These natural ingredients have received heightened attention given the multitude of medical articles demonstrating photoprotective, anti-inflammatory, and anti-aging effects with oral consumption and topical application. In this chapter, oatmeal and soy will be discussed with regards to their proposed mechanisms of action and clinical utility as cosmeceutical ingredients.

Colloidal oatmeal

Introduction and history

Avena sativa or common oat is a species of cereal grain and a member of the grass family *Gramineae*. Common oats contain beta-glucan, considered a heart healthy soluble fiber when consumed. Topical therapies are derived from dehulled oat kernels ground into a very fine powder and boiled to extract the colloidal material which is readily dispersible in water. Oatmeal has a long history of traditional folk use dating back to 2000 BC in Egypt and the Arabian Peninsula. Early descriptions of oatmeal as soothing, anti-pruritic, and cleansing have since been confirmed by scientific research demonstrating anti-inflammatory, antioxidant, and anti-histaminic effects. Oatmeal became available commercially in 1945 for various cutaneous conditions, especially pruritic inflammatory eruptions and burns.

Cosmeceuticals and Cosmetic Practice, First Edition. Edited by Patricia K. Farris.
© 2014 John Wiley & Sons, Ltd. Published 2014 by John Wiley & Sons, Ltd.

In 1989, the United States Food and Drug Administration (FDA) recognized the value of colloidal oatmeal as a safe and effective over-the-counter skin protectant. In 2003, the FDA codified oatmeal as a safe and effective agent in the *Skin Protectant Drug Products for Over-the-Counter Use* monograph (21 CFR Part 347). It identified colloidal oatmeal as the powder resulting from the grinding and processing of whole oat grain and characterized it as a skin protectant ingredient that "provides temporary skin protection and relieves minor skin irritation due to poison oak, poison ivy, poison sumac, and insect bites." A variety of colloidal oatmeal products including soaps, body washes, shaving gels, and moisturizers are available and are popular non-pharmaceutical options for treating dry, inflamed, or sensitive skin, as they are cosmetically stable and non-irritating. Oat-containing products may allow for a reduced need for topical prescription medications such as corticosteroids or calcineurin inhibitors for inflammatory or allergic-type skin conditions.

Mechanism of action

Oatmeal exerts its positive skin effects due to a combination of anti-inflammatory, antioxidant, anti-histaminic, skin barrier protection and repair, cleansing, and anti-infectious properties (Table 13.1). Modern colloidal oatmeal includes components of the whole oat kernel including polysaccharides, proteins, lipids, saponins, enzymes, flavonoids, vitamins, and a group of polyphenols called avenanthramides. Polysaccharides, the largest component (65–85%), and antioxidant enzymes such as saponins, vitamins, flavonoids, and prostaglandin synthesis inhibitors, have immunomodulatory activity. The anti-inflammatory properties are due to inhibition of arachidonic acid, cytosolic phospholipase A2, and tumor necrosis factor (TNF)-α pathways. Polysaccharides also form a gelatinous

Table 13.1 Components and mechanisms of oatmeal.

Components	Mechanisms
Polysaccharides	Barrier maintenance and repair; anti-pruritic, moisturization
Proteins	Barrier maintenance and repair; anti-pruritic, moisturization
Lipids	Barrier maintenance and repair; anti-pruritic, moisturization; cleanser
Fiber	Barrier maintenance and repair; anti-pruritic, moisturization
Beta-glucans	Barrier maintenance and repair; anti-pruritic, moisturization
Saponins	Antioxidant; immunomodulation; cleanser
Vitamins	Antioxidant; immunomodulation
Flavonoids	Antioxidant; immunomodulation
Polyphenols (Avenanthramides)	Antioxidant; immunomodulation; anti-inflammatory; anti-histamine; ultraviolet absorbent

hydrocolloid in water, leaving a protective film on the skin that physically retards water loss and helps to repair and maintain a proper epidermal barrier. The protein component (10–18%) acts as an emulsifier enhancing skin hydration and barrier function in concert with the polysaccharides. These properties give colloidal oatmeal its potent antipruritic effect. Oat proteins also have the ability to buffer both acids and bases to aid in barrier maintenance and repair after exposure to chemicals such as α-hydroxy acids, surfactants, bleaches, or other environmental insults. Lipids (3–9%) help to reduce transepidermal water loss (TEWL) promoting enhanced barrier repair, as well as absorb and solubilize aqueous debris, absorb dirt, oil, and sebaceous secretions concomitantly with saponins. Fiber (5%) and beta-glucans (5%) are responsible for the skin barrier protective and water-holding functions of colloidal oatmeal.

The oat components thought to have the most therapeutic importance are the phenolic compounds – such as the avenanthramides as well as vitamins A, B, E; all known to have potent antioxidant and anti-inflammatory effects. The avenanthramides have been shown to exhibit strong anti-inflammatory effects through inhibition of inhibitor of kappa B (IκB) degradation, decreased p65 phosphorylation, and nuclear factor kappa B (NF-κB) gene activity, and inhibition of the release of pro-inflammatory cytokines. Keratinocytes treated with avenanthramides showed a significant inhibition of TNF-α-induced NF-κB activity and a subsequent reduction of interleukin-8 (IL-8). IL-8 is a pro-inflammatory cytokine that is elevated in inflamed skin and is a potent chemotactic factor that can induce migration of neutrophils. Avenathramides have also been shown to inhibit histamine release in a dose-dependent fashion.

Topical application of a 3% formulation of avenathramides mitigated inflammation in a dose-dependent fashion in murine models of contact hypersensitivity (oxazolone-induced) and neurogenic inflammation (resiniferatoxin-induced) and reduced pruritogen (compound 48/80)-induced scratching in a murine itch model. In high concentration, the anti-inflammatory effects of avenanthramides can approach that of topical hydrocortisone 1%. Further, their antioxidant and anti-genotoxic activities are comparable to those of ascorbic acid and may harbor the potential for beneficial physiological effects.

Barrier dysfunction contributes to many dermatologic conditions, such as atopic dermatitis, and rosacea, and worsens with age and photodamage. Colloidal oatmeal has been shown to act as an emollient, humectant and occlusive, and to directly reduce TEWL. These benefits are due to starch and lipid components. The application of oatmeal extracts (*Avena rhealba*) to sodium laurel sulfate treated skin reduced irritation compared to vehicle, illustrating the anti-inflammatory effects of oats and suggesting potential benefits for the skin barrier.

Oatmeal extract also has antiviral properties, likely due to inhibitor effects on eicosanoid formation, expression of cytosolic phospholipase A2, and arachidonic acid metabolism in human keratinocytes. An open-label study of six children with mulloscum contagiosum treated with a zinc oxide cream containing colloidal oatmeal extracts (*Avena rhealba*) once daily for four weeks demonstrated significant improvements after four weeks of treatment. Further, oat seed extracts when applied to rye bread were shown to have a high degree of anti-fungal activity, preventing the formation of *Penicillium roqueforti* colonies in one study, and suggesting its use in food preservation.

Indications and clinical benefits

Oatmeal is widely used as a skin barrier protectant and moisturizer. It has become a standard part of many regimens both for routine dry skin care and the treatment of inflammatory and allergic skin disorders such as contact dermatitis, atopic dermatitis, rosacea, psoriasis, diaper rash, seborrheic dermatitis, burns, prickly heat, exfoliative erythroderma, and post-chemotherapy dermatologic toxicity (Figure 13.1).

Early studies reported benefits of colloidal oatmeal for management of dermatoses in pediatric and elderly patients, for whom the use of products with a well-established safety record is of particular concern. Colloidal grain suspensions of oatmeal are considered as adjuncts in atopic dermatitis therapy and may play a crucial role in decreasing the use of topical corticosteroids and calcineurin inhibitors.

Broader populations may also benefit, as a recent clinical study examining the benefits of a skin care regimen including a moisturizing cream and a body wash containing avenanthramides demonstrated improvement in all outcomes (eczema severity, itching, erythema, and scaling) as compared to baseline values. Matheson and colleagues reported that liquid paraffin with 5% colloidal oatmeal significantly decreased itching and the need for

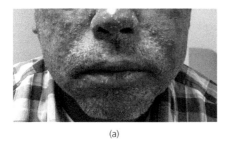
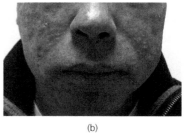

(a)   (b)

Figure 13.1 (a) A patient with severe granulomatous rosacea unwilling to begin oral therapies; (b) Clinical improvements seen as early as two weeks with use of a topical colloidal oatmeal preparation.

antihistamines in the management of patients with burn injuries, compared with liquid paraffin alone. In another study of adults, a colloidal oatmeal lotion was shown to be effective for controlling an acneiform eruption associated with epidermal growth factor receptor (EGFR) antagonists and tyrosine-kinase inhibitor (TKI) treatment (cetuximab, erlotinib, panitu-mumab and sorafenib) of various solid tumors with no associated toxicities. Hand-foot syndrome is another common, dose-limiting adverse effect of TKI therapy in which topical colloidal oatmeal may play a role in therapy.

Disorders such as post-inflammatory hyperpigmentation (PIH) are more common in patients with skin of color and require special treatment consideration. In a recent study the use of a moisturizer containing colloidal oatmeal to treat dry, ashy skin in subjects with Fitzpatrick Skin Types IV–VI demonstrated improvement in skin moisturization and brightness within one day of application. This study suggests that colloidal oatmeal-based may indirected prevent post-inflammatory hyperpigmentation by reducing inflammation.

Overall, colloidal oatmeal has anti-inflammatory, anti-irritant, antioxidant, and immunomodulatory effects. These properties make oatmeal a useful option for itchy and allergic conditions, as well as those with a compromised skin barrier such as eczema and rosacea.

Soy

Introduction and history

Soy (*Glycine max* L.), a member of the pea family *Fabaceae* and native to southeastern Asia, grows from 1–5 feet tall with clusters of three to five pods, each containing two to four beans. It has been used in traditional Chinese medicine for thousands of years. Large-scale soybean cultivation began in the US during World War II. Currently, the US produces almost 40% of the world's supply of soybeans.

Soy contains major and minor components, each with different roles in skin care (Table 13.2). Phospholipids (45–60%), essential fatty oils (30–35%) and several minor components including isoflavones, proteases soybean trypsin inhibitors (STIs) and Bowman-Birk inhibitors (BBIs) have the ability to reduce inflammation and may reduce skin pigmentation. Phytosterols help to restore barrier function and replenish moisture. Vitamin E is an antioxidant that helps protect the skin from environmental stressors such as free radicals. In addition, soy has been shown in vitro to stimulate collagen synthesis and initiate skin elastin repair thought to be due to the presence of isoflavones (genistein and daidzein).

Given the diverse combination of ingredients in soy, there is a broad therapeutic potential including reducing hyperpigmentation, enhancing

Table 13.2 Components and mechanisms of soy.

Components	Mechanism
Phospholipids	Anti-inflammatory; antioxidant; moisturization; barrier maintenance and repair
Essential fatty oils	Anti-inflammatory; antioxidant; moisturization; barrier maintenance and repair
Isoflavones	Anti-inflammatory; antioxidant; collagen stimulation; ultraviolet absorbent
Proteases	Depigmenting activity; hair reduction
Phytosterols	Barrier maintenance and repair; depigmenting activity; phytoestrogentic effects
Vitamins	Anti-inflammatory; antioxidant

skin elasticity, delaying hair regrowth, controlling oil production, moisturizing the skin, and improving the skin barrier. Soy may also improve the signs of photoaging and prevent skin cancers through the estrogenic and antioxidant effects of its metabolites.

Mechanisms of action

Antioxidant effects

Free radical formation is thought to be a major component in photoaging. These highly reactive compounds can act as initiators and/or promoters, cause DNA damage, activate procarcinogens, and alter the cellular antioxidant defense system. The primary metabolites of soy, the isoflavones (genistein and diadzein), have been identified in both animal and human cell cultures as phytoestrogens – plant compounds with a weak estrogenic effect – with a fourfold mechanism of action to fight the oxidative process.

Isoflavones inhibit chemical carcinogen-induced oxygen species, oxidative DNA damage, and proto-oncogenc expression. In particular, genistein has been shown to inhibit the initiation and promotion of skin carcinogenesis in mouse skin and ultraviolet B (UVB)-induced erythema in human skin. One study has confirmed topical genistein's photoprotective efficacy in vitro when pretreated and untreated human reconstituted skin was compared after exposure to UVB and after psoralen plus ultraviolet A (PUVA). These studies demonstrated that non-denatured soy extracts reduced UV-induced tymine dimer formation and might serve as a potent chemopreventive agent against photocarcinogenesis.

Phytoestrogen effects

Menopausal changes in the skin include a loss of collagen and measurable reduction in dermal thickness. Topical estrogen can reverse these changes since estrogen receptor levels are highest in the granular layer of the skin. Soy isoflavones have been investigated for their potential to stimulate collagen and increase levels of glucosaminoglycans, especially hyaluronic acid (HA) in aging skin. In vitro studies have demonstrated that genistein can increase collagen (COL1A2) gene expression in human fibroblasts and de novo collagen production while diadzein does not. Purified isoflavones stimulate collagen synthesis to a lesser extent than whole topical soy, suggesting that compounds other than isoflavones may necessary for the collagen stimulatory effect. In a 12 week, double-blind randomized clinical trial, a proprietary soy complex was found to stimulate in vitro collagen synthesis, in vivo elastin repair, and improved facial skin firmness and reduce laxity.

Hyperpigmentation

Phytosterols and small protein serine protease inhibitors, STIs and BBIs, have been shown to interfere with the transfer of melanosomes to keratinocytes in vitro and in vivo by reversibly inhibiting the protease-activated receptor-2 (PAR-2) pathway. Preclinical studies have demonstrated that modulation of PAR-2 activation by serine protease inhibitors present in soy extract can reduce melanosome transfer and distribution for a dose-dependent skin lightening effect in vivo. Thus, soy may be a clinically safer, although it probably less effective natural alternative to hydroquinone in patients who cannot tolerate the latter.

Reduction in Hair Growth

Soy has been used in topical body lotions that promise to reduce the frequency of shaving. The large proteins in soy smooth and soften the skin perhaps by acting as humectants and decreasing TEWL. Further, BBIs also inhibit ornithine decarboxylase, an enzyme involved in hair growth. Clinical studies have demonstrated a reduction in the appearance and texture of facial and leg hair and reduced irritation from shaving.

Indications and clinical benefits

Clinical studies have confirmed the efficacy of topical soy products for the treatment of hyperpigmentation and photoaging. In a 12-week, double-blind, placebo-controlled study of 68 patients, an active soy moisturizer containing non-denatured STIs, BBIs, vitamins and fatty acids produced superior improvement in facial skin tone, clarity, mottled hyperpigmentation, blotchiness, and fine lines as well as overall texture and appearance compared to vehicle alone. Clinical studies have also demonstrated improvement of dyschromias including post-inflammatory hyperpigmentation with the use of a daily soy moisturizer and a whole soy extract formulated with salicylic acid and retinal.

The effect of soybean phytosterols on skin barrier repair was assessed in patients with methyl nicotinate (MN)-induced erythema. MN-induced erthema was monitored by spectrophotmetry. Three days after tape stripping, the sites treated with a formulation containing soy phytosterols showed an appreciable recovery of barrier function compared to those treated with a vehicle control.

Adverse effects

Although there is some concern that oral consumption of phytoestrogens such as soy might increase the risk of breast and uterine cancer, epidemiologic data does not support this notion. On the contrary, soy ingestion appears to exert a protective effect against breast and prostate cancer that can be attributed to its antioxidant properties. In addition, although studies have demonstrated that soy does penetrate the stratum corneum reaching the epidermal and dermal layers, there is no evidence to suggest that topically applied soy products cause any sytemic effects.

Conclusion

Natural ingredients in cosmeceuticals now offer options for treating common dermatologic conditions. It is important for dermatologists to know what ingredients a product contains in order to best assess its capability to aid in medical therapy, cause potential harm, or interact with prescription therapies. For example, whether a cosmeceutical contains whole soy, the isoflavones genistein and daidzein, or soy protease inhibitors in the non-denatured form, will determine the potential depigmenting and/or anti-aging effects of soy. Further, the avenanthramide component appears necessary for much of the antioxidant and anti-inflammatory affects of colloidal oatmeal. Future studies are needed to determine both the biological and clinical behaviors of natural ingredients in cosmeceuticals in order to best guide proper therapeutic recommendations.

Further reading

Alexandrescu DT, Vaillant JG, Dasanu CA. Effect of treatment with a colloidal oatmeal lotion on the acneform eruption induced by epidermal growth factor receptor and multiple tyrosine-kinase inhibitors. *Clin Exp Dermatol* 2007; **32**: 71–74.

Fowler JF Jr, Woolery-Llyod H, Waldorf H, et al. Innovations in natural ingredients and their use in skin care. *J Drugs Dermatol* 2010; **9**: S72–S81.

Grais ML. Role of colloidal oatmeal in dermatologic treatment of the aged. *AMA Arch Derm Syphilol* 1953; **68**: 402–407.

Kurtz ES Wallo W. Colloidal oatmeal: History, chemistry and clinical properties. *J Drugs Dermatol* 2007; **6**: 167–170.

Paine C, Sharlow E, Liebel F, et al. An alternative approach to depigmentation by soybean extracts via inhibition of the PAR-2 pathway. *J Invest Dermatol* 2001; **116**: 587–595.

Pazyar N, Yaghoobi R, Kazerouni A, et al. Oatmeal in dermatology: A brief review. *Indian J Dermatol Venereol Leprol* 2012; **78**: 142–145.

Sur R, Nigam A, Grote D, et al. Avenanthramides, polyphenols from oats, exhibit anti-inflammatory and anti-itch activity. *Arch Dermatol Res* 2008; **300**: 569–574.

Wallo W, Nebus J, Leyden JJ. Efficacy of a soy moisturizer in photoaging: A double-blind, vehicle-controlled, 12-week study. *J Drugs Dermatol* 2007; **6**: 917–922.

Wei H. American Academy of Dermatology 1998 Awards for Young Investigators in Dermatology. Photoprotective action of isoflavone genistein: Models, mechanisms, and relevance to clinical dermatology. *J Am Acad Dermatol* 1998; **39**: 271–272.

Wei H, Saladi R, Lu Y, et al. Isoflavone genistein: Photoprotection and clinical implications in dermatology. *J Nutr* 2003; **133**: 3811S–3819S.

CHAPTER 14

Bioactive Peptides

Katie Rodan[1], Kathy Fields[1], and Timothy Falla[2]

[1] Stanford University, Stanford, CA, USA
[2] Rodan & Fields, LLC, San Francisco, CA, USA

Introduction

Naturally occurring bioactive active peptides, such as angiotensin, vaso-pressin, oxytocin and bradykinin, were first discovered over 40 years ago. The identification and application of peptides as dermatological thera-peutics followed shortly with the clinical development of wound healing and antimicrobial peptides such as GHK-copper and Magainin. However, despite many attempts, no bioactive peptide has been successfully devel-oped and approved as a topically applied therapeutic for any dermatological condition. Thus, the application of the technology was redirected towards the cosmetics industry with GHK-copper (Copper Tripeptide-1) and the Matrixyl (Palmitoyl Pentapeptide-3) being the first peptides to be included in skincare formulations. These first commercially applied peptide ingredi-ents targeted the stimulation of extracellular matrix components such as collagen and facets of wound healing such as cell proliferation. Since the early 2000s, numerous peptides have entered the market, creating a vast array of options for their inclusion in cosmetic dermatological products (Table 14.1). Here we define and characterize the ingredient class, role in nature, development process, clinical benefit, and limitations.

Definition of peptide

Peptides are short polymers of amino acid monomers linked by peptide bonds formed through covalent linkage of the carboxyl group of one amino acid with the amino group of the next. Every peptide has an N-terminus amino acid (unattached terminal amino group) and C-terminus amino acid (unattached terminal carboxyl group) at its ends (except for cyclic peptides). Because there are 21 naturally occurring amino acids in man, each with a unique chemical structure and reactivity, there exists a vast potential for peptide sequences based on the rationale that for each position in the sequence of a peptide there can be any one of 21 different amino

Cosmeceuticals and Cosmetic Practice, First Edition. Edited by Patricia K. Farris.
© 2014 John Wiley & Sons, Ltd. Published 2014 by John Wiley & Sons, Ltd.

Table 14.1 Summary of bioactive peptides marketed as ingredients in skin care products.

Company	Name	Activity	Premix products	Source
Atrium	Tripeptide-2	ECM stimulation via MMP-1 inhibition	ECM-protect®	Undisclosed
Atrium	Tripeptide-1	ECM stimulation via growth factor	Kollaren®	HGF
Atrium	Acetyl Tetrapeptide-2	Reduce loss of thymic factors	Thymulen®4	Thymopoieten
Atrium	Acetylpeptide-1	Melanin increase via MSH regulation	Melitane®	MSH agonist
Atrium	Nonapeptide-1	Tyrosinase activation inhibition	Melanostatine®	MSH antagonist
Evonik	Tetrapeptide-21	ECM stimulation	TEGO® PEP 4-17	ECM
Evonik	Tetrapeptide-30	Inflammation modulation	TEGO® PEP 4-EVEN	Innate immunity
Grant Industries	Palmitoyl Hexapeptide-14	Dermal repair	Matrix Rebuilder™	Innate immunity
Grant Industries	Oligopeptide-10	Dermal protection	InvisaSkin-64™	Innate immunity
Grant Industries	Tetrapeptide-14	Inflammation modulation	Granactive AR-1423™	Innate immunity
Grant Industries	Pentapeptide-21	UV protection	Granactive 1518™	Innate immunity
Lipotec	Acetyl Hexapeptide-38	Upregulate adipogenesis	Adifyline™	Undisclosed
Lipotec	Acetyl Dipeptide-3 aminohexanoate	Upregulate AMPs	Bodydefensine™	Innate immunity
Lipotec	Tripeptide-9 Citrulline	Metal chelation	deGlyage™	Undisclosed
Lipotec	Acetyl Hexapeptide-37	Upregulate aquaporin expression	Diffuporine™	Undisclosed
Lipotec	Acetyl Hexapeptide-30	Muscle relaxation by kinase inhibition	Inyline™	Undisclosed
Lipotec	Acetyl Tetrapeptide-22	Upregulate heat shock protein for protection	Thermostressine™	Undisclosed
Lipotec	Acetyl Hexapeptide-39	Inhibits adipocyte differentiation	Silusyne™	Undisclosed
Lipotec	Acetylarginyltryptophyl diphenylglycine	Elastase inhibition	Relastase™	Undisclosed
Lipotec	Palmitoyl Tripeptide-40	Upregulate melanin	Melatime™	Undisclosed
Lipotec	Tripeptide-1	Inhibits collagen glycation	Aldenine®, Trylagen™	Human serum
Lipotec	Tripeptide-10 Citrulline	Collagen fibrillogenesis	Decorinyl, Trylagen™	Decorin
Lipotec	Acetyl Tetrapeptide-5	Edema reduction by ACE inhibition	Eyeseryl®	Undisclosed
Lipotec	Pentapeptide-3	Botox-like via mimicking enkephalins	Leuphasyl®	Undisclosed
Lipotec	Acetyl Hexapeptide-3 (or -8)	Botox-like via SNARE inhibition	Argireline®	SNAP-25
Lipotec	Acetyl Octatapeptide-1	Botox-like via SNARE inhibition	SNAP-8	SNAP-25
Lipotec	Hexapeptide-10	Increases cell proliferation and laminin V	Serilesine®	Laminin
DSM/Pentapharm	Palmitoyl Dipeptide-5 Diaminobutyroyl	Dermal epidermal junction stimulation	Syn®-tacks	Waglerin 1
DSM/Pentapharm	Palmitoyl Tripeptide-5	Collagen synthesis via TGF-beta	Syn®-coll, Regu®-stretch, Regu®-CEA	Thrombospondin I

(continued)

Table 14.1 (*continued*)

Company	Name	Activity	Premix products	Source
DSM / Pentapharm	Dipeptide Diaminobutyroyl Benzylamide Diacetate	Botox-like via acetycholine receptor	Syn®-ake	Waglerin 1
DSM / Pentapharm	Oligopeptide-20	MMP inhibitor via TIMP	Pepha®-timp	TIMP-2
DSM / Pentapharm	Pentapeptide-3	Botox-like via acetycholine receptor	Vialox®	Undisclosed
PhotoMedex	Copper GHK / AHK	Wound healing	Brand example Neova®	Human serum
Sederma	Palmitoyl Tripeptide-38	ECM stimulation via signalling	Matrixyl® synthe'6	ECM
Sederma	Dipeptide-2	Lymph drainage via ACE inhibition	Eyeliss®	Rapeseed
Sederma	Palmitoyl Oligopeptide	Collagen synthesis via signalling	Eyeliss®, Matrixyl® 3000	Human serum
Sederma	Palmitoyl Tetrapeptide-7	Elasticity via IL6 reduction	Matrixyl 3000®, Rigin®	IgG / matrikine
Sederma	Palmitoyl Pentapeptide-3	Collagen stimulation via signalling	Matrixyl®	Procollagen
Sederma	Palmitoyl Oligopeptide	Retinoic acid-like activity	Biopeptide-CL™	Collagen
Sederma	Palmitoyl Oligopeptide	Increases collagen and HA	Biopeptide-EL™	Elastin

Notes:

Abbreviations

ACE	Angiotensin I converting enzyme
ECM	Extracellular matrix
HA	Hyaluronic acid
HGF	Hepatocyte growth factor
MMP	Matrix metalloproteinases
MSH	Melanocyte stimulating hormone
SNARE	Soluble NSF attachment receptor (NSF - N-ethylmaleimide sensitive factor)
TGF-beta	Transforming growth factor - beta
TIMP	Tissue inhibitor of MMP

Companies

Atrium Biotechnologies (Quebec City, Canada)
Grant Industries (Elmwood, NJ)
Evonik Industries AG (Essen, Germany)
Lipotec (Barcelona, Spain)
Pentapharm (Basel, Switzerland)
PhotoMedix (Montgomeryville, PA)
Sederma (Le Perray en Yvelines, France)

acids. This potential for diversity in structure allows peptides to be readily modified to target and adjust degree and specificity of bioactivity and bioavailability.

Peptides are distinguished from other proteins on the basis of size and typically contain fewer than 50 amino acids. As a result of this short length, they generally lack the more complex secondary and tertiary structures found in proteins. The shortest peptide is a dipeptide, consisting of two amino acids joined by a single peptide bond. Peptide bonds are strong and relatively resistant to heat, light and pH but are susceptible to protease degradation. Proteases are a large group of enzymes found in all organisms which catalyze the reaction of hydrolysis of the peptide bond. Some proteases detach the terminal amino acid from the peptide chain (exopeptidases, such as aminopeptidases, carboxypeptidase A) and others attack the internal peptide bond (endopeptidases, such as trypsin, chymotrypsin, pepsin, papain). The skin contains numerous proteases including collagenase, elastase and fibrinolysin. Skin conditions such as psoriasis and rosacea may be associated with a significant up-regulation in certain protease activity.

Role of peptides in skin

In the skin there are two primary sources of peptides. The first source is unique synthesis, and expression, as intact independent molecules for a specific purpose. The most significant example of this is peptides that have traditionally been referred to as antimicrobial peptides (AMPs) but, because we now understand their greater breadth of modulatory functionalities, are now termed "host defense peptides," "alarmins," or "innate immunity peptides." Throughout evolution these peptides have helped protect all living organisms and over 1200 unique sequences have been identified in nature. In mammals and other higher organisms these peptides have evolved to protect exposed and epithelial surfaces such as the gastrointestinal tract, the eyes and skin. Cathelicidins and human beta-defensins (hBDs) are the best characterized peptides expressed in human skin and these classes of innate immunity peptides exhibit a wide range of activities associated with protection against pathogens, wound healing modulation, angiogenesis and inflammation regulation. Such peptides can be expressed constitutively or induced upon challenge by pathogens, wounding or disease. In addition, certain skin conditions may modulate expression of such peptides or, conversely, their expression may be involved in the etiology of certain skin conditions. For example, it is well known that cathelicidins and hBDs are strongly induced in psoriatic lesions to the same level as if the skin were wounded. However, despite the presence of inflammation, there appears no up-regulation of these peptides in atopic dermatitis which has been linked to the propensity for *Staphylococcus aureus* colonization. In rosacea, an increase in the level of the cathelicidin LL-37 has been associated with inflammation and is believed, in part, to contribute to the pathology of this skin condition. Thus, modulation of peptides associated with innate immunity has created a wealth of possibilities for enhancing product formulations in the areas of topical anti-infectives, acne, rosacea and rejuvenation deriving from wound-healing activity.

The second source of bioactive peptides derives from the breakdown of a larger peptide or protein triggered by physiological events such as inflammatory disease, wounding, UV exposure or stress. During such events peptides are generated through proteolytic digestion of extracellular matrix proteins. These peptide fragments then act in a feedback loop to stimulate the healing process and the rebuilding of the extracellular matrix which plays a pivotal role in cellular migration, proliferations and gene regulation. Among these peptide sequences called matrikines are the hexapeptide VGVAPG derived from hydrolysis of elastin by elastase, the pentapeptide KTTKS derived from the proteolysis of a pro-collagen, and the tripeptide GHK derived from collagen 1. In vitro, the introduction of these peptides within the extracellular matrix has been shown to signal up-regulation of keratinocyte migration for wound healing and the promotion of chemotaxis and mitogenesis.

The development of peptide actives

Sequence origin

The amino acid sequence of peptides that has been used in dermatological and skin care products may come from the natural peptides described above or from the replication of short sequences that exist as a component of larger peptides and proteins but do not exist themselves as individual peptides in nature. This category includes sequences that may mimic a binding site, an active site for an enzyme or a ligand of an enzyme used to bind another molecule. These peptides are agonists and antagonists and so cause reactions to occur or prevent them from occurring, providing the possibility of reducing undesirable events such as inflammation, melanin production or neurotransmission or increasing desirable ones such as adipogenesis, aquaporin levels or DNA protection.

The advent of readily accessible and searchable protein and DNA databases has enabled scientists to significantly speed up and expand their ability to identify sequences of interest as well as structural motifs. Sequences and structures common to different proteins, binding sites and ligands can easily be compared to guide rational design and provide leads for potential bioactivities.

Peptide modification

The ultimate sequence of a peptide ingredient may be from what is seen in nature to enhance application in formulation. For example, the sequence of amino acids may be modified by substitution to improve the desired activity, to alter the solubility profile or to increase the ability of the peptide to reach its target. Such effects may be achieved by modifying the charge distribution, the hydrophobic and hydrophilic profile, or by varying the folding potential of the peptide. Oftentimes the ease of design and modification through peptide synthesis provides a significant advantage over the application of naturally derived peptide products.

Another common modification of naturally occurring peptide sequences is the reduction in the number of amino acids. If the desired bioactivity can be maintained in a subsection of the original sequence, then the overall length may be reduced and this can help with aspects of formulation, cost and skin penetration. Sequences may also be modified by the addition of a specific chemical group such as a fatty acid (e.g. a palmitic acid producing a palmitoyl group, often written PAL) to alter the chemical profile and properties of the peptide.

The development of combinatorial chemistry in which libraries of thousands of peptides can be synthesized, coupled with access to high throughput screening assays, has allowed researchers to cast a very wide net when seeking to optimize sequences for clinical benefits and product development. In addition, the advent of microarray analysis (mRNA quantitation for specific gene products) has provided both a validation tool for mechanism of action and a tool for early stage development to guide structural design.

Validation

A combination of in vitro assay and in vivo characterization has become the standard for the evaluation of potential active ingredients. When considering the value of a peptide for a particular benefit it is important that cell-based transcriptional data be supported by cell-based translational data as one is the validation of the other. In human studies the application of the peptide alone must be performed and the data presented from an endpoint and a mechanism of action perspective which should include both protein and mRNA readouts. This level of due diligence is of particular importance in evaluating peptide ingredients because, due to their size and susceptibility to protease degradation, in vitro data oftentimes will not translate to in vivo activity.

Clinical benefits

As described above, there have been many peptides developed to address a wide range of dermatological and skincare applications. One example of a peptide developed to target an anti-aging end-point is tetrapeptide-21, a skincare ingredient that has been fully characterized and published in a peer-reviewed journal.

The premise for the isolation of tetrapeptide-21 was based on the augmentation of extracellular matrix (ECM) production by carboxy terminal pro-peptides of type I collagen. The collagen synthesis inducing activity of these sub-fragments was located in a pentapeptide sequence comprising KTTKS (described above). Based on these observations it has been proposed that a regulation loop exists in which the release of peptides from the surrounding ECM stimulates the activity of fibroblasts. This line of reasoning was extended to identify peptide sequences with the potential for the regulation of ECM biosynthesis with the hypothesis that highly repetitive sequences in ECM components, such as collagen, may have a high potential in a signaling role at the time of collagen breakdown. Collagen protein sequences were assessed for frequent occurrence of repetitive tetrapeptide sequences.

In vitro validation at translational and transcriptional level

Initial screening of 15 multiply occurring tetrapeptide sequences was performed with human dermal fibroblasts incubated with 50 ppm of tetrapeptide for 24 and 48 hours and the supernatants assessed for total soluble collagen. Tetrapeptide-21 (GEKG), a sequence found many times in collagens I through V, proved to induce collagen production at both time points. When retested using primary human dermal fibroblasts exposed to 1 ppm and 10 ppm peptide for 24 hours, the tetrapeptide increased collagen synthesis by 80% and 170% respectively ($p < 0.01$).

The upregulation of collagen was confirmed at the mRNA level, which was analyzed by RT-PCR. The main skin collagen COL1A1 was increased 2.8-fold by Tetrapeptide-21 at 1 ppm. In addition, also at 1 ppm, there was a 24-fold increase in fibronectin and 5.7-fold increase in hyaluronic acid synthase (HAS1).

In vivo proof of concept

In order to determine if these modulatory effects could be replicated in vivo, Tetrapeptide-21 was administered topically to the skin of 10 healthy volunteers in a double-blind, randomized, placebo-controlled study once a day for a period of 8 weeks, using a vehicle-only control or the same vehicle containing 50 ppm peptide.

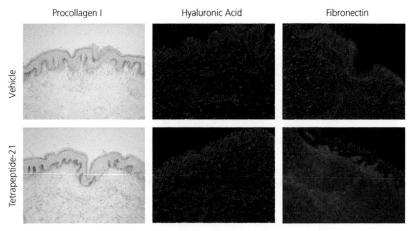

Figure 14.1 Ten healthy human volunteers (six female and four male, 40–65 years, average age 48.2; with 45.0 for women and 54.0 for men) were enrolled after written informed consent into a double-blind, placebo-controlled study. After treatment with 50 ppm GEKG or O/W vehicle (= placebo 1) for 60 days on buttock skin, biopsies were taken for immunohistochemical assessment of procollagen I (red), hyaluronic acid (red) and fibronectin (green).

RNA was extracted from biopsies of treatment areas, primarily buttock skin, reverse transcribed and gene expression analyzed by RT-PCR. Expression of COL1A1 was significantly increased under both treatments after 8 weeks resulting in a 2.0-fold increase for the placebo treated areas and a 3.1-fold rise for the tetrapeptide-containing vehicle as compared to the untreated skin. The difference between the two treatment arms was significant ($p = 0.02$, Wilcoxon signed rank test).

Immune-histochemistry sections were stained with monoclonal antibodies for collagen 1, hyaluronic acid and fibronectin (Figure 14.1). All showed a visible up-regulation.

Skin elasticity was measured and calculated as resilient distension (R1) at the start and the end of the eight-week study. Tetrapeptide-21 improved in vivo R1 to 34.1% ($p = 0.002$ paired t-test versus baseline). In a second study, enrolling 60 volunteers, the skin physiological effects of Tetrapeptide-21 were determined with respect to resilient distension (R1), skin volume and skin roughness after 8 weeks of twice-daily application at 10 ppm or 100 ppm. Skin elasticity on the inner forearm increased to 41.3 % for 10 ppm Tetrapeptide-21 over eight weeks. To assess the anti-aging effect of the tetrapeptide, photographs were taken of the subjects' skin before and after the eight-week application period using Visioscan™. A reduction in skin volume could be observed for 10 ppm and 100 ppm Tetrapeptide-21 resulting in a decrease of 8% and 12.2% respectively. Smoothness was improved by 19% after treatment with 10 ppm and even

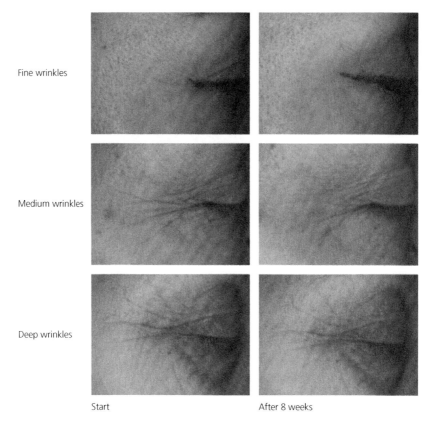

Fine wrinkles

Medium wrinkles

Deep wrinkles

Start　　　　　　　　　　　　After 8 weeks

Figure 14.2 In a facial wrinkle study (N = 30), the effects of 50 ppm GEKG on facial wrinkles as compared with a O/W vehicle were assessed. Representative examples of periorbital wrinkles are given before and after a twice daily, 8-week treatment.

further increased to 41.9% by 100 ppm peptide. When this study was repeated using the application of 10 ppm Tetrapeptide-21 (twice daily for 8 weeks) in the periorbital region, an aesthetic improvement in fine lines and wrinkles could be observed (Figure 14.2). In addition, this was associated with a corresponding statistically significant ($p < 0.01$) improvement in skin roughness as determined by the Primos Pico system.

Conclusion

Advantages of peptide technology for dermatological application

Peptides from a variety of sources within the body elicit a wide range of effects within and on the skin. Because of this fact, their use as topical therapeutics and cosmeceutical skincare ingredients makes a great deal of sense as peptides applied to the skin should be treated by the body in the same way as host peptides. As a result, they are non-immunogenic, being based primarily on short naturally occurring sequences and being composed of naturally occurring amino acids. In addition, they do not tend to be chemically active as their activity is biologic in nature (i.e. signaling and binding) which in both theory and practice reduces the potential for irritancy or side effects.

Importantly, peptide synthesis provides an opportunity and ability to create "designer" skincare ingredients that has not previously existed. Through synthesis and screening of the virtually endless combination of amino acid sequences and optimization of the chemical structure of the potential peptide ingredients for activity, delivery and formulation, peptides have opened a world of possibilities for the future of both drug actives and cosmetic ingredients.

Disadvantages of peptide technology for dermatological application

The most significant disadvantages to the use of peptides in treating the skin lie in delivery and access to the target. To deliver a molecule over 500 mw across the outer layers of the skin is extremely difficult, as evidenced by the field of transdermal drug delivery which has applied vast resources to address this very issue. Without assistance from penetration enhancers such as electrical current and injection strategies or delivery systems such as targeted liposomes or nanoparticles, it is unlikely that a peptide over 500 mw will reach a dermal or even an epidermal target. This is due first of all to the physical nature of the skin and also to the presence of proteases.

Peptide synthesis, although not a complicated or difficult process, can be expensive. Production by synthetic means (solid phase or solution phase chemistry) using amino acids derived from plants is the standard process used for both therapeutic and ingredient peptides. Recombinant production of peptides has been studied for many years and although it would be more cost effective, the end product is unlikely to be as pure as is currently available synthetically.

The future

To fully exploit this technology a rational approach must be taken with the design, development and validation of bioactive peptides. This would take into account the proposed mechanism of action and the location where that activity takes place. Targets that are located on the surface of the skin are easily accessible and provide a viable application for peptides. For example, a currently marketed peptide, Oligopeptide-10, was designed to bind lipoteichoic acid (the toxin on the surface of Gram-positive bacteria) which contributes to inflammation in acne and rosacea. The binding of this toxin can occur very near the surface of the skin and therefore does not require dermal penetration. Another example is Tetrapeptide-14 which is able to down-regulate IL8 in keratinocytes which in turn reduces MMP-1 expression in fibroblasts. In this case, the peptide does not need access to the fibroblast but operates through signaling. These strategies avoid the key disadvantage of peptides. When the peptide target is within the lower layers of the skin, then the data supporting the application of that peptide to dermatologic or skin care use must be comprehensive, as described above.

The true potential of validated peptide technology in dermatology may be in combination with activities derived from traditional ingredients and OTC therapeutics. Peptides are tailored to deliver a specific activity at a specific target through a specific binding process. For a formulated product to provide outstanding performance, this activity should be complemented by other technologies designed to address the clinical endpoint as broadly and comprehensively as possible either in the same product or in companion products. In-depth analysis of ingredient activities, for example, microarray data, can provide an excellent tool for compatibility analysis.

In the body, and particularly in the skin, peptides are produced quickly in response to a trigger event and are quickly degraded. They are the foot soldiers of many biological systems. And perhaps that is the most attractive aspect of bioactive peptides – their ability to mimic the skin's natural biological processes.

Further reading

Abu NH, Heard CM. Topically applied KTTKS: A review. *International Journal of Cosmetic Science* 2011; **33**: 483–490.

Farwick M, Grether-Beck S, Marini A, et al. Bioactive tetrapeptide GEKG boosts extracellular matrix formation: In vitro and in vivo molecular and clinical proof. *Exp Dermatol* 2011; **20**: 602–604.

Fields K, Falla TJ, Rodan K, et al. L bioactive peptides: Signaling the future. *Journal of Cosmetic Dermatology* 2009; **8**: 8–13.

Katayama K, Seyer JM, Raghow R, et al. Regulation of extracellular matrix production by chemically synthesized subfragments of type I collagen carboxy propeptide. *Biochemistry* 1991; **30**: 7097–7104.

Nakatsuji T, Gallo RL. Antimicrobial peptides: Old molecules with new ideas. *Journal of Investigational Dermatology* 2012; **132**: 887–895.

Yamasaki K, Gallo RL. Rosacea as a disease of cathelicidins and skin innate immunity. *J Investig Dermatol Symp Proc* 2011; **15**: 12–15.

Zhang L, Falla TJ. Cosmeceuticals and peptides. *Clinics in Dermatology* 2009; **27**: 485–494.

Zhang L, Falla TJ. Potential therapeutic application of host defense peptides in antimicrobial peptides. *Methods Molecular Biology* 2010; **618**: 303–327.

CHAPTER 15

Growth Factors in Cosmeceuticals

Sabrina G. Fabi[1] and Hema Sundaram[2]

[1]Goldman, Butterwick, Fitzpatrick, Groff & Fabi, Cosmetic Laser Dermatology, San Diego, CA, USA
[2]Sundaram Dermatology Cosmetic & Laser Surgery, Rockville, MD, and Fairfax, VA, USA

Introduction

The skin's mechanical, protective and restorative properties decline with age. Daily exposure to extrinsic, environmental stressors including ultraviolet (UV) light and cigarette smoke causes increased oxidative stress and consequent tissue damage due to antioxidant depletion, coupled with increased production of reactive oxygen species (ROS – also known as free radicals). Multiple biochemical pathways triggered by ROS overload result in suppression of transforming growth factor beta (TGFβ-R2), over-expression of matrix metalloproteinases (MMPs) which are collagenases, and increased inflammation through the nuclear factor kappa beta (NFkB) pathway. UV rays also cause direct damage to the skin's structural proteins.

These effects exacerbate the skin's intrinsic deterioration, which is related to a progressive, age-related decline in antioxidant capacity coupled with increased production of reactive oxygen species from oxidative metabolism in the cells of the skin. This contributes to ROS overload and the biochemical effects described above. Analysis of aging cells reveals progressive telomere shortening, which also contributes to tissue damage. Figure 15.1 shows a summary of major pathways involved in the skin aging process.

Aging of the skin, due to these extrinsic and intrinsic factors, results in intracellular and extracellular damage and the breakdown of the collagen and elastin network in the dermis. This manifests as xerosis, loss of elasticity, atrophy, dyschromia, and fine and deep rhytides. The search for safe, non-invasive treatments to slow or reverse these changes in aging skin remains challenging.

Research into the pathophysiology of photodamaged skin has revealed a correlation with certain aspects of acute and chronic wound healing. Specifically, some of the biochemical changes that occur during intrinsic and extrinsic skin aging are similar to the changes that occur during wound

Cosmeceuticals and Cosmetic Practice, First Edition. Edited by Patricia K. Farris.
© 2014 John Wiley & Sons, Ltd. Published 2014 by John Wiley & Sons, Ltd.

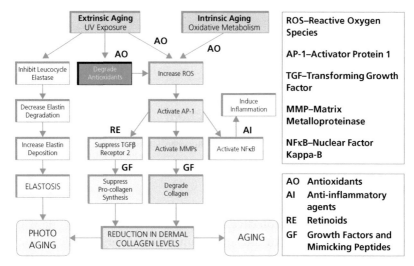

Figure 15.1 Simplified overview of extrinsic and intrinsic biochemical pathways of skin aging. Source: Courtesy of SkinMedica, Inc.

formation and its aftermath. Therefore, an understanding of the wound healing process may enhance the understanding of skin aging and the interventions that can be attempted to slow or even reverse this process.

Growth factors and cytokines (hereafter referred to as GFs) comprise a large group of regulatory proteins that attach to cell surface receptors to mediate inter- and intracellular signaling pathways that control cell growth, proliferation and differentiation. In the skin, they are naturally produced by fibroblasts, keratinocytes, lymphocytes and mast cells. GFs are chemical messengers that regulate specific, vital cellular activities such as cell proliferation, chemotaxis, and formation of the extracellular matrix. Tables 15.1 and 15.2 show the major mechanisms of action of key and supplemental GFs and cytokines.

When the skin is wounded, GFs accumulate at the site of injury and interact synergistically to initiate and coordinate wound healing. GFs can reverse the effects of collagenases, increase collagen levels, and reduce tissue inflammation. Topical application of human or animal-derived growth factors in clinical studies has been shown to reduce the signs and symptoms of skin aging. Results include a statistically significant reduction in fine lines and wrinkles and an increase in dermal collagen synthesis.

GFs may be derived from a variety of sources including humans, animals, microbes, yeast and plants. Topical GFs have emerged as an intriguing therapeutic modality that can be harnessed for aesthetic and medical purposes. It is postulated that topically applied GFs and cytokines can act together to produce the desired effects. As our understanding of the mechanisms of action of GF formulations increases, so does our ability to fully apply their potential benefits in the clinical setting.

Table 15.1 Key growth factors and cytokines.

• Vascular Endothelial Growth Factor VEGF
– Chemotactic and mitogenic to endothelial cells and promotes angiogenesis
– Believed to increase blood vessel permeability to improve tissue nutrition
• Platelet Derived Growth Factor PDGF AA, PDGF BB
– Chemotactic and mitogenic to fibroblasts
– Believed to regulate cell growth and division in wound healing
• Transforming Growth Factor TGFβ1, TGFβ2, TGFβ3
– Chemotactic and mitogenic to fibroblasts
– Regulates matrix protein including collagen and proteoglycans
• Tissue Inhibitor of Metalloproteinases TIMP1, TIMP2
– Regulates activity of enzymes preventing breakdown of collagen and hyaluronic acid

Source: Sundaram et al. (2009). Reproduced with permission of the Journal of Drugs in Dermatology.

Table 15.2 Supplemental growth factors and cytokines.

• Fibroblast Growth Factors bFGF (FGF-2), FGF-4, FGF-6, KGF (FGF-7), FGF-9
– Believed to promote skin cell growth and tissue repair
• Hepatocyte Growth Factor HGF
– Believed to promote three dimensional tissue growth
• Insulin Like Growth Factor IGF1, IGFBP1, IGFBP2, IGFBP3, IGFBP6
– Believed to promote cell growth and multiplication
• Placenta Growth Factor PLGF
– Believed to promote endothelial cell growth
• Bone Morphogenetic Protein BMP7
– Believed to promote development of nerve cells in developing tissue
• Interleukins: 15 Different Interleukins including IL10 and IL13
– Believed to plan a critical role in inflammation and wound healing
• Colony Stimulating Factors GCSF, GM-CSF, M-CSF
– Believed to induce secretion of other cytokines

Source: Sundaram et al. (2009). Reproduced with permission of the Journal of Drugs in Dermatology.

Pathophysiology of skin aging

Intrinsic and extrinsic skin aging are cumulative processes that occur simultaneously. Over time, they result in reduced dermal collagen levels and also elastosis. Histological evaluation of sun-damaged skin shows flattening of the dermoepidermal interface with loss of dermal papillae, a decrease in dermal fibroblast activity, a decrease in dermal thickness, diminished dermal vascularity, and haphazardly arranged, fragmented elastin fibers. A decrease in total elastin content and reduced ability to synthesize type I procollagen has been observed in sun-damaged skin when compared to young skin. Photodamaged skin shows a statistically significant decrease (20%) in total collagen in comparison to sun-protected skin, and both sun-protected and photodamaged skin show a reduction in mean epidermal thickness with age. Moreover, intrinsic aging causes decreased production and levels of growth factors in the skin.

Comparison of skin aging with wound formation and healing

Some biochemical changes during intrinsic and extrinsic skin aging are similar to those that are observed when a wound occurs. GFs are known to be crucial to the complex, multi-step process of wound healing. GF levels in the body peak in youth and decline thereafter. It can therefore be hypothesized that skin aging is analogous to a wound that is sufficiently extensive to overwhelm the skin's inherent repair mechanisms, which become attenuated with age. This provides a rationale for topical application of GFs that are responsible for wound healing, with the aim of replenishing the skin's own depleted levels and slowing or even reversing skin aging. The rationale can be extended to iatrogenic skin wounding, such as during laser and other skin rejuvenation procedures; the hypothesis being that topical GFs may also facilitate healing in this situation and perhaps even enhance the ultimate results.

The wound healing response is initiated once skin injury has occurred, to promote new cell growth and to decrease wound contraction and scarring. Wound healing is commonly divided into four phases: hemostasis, inflammation, proliferation and remodeling. Different phases are controlled by GFs, as is transition from one phase to the next. The parallel between skin wounding and skin aging is heightened by the fact that the initial inflammation seen in wounded skin is ROS-mediated, just like the changes seen in aging skin. It is noteworthy that, while intrinsic aging is not associated with inflammation, acute photodamage is associated with ROS-mediated inflammation. The proliferative phase, known as the granulation phase, is marked by angiogenesis, fibroplasia, and extracellular matrix deposition, all leading to re-epithelialization. The remodeling phase, also known as the maturation phase, is the final stage of wound healing after granulation and wound re-epithelialization or post-inflammatory desquamation of sun-burned skin. During this stage of wound repair, deposition and remodeling of the ECM occur and low strength, relatively less organized type III collagen and elastin structures produced during the initial wound healing process are replaced by stronger type I collagen and structured

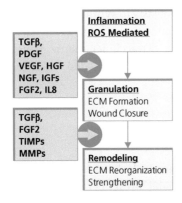

Figure 15.2 Key GFs that are active during wound healing. GF are part of a complex cellular communication network and work in harmony with each other.

elastin fibers to restore strength and resilience to the dermis. This remodeling phase can last for several months. Figure 15.2 shows key GFs that are active during the three main stages of wound healing: initial, ROS-mediated inflammation, followed by subsequent wound granulation, and finally wound remodeling.

The balance between the development of inflammation and its resolution involves growth factors and cytokines including PDGF, VEGF, HGF, TGF-β, EGF, G-CSF, KGF, IL-6, and IL-8, and results in successful wound healing.

Growth factors and cytokines in skin aging

Wound healing is dependent upon complex interactions between various GFs. GFs relevant to wound healing may induce new collagen, elastin, and glycosaminoglycan formation and mediate angiogenesis. If some of these agents are provided to the cells in aging skin that are responsible for extracellular matrix production and remodeling, they may mediate skin rejuvenation.

Studies have shown minimal penetration of intact stratum corneum by hydrophilic molecules larger than 500 Da molecular weight. GFs are large, hydrophilic molecules with greater than 15,000 Da molecular weight. Thus, it is unlikely that GFs could penetrate the intact epidermis in sufficient quantity to produce clinically significant effects. It is believed that one mechanism by which GFs might exert their effects in the dermis is via penetration of hair follicles and sweat glands. Aging skin may also permit better penetration, since its barrier function is somewhat compromised. Once GFs have penetrated the stratum corneum, they can interact with specific receptors on keratinocytes and initiate a cytokine signaling cascade that affects fibroblasts and other cells in the dermis. This epidermal-dermal communications during wound healing may mirror the effects of exogenous, topically applied GFs. Amplification of the initial effect of topical

GFs may occur as keratinocytes stimulate fibroblasts to synthesize growth factors that in turn stimulate keratinocyte proliferation (Figure 15.3). The resultant collagenesis and remodeling of the extracellular matrix have been observed histologically (Figure 15.3) and can be correlated with the clinical results that are detailed below.

Clinical benefits and indications

Topical human GFs that are commercially available have been derived from cultured fibroblasts harvested from neonatal foreskin (TNS Recovery Complex™, SkinMedica Inc., Carlsbad, CA), and from processed skin cell proteins (PSP™, Neocutis, Lausanne, Switzerland), containing a mixture of cytokines, growth factors and antioxidants harvested from fetal cell lines. GFs derived from the secretions of the snail *Cryptomphalus aspersa* (SCA) are also commercially available (Tensage™, Biopelle, Inc., Ferndale, MI, manufactured by Industrial Farmaceutica Cantabria, SA).

In a clinical study, a mixture of multiple GFs derived from human fibroblasts (TNS Recovery Complex) was applied topically to 14 patients twice daily for 60 days with the aim of stimulating dermal remodeling. Patients were evaluated for clinical grading of photodamage on a nine-point scale, by optical profilometry and with a punch biopsy of the treated skin for

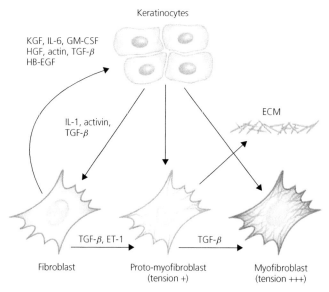

Figure 15.3 Proposed mechanism of action and signaling cascade for GFs and cytokines.

Collagen Deposition in Epidermis

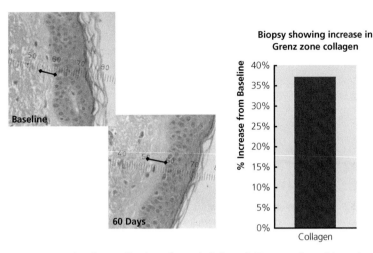

Figure 15.4 Results after application of a topical Growth Factor and cytokine mixture (TNS Recovery Complex, SkinMedica) twice daily for 60 days in 14 patients. The black bars on the photomicrographs show the thickness of the Grenz zone of the dermis. The bar graph shows a mean increase of over 35% in thickness of the Grenz zone in the 14 patients studied. Source: Fitzpatrick & Rostan.

evaluation of changes in Grenz zone thickness and histopathology. Some 78.6% of patients with photodamaged skin showed clinical improvement at 60 days (Figure 15.4). Microscopic evaluation revealed that 37% showed new collagen formation in the Grenz zone, and 27% showed epidermal thickening (Figure 15.4).

A randomized, vehicle-controlled double-blind study of the same GF mixture in 60 patents with a mean age of 55 and facial photodamage (mild to moderate in 48 subjects and severe in 12 subjects) showed improvement in periocular fine rhytids, skin tone and texture and hyperpigmentation. ($p = 0.012$ at 3 months) (Figure 15.5). Patient and physician assessments were performed at baseline and at 3 and 6 months. Optical profilometry of silicone skin surface impressions showed improvements in skin roughness ($p = 0.045$ at 3 months) (Figures 15.6 and 15.7).

A single center study evaluated the clinical, histologic, and ultrastructural changes from multiple human-derived GFs from PSP (Biocream, Neocutis, Lausanne, Switzerland). Twelve subjects applied the cream twice a day to the entire face for 6 months. Pre- and post-treatment punch biopsies were taken from the preauricular skin. Further evaluations included photographic and clinical assessment of facial skin for wrinkles. Clinical improvement of periorbital and perioral wrinkles by 33% and 25% on average, respectively, was noted. Histologic evaluation demonstrated moderate changes in the epidermal thickness as well as an increased fibroblast

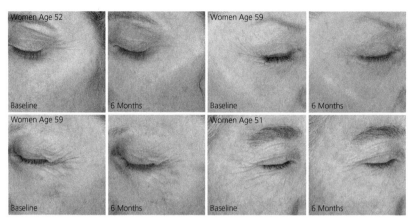

Figure 15.5 Clinical results after application of a topical human-derived Growth Factor and cytokine mixture (TNS Recovery Complex) twice daily for 60 days in 60 patients. Improvement in fine rhytids and mottled hyperpigmentation is seen.

Skin Surface Impression of Periorbital Area

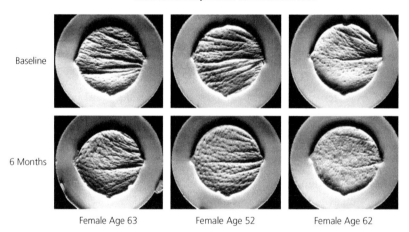

Figure 15.6 Silicone skin surface impressions from the periocular region of patients treated with the topical human-derived GF mixture. There is a visible reduction in number and depth of rhytids after 6 months of use.

density in the superficial dermis at the end of the 6-month treatment period. Electron microscopy corroborated changes seen histologically by showing findings consistent with new collagen formation.

In a two-center, double-blind, randomized 14-week study, 25 patients with moderate to severe facial photodamage were treated for 12 weeks with an emulsion containing 8% SCA and a liquid serum containing 40% SCA (Tensage) on one side of the face, and with a placebo cream on the contralateral side. Silicone skin impressions of periocular rhytides were performed at baseline and after 12 weeks of treatment. Patient and

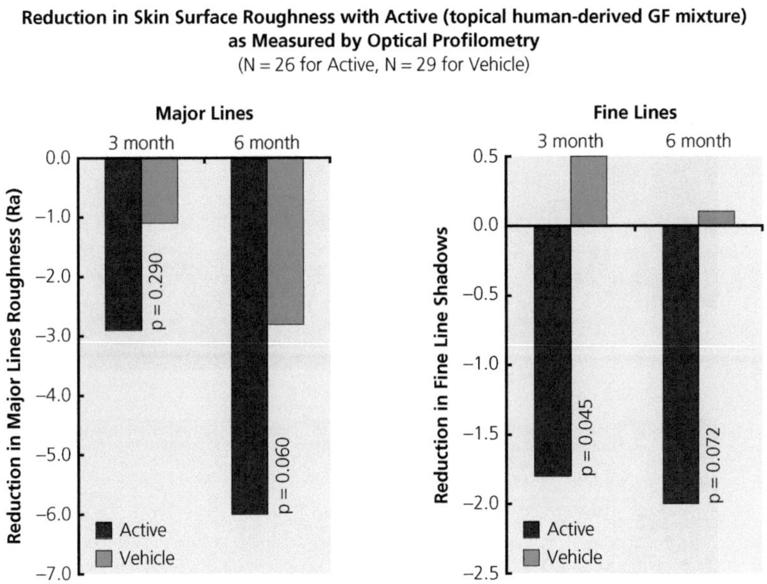

**Reduction in Skin Surface Roughness with Active (topical human-derived GF mixture)
as Measured by Optical Profilometry**
(N = 26 for Active, N = 29 for Vehicle)

Figure 15.7 Optical profilometry analysis of the silicone skin surface impressions. A statistically significant reduction in fine and coarse rhytids is seen at 3 months and a trend towards significance at 6 months.

physician assessments were also performed at baseline and at 8, 12 and 14 weeks. At 12 weeks, there was significant improvement in coarse periocular rhytides on the side treated with the GF active ($p = 0.03$). Skin texture was also improved at 8 and 12 weeks and remained improved 2 weeks after discontinuing the product (14 weeks) (Figure 15.8).

New developments

An interesting new development is the generation of GFs from cultured neonatal human dermal fibroblasts that demonstrate multipotent behavior under conditions of hypoxia that simulate the fetal environment. These fibroblasts express and secrete GFs including KGF, VEGF and IL-8, together with stem cell-associated proteins. It is hypothesized that this may induce a more regenerative pattern of collagenesis, with higher expression of Types III and V relative to Type I collagen, as is seen in the fetus where skin healing is scarless. An open-label comparative study of a lotion containing conditioned cultured medium produced by these multipotent fibroblasts (ReGenica, Suneva Medical) was performed in 49 subjects receiving ablative Erbium laser resurfacing of the periocular and perioral regions. At day 7, following laser resurfacing, there was greater reduction than with placebo lotion in periocular and perioral

Baseline

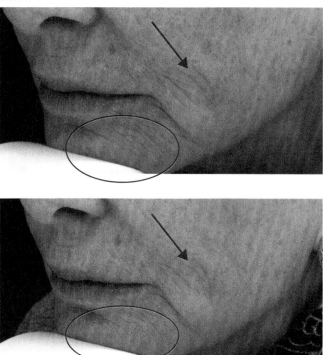

14 weeks, Left side Active

Figure 15.8 Clinical results after application of a topical animal-derived Growth Factor and cytokine mixture (Tensage) for 14 weeks in 25 patients. Caucasian female at baseline (top) and 14 weeks (bottom). The left side of the face received the GF active; the right side received placebo cream. Courtesy of Joel Cohen, MD.

erythema, as determined by blinded clinical evaluation of photographs and by mexameter measurements. There was also a statistically significant reduction in rescue petrolatum use in subjects treated with the active lotion ($p = 0.0004$). A split-face evaluation of 42 subjects undergoing combination ablative and non-ablative laser procedures showed a more rapid return to normal skin barrier function with gel containing the active GF formulation, as measured by transepidemal water loss readings (p less than or $= 0.05$).

Safety and efficacy considerations

All topically applied products carry the risk of irritant or allergic contact dermatitis. Since some malignant cells may have receptors for certain GFs, and some GFs may increase cellular proliferation, there has been discussion as to whether GFs have the potential for tumorigenesis or promotion of cellular atypia. Studies of the effects of specific GFs on animal skin and on human tumor cells have shown mixed results. The validity of extrapolating these data to topical application of GF mixtures to human skin remains to be clarified.

In one study, EGF, TGF-α and suramin (growth factor inhibitor) were applied to murine skin for nine days before the mice were sacrificed. It was found that TGF-α increased creatine phosphokinase (CPK) activity. EGF and TGF-α both induced a transition from the CPK MM to CPK BB isoenzyme. The significance of these findings is that the phosphocreatine/CPK system is believed to play an important role in the normal physiology of skin and in pathophysiological conditions such as psoriasis and carcinogenesis. Histopathological evaluation showed abnormal differentiation and distribution of keratinocytes. In a study of human tumor cells using the reverse-transcriptase polymerase chain reaction, VEGF expression was found in all 15 cell lines that were examined, while the VEGF receptor, KDR, was detected only in three melanoma cell lines. Exogenously added VEGF (10 ng/mL) was able to stimulate up to 40% increased proliferation in these melanoma cells. Conversely, Graeven et al. found exogenous VEGF had no significant effects on melanoma cell proliferation or on production of a transcriptional target for VEGF. Another study of human tumor cells, including squamous cell carcinomas of the head and neck and melanomas, found that VEGF treatment of tumor cells expressing the receptor, VEGFR-1, actually inhibited cell proliferation and migration.

To date, there are no data or reports that indicate that topical GFs might have either a stimulatory or inhibitory role in human carcinogenesis. An evidence-based approach requires controlled studies of GFs that are applied topically to intact human skin, rather than anecdotal reports or animal studies that employ supraphysiological concentrations of GFs. It is debatable whether the effects of applying high concentrations of one or a few GFs can be extrapolated to the clinical situation where lower concentrations of mixtures containing multiple GFs are utilized. Production and activity of the body's endogenous GFs are closely controlled by positive and negative feedback mechanisms. Naturally secreted GF mixtures may be in a similar state of physiological balance and also subject to some of the same control mechanisms.

Like many proteins, GFs are inherently unstable when not in their physiologic environment. Formulations that contain surfactants, oils and other excipients are likely to denature and inactivate the proteins. Therefore, the clinical efficacy of a GF mixture can only be evaluated accurately by studies that utilize the complete formulation, rather than the individual components.

Conclusion

Growth factors and cytokines (GFs) upgrade cell healing and regeneration. Topical growth factors have been shown to stimulate new collagen formation and to thicken the epidermis, resulting in clinical improvement in rhytides and skin roughness. GFs may also function synergistically with antioxidants and retinoids. An evidence-based approach to evaluating the clinical effects of GFs, including their activity when combined with other anti-aging actives, requires further controlled studies, which should ideally be vehicle-controlled. As with all cosmeceutical manufacturing processes, the stability and quality of GF products remain a priority.

Further reading

Babu M, Wells A. Dermal-epidermal communication in wound healing. *Wounds* 2001; **13**:183–189.

Eming SA, Krieg T, Davidson JM. Inflammation in wound repair: molecular and cellular mechanisms. *J Invest Dermatol* 2007; **127**: 514–525.

Fabi SG, Peterson JD, Kiripolsky MG, Cohen J, Goldman MP. The effects of filtrate of the secretion of the cryptomphalus aspersa (SCA) on photoaged skin. *J Drugs Dermatol* 2013; **12**(4): 453–457.

Fitzpatrick RE. Endogenous growth factors as cosmeceuticals. *Dermatol Surg* 2005; **31**:827–831 [discussion 831].

Fitzpatrick RE, Rostan EF. Reversal of photodamage with topical growth factors: A pilot study. *J Cosmet Laser Ther* 2003; **5**: 25–34.

Hussain M, Phelps R, Goldberg D. Clinical, histologic, and ultrastructural changes after use of human growth factor and cytokine skin cream for the treatment of skin rejuvenation. *J Cosmet Laser Ther*, **10**:2,104–109.

Kellar R, Hubka M, Lawrence A Rheins, Fisher G., Naughton G. Hypoxic conditioned culture medium from fibroblasts grown under embryonic-like conditions supports healing following post-laser resurfacing. *J Cosmet Dermatol* 2009; **8**: 190–196.

Liu B, Earl HM, Baban D, et al. Melanoma cell lines express VEGF receptor KDR and respond to exogenously added VEGF. *Biochem Biophys Res Commun* 1995; **217**: 721–727.

Mehta RC, Fitzpatrick RE. Endogenous growth factors as cosmeceuticals. *Dermatol Ther* 2007; **20**(5): 350–359. Review.

Moulin V. Growth factors in skin wound healing. *Eur J Cell Biol* 1995; **68**(1):1–7.

Sundaram H, Mehta RC, Norine JA, Kircik L, Cook-Bolden FE, Atkin DH, Werschler PW, Fitzpatrick RE. Topically applied physiologically balanced growth factors: a new paradigm of skin rejuvenation. *J Drugs Dermatol.* 2009; **8**(5 Suppl. Skin Rejuvenation): 4–13. Review.

Zemtsov A, Montalvo-Lugo V. Topically applied growth factors change skin cytoplasmic creatine kinase activity and distribution and produce abnormal keratinocyte differentiation in murine skin. *Skin Res Technol* 2008; **14**(3): 370–375.

Zimber M, Mansbridge J, Taylor M, Stockton T, Hubka M, Baumgartner M, Rheins L, Hubka K, Brandt E, Kellar R, Naughton G. Human cell-conditioned media produced under embryonic-like conditions result in improved healing time after laser resurfacing. *Aesth Plast Surg* 2012; **36**(2): 431–437.

CHAPTER 16

Resveratrol and Synthetic Sirtuin Activators

Patricia K. Farris
Tulane University School of Medicine, New Orleans, LA, USA

Introduction

The observation that dietary restriction (DR) extends lifespan and reduces age-related illnesses led to the discovery of a family of enzymes called sirtuins. Sirtuins are encoded by silent information regulator (SIR) genes. SIR genes are found in virtually all species and control the function of other genes. The Sir family of genes was first discovered in the yeast *Saccharomyces cerevisiae*. This novel gene was named silent mating type information regulator-2 (Sir2) and was later identified in both the fruit fly and roundworm. In these organisms, Sir2 is important in the regulation of a variety of metabolic pathways including those that influence aging and longevity. Seven sirtuin genes (SIRT1–SIRT7) have now been identified in mammals. The first gene, silent mating type information regulation-2 homolog (SIRT1), is considered to be biologically equivalent to Sir2. Each SIRT gene encodes for a unique sirtuin enzyme that is numbered accordingly. Accordingly, the product of SIRT1 gene is SIRT1 enzyme.

Mammalian sirtuins are found in the nucleus, cytoplasm, and in mitochondria. SIRT1, SIRT2, SIRT6 and SIRT7 are found in the nucleus, while SIRT1 and SIRT2 are also located in the cytoplasm. SIRT3, SIRT4 and SIRT5 are found in mitochondria. In addition to being present in different cellular compartments, sirtuins are expressed at varying degrees in different tissues. SIRT1 is perhaps the most well studied of all sirtuins. It is expressed in a variety of tissues including the hypothalamus, heart, pancreas, kidney, liver, skeletal muscle, and fat. SIRT2 is most plentiful in fatty tissue, but is also found in the brain and nervous system. SIRT3 is found in skeletal muscle, brown and white adipose, kidney, liver and heart. SIRT4 is found in the pancreas and SIRT5 is expressed in the heart, brain, muscle, kidney and liver. SIRT6 is found in heart, brain, muscle, kidney and liver while SIRT7 is found in the heart and adipose tissue (Table 16.1).

Table 16.1 Sirtuins and their site of effect.

Sirtuin	Site of effect	
Sirtuin 1	Nucleus, cytoplasm	Hypothalamus, heart, pancreas, kidney, liver, skeletal muscle, and fat
Sirtuin 2	Nucleus, cytoplasm	Fat, brain, nervous system
Sirtuin 3	Mitochondria	Skeletal muscle, brown and white adipose, kidney, liver and heart
Sirtuin 4	Mitochondria	Pancreas
Sirtuin 5	Mitochondria	Heart, brain, muscle, kidney and liver
Sirtuin 6	Nucleus	Heart, brain, muscle, kidney and liver
Sirtuin 7	Nucleus	Heart and adipose tissue

The majority of sirtuin enzymes are classified as class III histone deacetylases. These enzymes deacetylate lysine residues on various proteins in a reaction that is nicotinamide adenine dinucleotide (NAD+) dependent. Once the acetyl group is removed from the acetyl lysine residue in a histone, it is transferred to the ADP-ribose moiety of NAD+. In general, when histone is deacetylated, transcription does not occur. Hence, sirtuins function primarily as gene silencers. In addition, some sirtuins participate in non-histone deacetylase reactions while others possess mono-ribosyltransferase (mono-ADP-ribosyltransferases) activity.

The expression of sirtuin genes is influenced by changes in the environment and diet. Caloric restriction changes the expression of sirtuins in a way that improves the adaptive capabilities of organisms to stressful environments and enhances longevity. It has been shown that caloric restriction in mice that are SIRT1 deficient does not extend lifespan. Data in humans also validates the role of sirtuins. In healthy humans, serum was collected before and after caloric restriction or alternate day fasting. When added to cultured cells, the serum collected after caloric restriction or fasting had increased in SIRT1 expression. Studies looking at SIRT1 in overweight human volunteers demonstrated that restricting caloric intake by 25% or by 12.5% with an increase in exercise of 12.5%, increased the expression of SIRT1 compared to controls that were fed 100% of energy requirements. It is also of interest that in a study of obese women, who followed a 10-week diet of either low-fat (high-carbohydrate) or a moderate-fat (low-carbohydrate) hypoenergetic diet, there was an increase in the expression of five genes including SIRT3 in adipose tissue in those women on the moderate-fat diet. The two diets induced similar weight loss and profiles for most biologic variables, except lipid profiles.

It appears that changes in sirtuin expression caused by dietary restriction, and the biologic effects they mediate, are adaptive responses to dietary stress. Sirtuins are known to modulate cell survival, DNA repair, gluco-neogenesis, cell-cycle regulation, lipid metabolism, insulin sensitivity, fat mobilization, and lifespan. Fasting induces SIRT1 expression in the liver, skeletal muscle, and white adipose tissue. In the liver, SIRT1 promotes glu-coneogenesis by increasing the transcription of key gluconeogenic genes through the deacetylation of PGC-1α and FOXO1. In addition to promot-ing gluconeogenesis, sirtuin activation increases insulin sensitivity. These combined biologic effects of SIRT1 are adaptive mechanisms that help to maintain blood glucose levels during fasting. Hepatic SIRT1 regulates lipid homeostasis by positively regulating peroxisome proliferators-activated receptor alpha (PPARα), a nuclear receptor that mediates adaptive response to fasting and starvation. PPARα promotes lipolysis and free fatty acid mobilization that can be used as an energy source during fasting.

Resveratrol: a sirtuin activator

In view of the importance of sirtuins and their role in health and longevity, there has been a great deal of interest in identifying molecules that can mimic their effects. A screening of potential compounds led to the discovery that resveratrol was among the most potent sirtuin-activating molecules. Resveratrol (3,4,5-trihydroxystilbene) is a polyphenolic antioxidant that is found in various berries, nuts, and other plant sources. Grapes and red wine contain high concentrations of resveratrol and are frequently cited as nutri-tional sources. Resveratrol from red wine consumption has been linked to the low incidence of heart disease seen in the French paradox peaking scientific interest in its health benefits. Resveratrol has been studied exten-sively in animal models and has been shown to improve insulin resistance and cardiovascular health, protect neurons from degeneration, reduce inflammation, prevent cancer and increase longevity. Since metabolic syn-drome and caloric restriction lie on opposite ends of the spectrum, it is no surprise that resveratrol has been proposed as a pharmacologic agent for treating metabolic syndrome. Subsequently numerous in vitro and ani-mal studies have demonstrated that resveratrol reduces fat accumulation, improves insulin sensitivity and improves glucose homeostasis. Since these are major components of metabolic syndrome, future studies will clarify if these beneficial effects of resveratrol can be reproduced in humans.

Resveratrol: photoprotection and chemoprevention

Resveratrol has important biologic activity in the skin including photo-protection and chemoprevention. As an antioxidant, resveratrol has been shown to reduce UVA-induced oxidative stress and to increase cell viability after UVA exposure. Resveratrol exerts antitumor activity by affecting all three pathways of carcinogenesis, including initiation, promotion, and progression. Hairless mice that received pretreatment with topical resveratrol 30 minutes before UVB exposure or 5 minutes after UVB exposure demonstrated inhibition of tumorigenesis. After 28 weeks of UVB exposure, there was both a delay in onset and reduced incidence in tumor formation in both groups of resveratrol-treated mice. Since post treatment delivered protective effects similar to pretreatment, the benefits of resveratrol are not believed to be due to sunscreen effects. Resveratrol exerts antitumor activity in part by down-regulating the expression and function of survivin, a member of the inhibitor of apoptosis gene family. Resveratrol also induces apoptosis by increasing the expression of tumor suppressor genes, including P-53. Resveratrol has also been shown to act as a sensitizer to enhance the therapeutic effect of ionizing radiation against cancer cells.

Resveratrol as an anti-aging agent

Resveratrol has significant potential as a topical agent for treating aging skin. In a comparative study, the antioxidant capacity of a commercially available skin care product containing 1% resveratrol (FAMAR, Athens, Greece) was found to be more potent than a 1% idebenone cream (Prevage MD, Allergan, Inc., Irvine, CA). Using the oxygen radical absorbance capacity test (ORAC), the resveratrol skin care product had a 17-fold greater antioxidant capacity than the idebenone product. Resveratrol down-regulates transcription factors activator protein 1 (AP-1) and nuclear factor kappa beta (NF-kB) that are important in the pathogenesis of skin aging. AP-1 is responsible for the synthesis of collagen-degrading metalloproteinases (MMPs) and NF-kB is responsible for the synthesis of a variety of inflammatory mediators. Hence, down-regulation of these transcription factors preserves dermal collagen and reduces inflammation that contributes to skin aging. Resveratrol also acts as a skin lightening agent and appears to work synergistically with other skin-lightening compounds. Its ability to inhibit tyrosinase is believed to be due to the double bond of the stilbene structure. These combined effects make resveratrol of interest as a topical ingredient for treating photodamaged skin.

A recent study evaluated the benefits of a nutraceutical containing a resveratrol-procyanin blend for treating photoaged skin. This commercially available supplement contained a blend of 8 mg of resveratrol and 14.63 mg procyanidins (Revidox®, GMC Pharma, Milan; Actafarma, Laboratorios, Madrid). In a double-blind, placebo-controlled study of 50 patients, subjects took the supplements for 60 days after which a statistically significant improvement was observed in skin and plasma antioxidant capacity, skin hydration, elasticity, wrinkles and brown spots compared to placebo control.

Resveratrol as a phytoestrogen

After menopause, the lack of estrogen profoundly affects the skin. Low estrogen levels combined with age-related changes accelerate skin aging. The skin becomes thin, wrinkled and fragile due to a loss of dermal collagen. Fibroblasts become sparse and collagen production decreases after menopause. The stilbene chemical structure of resveratrol is chemically related to the synthetic estrogen diethylstilbestrol. Thus it is no surprise that resveratrol functions as a phytoestrogen acting as a natural estrogen β receptor (ERβ) agonist. ERβ is an important target for preventing photoaging and skin tumor growth. ERβ agonists have been shown to reduce the level of inflammatory markers associated with photoaging and inhibit metalloproteinase expression. Thus resveratrol holds great potential as a cosmeceutical active that may provide natural estrogenic effects to aging skin.

Delivery of resveratrol

Bioavailability of resveratrol after oral administration is poor. It has been suggested that only small amounts of circulating resveratrol are necessary for skin benefits since the molecule is highly lipophilic. Topical application has been successful and is proposed as an alternative method for delivering resveratrol to the skin. Topical formulations including hydrogels and nanosuspensions have been used with some success. Recent studies evaluated several stabilizers and surfactants to produce a stable nanosuspension of resveratrol identifying two non-ionic stabilizers that worked well. These nanosuspensions were stable at room temperature for 30 days making them amenable for cosmeceutical formulations. Although many nutriceuticals and cosmeceuticals that contain resveratrol are being sold as anti-aging remedies, further studies are required to determine optimal dosing, delivery and duration of therapy.

Synthetic sirtuin activators (STACs)

In 2007, synthetic compounds (SRT1720, SRT2183) similar in structure to resveratrol were screened for SIRT1 activating activity. These synthetic compounds, now referred to as STACs, were shown to activate SIRT1 at submicromolar concentrations and increased SIRT1 catalytic activity several hundredfold. When administered orally, these small molecule activators of SIRT1 improved metabolic parameters in mice fed high-fat diets and in diabetic animal models. Ongoing research on these and other molecules may provide us with synthetic alternatives offering superior clinical benefits.

Sirtuins, resveratrol and STACs: the controversy

Although there is ongoing controversy surrounding resveratrol, the most recent studies published confirm that this polyphenol does in fact up-regulate SIRT1. While here is still some degree of skepticism about sirtuins and their ability to extend lifespan in humans, research is ongoing in this area. Since resveratrol exerts its activity by modulating numerous cell-signaling pathways and directly binding target molecules, it is clear that its activity does not rely solely on sirtuin activation (Table 16.2).

Yeast biopeptides as sirtuin activators

A unique active that has been shown to increase sirtuin expression are yeast biopeptides from *Kluyveromyces*. In vitro studies have demonstrated that these biopeptides activate SIRT1 in human epidermal cells and dermal fibroblasts. They also have been shown to decrease UVB-mediated cell senescence and DNA fragmentation. A commercially available product containing 1% yeast biopeptides, an extract of *aframomum angustifolium*

Table 16.2 Biologic effects of resveratrol.

Sirtuin-activator	Modulates cell survival, DNA repair, gluconeogenesis, cell-cycle regulation, lipid metabolism, insulin sensitivity, fat mobilization, lifespan
Antioxidant	Reduces UVA induced oxidative stress, increases cell viability after UVA
Chemoprevention	Inhibits tumor initiation, promotion, and progression. Inhibits survivin, induces apoptosis through P-53 expression
Anti-aging	Inhibits transcription factors AP-1 and NF-kB, Phytoestrogen effects
Anti-inflammatory	Inhibits NF-kB, inhibits Cox 1 and Cox 2
Phytoestrogen	Natural estrogen beta receptor agonist

seeds and nine other anti-aging ingredients, was tested on 33 female subjects with photodamage. After daily application to the face and neck for 4 weeks, skin hydration was improved as were fine lines and wrinkles, pigmentation, radiance, and skin texture. While the study does not specifically determine the efficacy of the yeast biopeptides for treating aging skin, this product has multiple beneficial ingredients offering a complementary approach to treating aging skin.

Conclusion

Nutriceuticals and cosmeceuticals containing resveratrol are now widely available. They are embraced by consumers as products that may slow aging and prevent age-related diseases. Resveratrol is a potent antioxidant that offers photoprotection, chemoprevention, health and anti-aging benefits making it of interest to dermatologists and other clinicians. Further research is warranted to delineate the full potential of this unique polyphenolic compound.

Further reading

Aziz MH, Reagan-Shaw, S, Wu J, Longley BJ, Ahmad N. Chemoprevention of skin cancer by grape constituent resveratrol: Relevance to human disease. *FASEB J* 2005; **19**: 1193–1195.

Barger JL, Kayo T, Vann JM, Arias EB, Wang J, Hacker TA, et al. A low dose of dietary resveratrol partially mimics caloric restriction and retards aging parameters in mice. *PLoS One* 2009; **3**: e2264.

Baur JA. Resveratrol, sirtuins and the promise of a DR mimetic. *Mech Ageing Dev* 2010; **131**: 261–269.

Baxter RA. Anti-aging properties of resveratrol: review and report of a potent new antioxidant skin care formulation. *J Cosmet Derm* 2008; **7**: 2–7.

Buonocore D, Lazzeretti A, Tocabens P, et al. Resveratrol-procyanidin blend: nutraceutical and anti-aging efficacy evaluated in a placebo-controlled, double-blind study. *Clin Cosm Invest Derm* 2012; **5**: 159–165.

Dali-Youcef N, Lagouge M, Froelich S, et al. The "magnificent seven": Function, metabolism and longevity. *Ann Med* 2007; **39**: 335–345.

Frescas D, Valenti L, Acoili D. Nuclear trapping of the Forkhead transcription factor FOX01 via Sirt-dependent deacetylation promotes expression of glucogenetic genes *J Biol Chem* 2005; **280**; 20589–20595.

Huber JL, McBurney MW, Distefano PS, McDonagh T. SIRT1-independent mechanisms of the putative sirtuin enzyme activators SRT1720 and SRT2183. *Future Med Chem* 2010; **2**: 1751–1759.

Kundu JK, Shin YK, Surh YJ. Resveratrol modulates phorbol ester-induced pro-inflammatory signal transduction pathways in mouse skin in vivo: NF-kappa B and AP-1 as prime targets. *Biochem Pharmacol* 2006; **72**: 1506–1515.

Marques FZ, Markus MA, Morris BJ. Resveratrol: Cellular actions of a potent natural chemical that confers a diversity of health benefits. *Int Journ Biochem Cell Biol* 2009; **41**: 2125–2128.

Moreau M, Neveu M, Stéphan S, et al. Enhancing cell longevity for cosmetic application: a complementary approach. *J Drugs Dermatol* 2007; **6**: 14–19.

Ndiaye M, Philippe C, Mukhtar H, Ahmad N. The grape antioxidant resveratrol for skin disorders: Promise, prospects and challenges. *Arch Biochem Biophys* 2011; **508**(2): 164–170.

Pirola L, Fröjöd S. Resveratrol: One molecule, many targets. *IUBMB Life* 2008; **60**: 323–332.

CHAPTER 17

Skin Aging, Glycation and Glycation Inhibitors

Patricia K. Farris
Tulane University School of Medicine, New Orleans, LA, USA

Introduction

Aging is a multifactorial process that includes intrinsic and extrinsic factors. Although sun exposure, cigarettes and pollution are known to contribute to extrinsic aging, recent studies have focused on nutrition as an environmental factor that can influence aging by altering gene expression. It is known that caloric restriction prolongs longevity and reduces the incidence of age-related illnesses. The exact mechanism whereby caloric restriction influences aging is still the subject of ongoing research but potential upstream targets include down-regulation of mTor signaling and up-regulation of Sir1 gene expression. Although the health benefits of caloric restriction are well documented, it is generally regarded as an unrealistic approach to improving health and longevity. Alternatively rather than change the quantity of our nutritional intake, improving the quality of foods represents a more realistic approach.

This chapter will discuss the importance of restricting dietary sugars in improving general health and appearance. The glycation theory of aging has gained favor in recent years due to a growing body of science demonstrating that diets high in added sugars and refined carbohydrates contribute to the development of metabolic syndrome, type II diabetes and other age-related illnesses. The role of dietary sugars in skin aging and the use of nutritionally derived compounds to inhibit glycation will be reviewed. The emerging category of anti-glycation skin care products will also be discussed.

Sugar and advanced glycation end products

Glycation was first described by Maillard who observed that amino acids heated in the presence of reducing sugars caused a characteristic browning

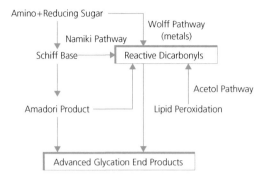

Figure 17.1 Multiple pathways to reactive dicarbonyls and advanced glycation end products (AGEs). Source: Adapted from Peng X, Ma J, Chen F, Wang M. 2011. Reproduced with permission of the Royal Society of Chemistry.

of foods. The Maillard reaction contributes not only to the color of food but also to the odor and flavor, making it vitally important to food science. In the late 1960s, physicians determined that the Maillard reaction also occurred in diabetics through a process called glycation. The most notable byproduct of glycation in diabetics is glycated hemoglobin or hemoglobin A_{1c}. Hemoglobin A_{1c} is now used as an indicator of long-term glycemic control and can be used to assess the risk for complications in patients with diabetes mellitus. Glycation of proteins in diabetics occurs in many tissues causing common diabetic complications such as cardiovascular disease, nephropathy, retinopathy and neuropathy.

The chemical process of glycation is now well defined. Glycation occurs through a non-enzymatic process that ultimately results in the irreversible formation of advanced glycation end products (AGEs) (Figure 17.1). The first step of glycation occurs when the aldehyde or ketone group of a reducing sugar binds to the free amino groups on proteins, forming unstable Schiff bases. These Schiff bases then undergo Amadori rearrangement, forming Amadori products. Further modification yields highly reactive dicarbonyl compounds that act as AGE precursors. Dicarbonyls can also be formed by oxidative fermentation of Schiff bases (Namiki pathway), metal-catalyzed auto-oxidation of glucose (Wolff pathway) or lipid peroxidation (Acetol pathway). Once formed, these dicarbonyl compounds interact with various intracellular and extracellular proteins resulting in the formation of stable yet irreversible AGEs. Some AGEs such as pentosidine have a yellowish brown color that can be detected by autofluorescence in tissues including the skin.

Glycation and aging skin

We now know that glycation occurs as part of intrinsic and extrinsic skin aging. Glycation starts in the mid-thirties and affects both collagen and elastin molecules. Extrinsic factors such as sun exposure accelerate AGE deposition found in areas of solar elastosis. It is believed that these advanced glycation end products cause the yellow appearance of actinically damaged skin. Cross-linking of collagen and elastin fibers render them stiff and inelastic, causing loss of skin suppleness and contributing to the aging phenotype. Once deposited in the tissues, glycated collagen and elastin cannot be broken down, so prevention remains the best strategy. The rate of glycation can be altered by lowering the intake of dietary sugars and maintaining tight glycemic control.

In addition to their direct effects on tissues, glycated proteins increase oxidative stress and up-regulate inflammation by binding to receptors for AGEs (RAGE). RAGEs are cell surface receptors in the immunoglobulin family and are expressed primarily in heart, lung and skeletal muscle. AGEs induce post-receptor signaling, activating the transcription factor nuclear factor kappa beta (NF-κβ). NF-κβ increases the production of pro-inflammatory cytokines that contribute to skin aging and inflammation. AGEs themselves up-regulate oxidative stress in a process called glycoxidation that further promotes the formation of AGEs.

Glycation inhibitors

Glycation can be inhibited in early and late stages. AGE inhibitors can block sugar attachment to proteins, attenuate oxidative stress and glycoxidation by scavenging dicarbonyls, free radicals and nitrogen species produced by glycation. Metal ions are known to be important in the formation of AGEs so metal chelators are also helpful. Late stage anti-glycation strategies include inhibiting cross-linking and blocking RAGEs. All of these approaches have significant potential to inhibit AGE formation. Cosmeceuticals have been marketed with the aim of preventing skin glycation. These products contain a variety of active ingredients including plant extracts, algae extracts and other naturally occurring antioxidants that have demonstrated glycation-inhibiting activity in vitro.

Glycation inhibitors from botanical sources

Botanical extracts are among the most popular cosmeceutical ingredients (Table 17.1). They are popular with consumers who view them as natural and valuable to cosmetic chemists since they contain a plethora of beneficial ingredients including antioxidants. In an interesting study, vegetable extracts known in folklore to be helpful in treating diabetes were tested on living human skin explants ex vivo for their ability to inhibit methylglyoxal-induced glycation. Extract of kudzu root, *Pueraria*

Table 17.1 Botanicals that inhibit glycation.

Rosemary
Sage
Marjoram
Tarragon
Ginger
Allspice
Cinnamon
Green Tea
Turmeric
Pomegranate
Apple
Blueberry

lobata and the leaves of the Hardy rubber tree, *Eucommia ulmoides*, were tested against aminoguanidine hydrochloride, a potent glycation inhibitor. Kudzu root contains the isoflavone puerarin and the Hardy rubber tree leaf chlorogenic acid. All three agents proved effective when topically applied to human skin and prevented AGE formation. Although these particular extracts are not found in skin care products, this study provides a valuable model for testing the ability of botanical extracts and other compounds to inhibit skin glycation.

Cosmeceutical ingredients

Green tea (*Camellia sinensis*)
Green tea has been used extensively for medicinal purposes. Green tea polyphenols (GTPs) include (-)epigallocatechin 3-O-gallate (EGCG), (-)epicatechin 3-O-gallate (ECG), (-) epigallocatechin (EGC) and (-)epigallocatechin (EGC) and are among the most potent antioxidants. GTPs have been shown to inhibit glycation. Animal studies have confirmed that ingestion of green tea extract effectively blocks collagen cross-linking and inhibits AGE accumulation associated with aging. Green tea extract inhibits glycation and cross-linking of tail tendon collagen in diabetic rats and it has been suggested that GTPs may have therapeutic value in treating diabetic complications. It is also of interest that recent studies have demonstrated that tea polyphenols may also scavenge intermediate reactive carbonyl species, suggesting that antioxidant properties may not be only mechanism whereby GTPs can inhibit AGE formation. Studies have demonstrated that topical green tea extract protects against UV-induced inflammation, oxidative stress and inhibits carcinogenesis, making it a valuable ingredient for protecting and treating aging skin.

Silymarin (*Silybum marianum*)

Silymarin is a flavonoid complex that can be extracted from the seeds of the milk thistle plant. Silymarin contains the antioxidants silybin A and B, isosilibybin A and B, silychristin and silydianin. These flavanoid antioxidants have been touted as a treatment for liver and gallbladder disease since ancient times. Benefits of silymarin have been observed with systemic and topical administration. Recent studies have demonstrated that oral administration of silymarin to streptozotocin (STZ) induced diabetic mice inhibited late stage glycation by trapping reactive carbonyl species and blocking cross-linking. This study also found that silymarin reduced AGE accumulation, cross-linking of tail collagen and anti-inflammatory mediators. Topically applied silymarin has been shown to have photoprotective effects, including preventing UV-induced carcinogenesis, oxidative stress and immunosuppression. Thus silymarin holds promise as a cosmeceutical ingredient offering a multi-mechanistic approach to treat aging skin.

Phloretin and phloridzin (apple)

Apples are known to have numerous health benefits including prevention of cancer, heart disease and diabetes. Phloretin is a flavonoid found exclusively in apples and apple products. Phloridzin is the glucosidic form of phloretin and recent studies have shown that both compounds have anti-diabetic effects. These compounds inhibit intestinal absorption of glucose and prevent AGE formation by trapping reactive dicarbonyl compounds. Topical phloretin in combination with vitamin C and ferulic acid has been shown to confer photoprotective effects on skin and improve the appearance of photoaging. Accordingly, phloretin remains of interest as a cosmeceutical active for photoprotection, inhibiting glycation and treating aging skin.

Quercetin

Quercetin is one of the most plentiful flavonols in our diet. It is found in green and black tea, capers, red apples, red onions, red grapes and some berries. Like other flavonoids, quercetin has broad biologic activity, including anti-inflammatory and chemoprevention. Quercetin has been shown to inhibit glycation of DNA in experimental models. In vitro studies demonstrating rejuvenating effects on fibroblasts and tyrosinase-inhibiting activity make this polyphenol unique as an anti-aging ingredient. Cosmeceuticals containing quercetin are marketed for treating photoaging although well-designed clinical studies have not been performed.

Blueberry

Blueberry extract contains antioxidant flavonoids and has been shown to inhibit glycation in experimental models. Cosmeceuticals containing

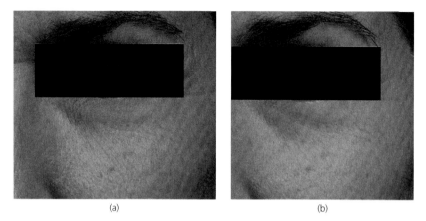

(a)   (b)

Figure 17.2 (a) and (b) Before and after using a cosmeceutical containing 4% blueberry extract, 30% proxylane and 0.2% Phytosphingosine for 12 weeks. (SkinCeuticals A.G.E. Interrupter). Note improvement in wrinkles, laxity, creping and skin texture. Source: Courtesy of SkinCeuticals.

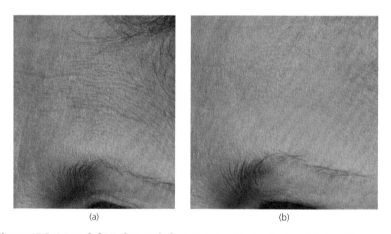

(a)   (b)

Figure 17.3 (a) and (b) Before and after using a cosmeceutical containing 4% blueberry extract, 30% proxylane and 0.2% phytosphingosine for 12 weeks. (SkinCeuticals A.G.E. Interrupter). Note improvement in skin texture, fine lines and forehead wrinkles. Source: Courtesy of SkinCeuticals.

blueberry extract in combination with other skin rejuvenating ingredients have been shown to improve skins appearance (Figures 17.2 and 17.3). In a clinical study a proprietary cosmeceutical product containing blueberry extract and C-xyloside was evaluated for its ability to inhibit glycation and improve mild to moderate photoaging in type II diabetic females. C-xyloside stimulates glycosaminoglycan products and blueberry extract was chosen for its anti-glycation properties. After 12 weeks of applying the test product twice daily, investigators found significant improvement over baseline in skin hydration, skin thickness, fine lines, firmness, radiance, creping and overall appearance. AGE inhibition was measured by skin autofluorescence and remained unchanged throughout the study. Although inhibition of glycation was not documented with the test product during the 3-month study, the authors suggest a longer study might be necessary to document changes in AGE accumulation. This study design serves as an excellent template for in vivo testing of anti-glycation cosmeceuticals.

Pomegranate

Pomegranate is an ancient fruit with medical and cosmetic application. The peel of this fruit is known for its astringent properties and pomegranate seed oil is rich in hydrating fatty acids. Pomegranate contains polyphenolic compounds that are found in the seed oil, juice and peel. These polyphenols have potent antioxidant, anti-glycating, anti-inflammatory and anti-cancer activity. Pomegranate seed oil stimulates keratinocyte proliferation in culture while pomegranate peel extract stimulates procollagen 1 production and inhibits metalloproteinases. A more recent study demonstrated that an isolate of a polysaccharide fraction from pomegranate rind inhibited tyrosinase, neutralized free radicals and inhibited AGE formation. The authors suggest that this byproduct in the process of fruit juice production may be valuable as a raw material for ingredients useful in the cosmetic industry. Pomegranate extract is found in a variety of cosmeceuticals designed to rejuvenate aging skin and lighten pigmentation.

Herbs and spices

In a comparative study, extracts of 24 herbs and spices were tested for their ability to inhibit glycation of albumin in vitro. In general, spice extracts were more potent inhibitors of glycation than herbal extracts with ginger, cinnamon, allspice and cloves being among the most potent. Sage, marjoram, tarragon and rosemary extracts were also effective but to a lesser degree. Glycation-inhibiting botanicals of interest in cosmeceuticals will be discussed below.

Rosemary (*Rosmarinus officinalis L*)

Rosemary is a common household herb that is known for its unique fragrance and flavor. Rosemary contains phenolic compounds including carnasol, rosmanol, caffeic acid, rosmarinic acid, carnosic acid and ursolic acid. Rosemary extract has a potent antioxidant that has antibacterial activity and inhibits UV-induced metalloproteinases. An alcoholic extract of rosemary leaves, Rosm1, was shown to inhibit oxidative alterations to skin surface lipids and protect skin from free radical damage. In addition, in vitro studies confirm the ability of rosemary extract to inhibit collagen glycation, making it of interest as an anti-glycation cosmeceutical active.

Turmeric (*Curcuma longa*)

Curcuma longa is a medicinal herb that has long been used in Chinese medicine. The roots of *Curcuma longa* are ground into a power, yielding the spice turmeric. Turmeric is used as flavoring for foods such as curry. Turmeric contains the active ingredient curcumin, a polyphenolic antioxidant that gives it a yellow color. Curcumin has diverse biologic activity including antibacterial, chemopreventative, chemotherapeutic, wound-healing, anti-inflammatory and anti-proliferative effects. In spite of the multitude of beneficial effects, medicinal use of curcumin in humans is limited by its poor bioavailability after ingestion. Studies are underway to improve absorption and maintain biologic activity of curcumin using nanoparticles, liposomes and other delivery systems. Studies have demonstrated that curcumin has anti-glycation activity. Animal studies have shown that curcumin administered orally improves insulin sensitivity, lowers blood glucose, reduces inflammation and inhibits AGEs and collagen cross-linking in diabetic rats.

Topical curcumin gel has been studied in the clinical setting. Curcumin gel was used to treat patients with psoriasis where it was shown to inhibit phosphorylase kinase activity in psoriatic skin. In a large study uncontrolled of 647 psoriatic patients, topical steroids used in conjunction with curcumin gel resulted in over 70% of the patients achieving complete clearing after 16 weeks of treatment. A higher concentration of the same curcumin gel was shown to prevent and decrease scar tissue formation following surgery in a study of 220 patients. The same investigators treating patients with photodamage with topical curcumin gel demonstrated clinical improvement of many parameters of photoaging, including actinic keratoses, lentigenes, skin texture and decreased appearance of wrinkles after 3–6 months. Curcumin has multiple mechanisms whereby it might improve photoaged skin including acting as an antioxidant, anti-inflammatory, inhibiting activator protein 1 (AP 1) and preventing glycation.

Glycation inhibitors from marine sources

There is growing interest in marine life as a resource for cosmeceutical actives. Brown algae contain phlorotannins that are polyphenolic antioxidants with diverse biologic activity. Algal phlorotannins include phloroglucinol, diphlorethohydroxycarmalol, eckol and dieckol and are plentiful in the brown seaweed *Eckolonia cava*. These compounds are potent antioxidants and exhibit anti-inflammatory activity mediated by down-regulating NF-kB. Extracts of *E. cava* are metalloproteinase and tyrosinase inhibitors and inhibit activator protein 1 (AP-1), making them of interest for treating aging skin. Phloroglucinol, the constituent unit of phlorotannins, has been shown to inhibit glycation in vitro. In addition, the algal polysaccharide fucoidan can block receptors for AGEs, inhibiting AGE accumulation and further tissue damage by AGEs. The carotenoid astaxanthin found in red algae has also been shown to inhibit glycation. Thus, marine-based ingredients may be of interest as AGE inhibitors blocking both early and late stage reactions.

Other important glycation inhibitors

Alpha lipoic acid (ALA)

Alpha lipoic acid is a naturally occurring antioxidant that is both fat- and water-soluble. ALA and its reduced form dihydrolipoic acid (DHLA) scavenge free radicals, help regenerate vitamin E and C, chelate metals and have anti-inflammatory activity. Studies in STZ-induced diabetic rats demonstrate that oral supplementation with ALA decreased AGEs in both serum and renal tissue and inhibited RAGE expression by reducing oxidative stress. Animal studies using fructose-fed rats demonstrate that collagen abnormalities including collagen cross-linking and reduction of collagen production caused by a high sugar diet were mitigated by simultaneous administration of oral alpha lipoic acid. Cosmeceuticals containing alpha lipoic acid are plentiful and generally marketed as antioxidants with anti-aging benefits. There are a limited number of studies on cosmeceuticals containing alpha lipoic acid. In a randomized, placebo-controlled, double blind study, 33 women used a 5% alpha lipoic acid cream on half of their face for 12 weeks and vehicle on the other side. The vehicle contained 0.3% co-enzyme Q10 and 0.03% acetyl-L-carnotine. Laser profilometry showed a statistically significant improvement in periorbital wrinkles on the alpha lipoic acid-treated side compared to vehicle control. Clinical and photographic evaluation showed significant improvement in overall global assessment of skin aging in the group using the lipoic acid cream.

Carnosine

Carnosine is the dipeptide beta-alanine-L-histidine and is found in muscle and the brain. It acts as an intracellar buffer scavenging carbonyl compounds and protecting proteins from cross-linking. Carnosine is a versatile antioxidant that exhibits zinc and copper chelating activity and competes with glucose to inhibit protein glycation. This dipeptide has been shown to delay senescence in cultured human fibroblasts and delay aging in senescence-accelerated mice. Carnosine supplements are widely available and have been proposed to treat Alzheimer's disease, prevent diabetic complications and as an anti-aging agent. Studies have shown that oral supplementation with carnosine can improve the skin's appearance including fine lines and wrinkles when compared to placebo control. In view of these biologic effects, cosmeceuticals containing carnosine have been developed for preventing glycation and treating aging skin.

Conclusion

Anti-glycation skin care products represent a new niche in cosmeceuticals. These products are sold both in the mass and the prestige markets and contain a variety of innovative botanical antioxidants and other glycation inhibitors. The importance of glycation and its role in skin aging is an emerging concept that is gaining favor among aesthetic physicians and consumers. The use of functional foods, supplements or topical skin care products to prevent glycation may represent a new strategy for our patients desiring skin rejuvenation.

Further reading

Babizhayev MA, Deyev AI, Savel'yeva El, et al. Skin beautification with oral non-hydrolized versions of carnosine and carcinine: Effective therapeutic management and cosmetic skincare solutions against oxidative glycation and free-radical production as a causal mechanism of diabetic complications and skin aging. *J. Dermat Treat* 2012; **23**(5): 345–385.

Beitner H. Randomized, placebo-controlled, double blind study on the clinical efficacy of a cream containing 5% alpha lipoic acid related to photoageing of facial skin. *Br J Derm* 2003; **149**: 841–849.

Danby FW. Nutrition and aging skin: Sugar and glycation. *Clin Dermatol* 2010; **28**: 409–411.

Dearlove RP, Greenspan P, Hartle DK, et al. Inhibition of protein glycation by extracts of culinary herbs and spices. *J Med Food* 2008; **11**: 275–281.

Draelos ZD, Yatskayer MS, Raab MS, Oresajo C. An evaluation of the effect of a topical product containing C-xyloside and blueberry extract on the appearance of type II diabetic skin. *Journ Cosmet Dermatol* 2009; **8**: 147–151.

Gasser P, Arnold F, Peno-Massarino L, et al. Glycation induction and antiglycation activity of skin care ingredients on living human skin explants. *Int J Cos Sci* 2011; **33**: 366–370.

Heng MC. Curcumin targeted signaling pathways: basis for anti-photoaging and anti-carcinogenic therapy. *Int J Dermatol* 2010; **49**: 608–622.

Jeanmarie C., Danoux L, Pauly G. Glycation during human dermal intrinsic and actinic ageing: an in vito and in vitro model study. *Br J Derm* 2001; **145**: 10–18.

Peng X, Ma J, Chen F, Wang M. Naturally occurring inhibitors against the formation of advanced glycation end-products. *Food Funct* 2011; **2**: 289–301.

Reddy VP, Garrett MR, Perry G, Smith MA. Carnosine: A versatile antioxidant and antiglycating agent. *Sci Aging Knowledge Environ* 2005; **18**: pe12.

Rout S, Banerjee R. Free radical scavenging, anti-glycation and tyrosinase inhibition properties of a polysaccharide fraction isolated from the rind from *Punica granatum*. *Bioresource Technology* 2007; **98**(16): 3159–3162.

Semba RD, Nicklett EJ, Ferrucci L. Does accumulation of advanced glycation end products contribute to the aging phenotype? *J Gerontol A Biol Sci Med Sci* 2010; **65**: 963–975.

Ulrich P, Cerami A. Protein glycation, diabetes, and aging. *Recent Prog Horm Res* 2001; **56**: 1–21.

Yamauchi M, Prisayanh P, Haque Z, Woodley DT. Collagen cross-linking in sun-exposed and unexposed sites of aged human skin. *J Invest Dermatol* 1991; **97**: 938–941.

CHAPTER 18

Essential Ions and Bioelectricity in Skin Care

Ying Sun[1], Elizabeth Bruning[1], Susan H. Weinkle[2], and Samantha Tucker-Samaras[1]

[1]Johnson & Johnson Consumer Companies, Inc., Skillman, NJ, USA
[2]University of South Florida, Tampa, FL, USA

Ion flow and bioelectricity

Bioelectricity is the electrical phenomena of all life processes, and it is represented in the forms of non-uniform distribution and directional migration of ions in various parts of the body. Trans-membrane potential is a well-known example of bioelectricity. In humans, bioelectricity is used as a signaling process to direct physiological activities at a cellular level. As such, biological cells use bioelectricity to function, trigger internal changes, store metabolic energy, and to signal one another through cell-to-cell communication. This innate electrical signaling system regulates physiological functions on the cellular level by using the movement of ions with a small positive or negative electrical charge, such as sodium ion (Na^+), potassium ion (K^+), chloride ion (Cl^-) and calcium ion (Ca^{2+}), in and out of cells to create a concentration gradient and consequently an electric potential gradient. An asymmetrical concentration of these ions inside and outside of a cell causes an electrical trans-membrane potential across cell membranes. Similarly, a trans-membrane potential exists for the living epidermis.

It is well known that low-level electrical signals are involved in wound healing. In skin wounds, healing is accomplished by cell migration to the wound site and transportation of essential ions and proteins to the wound. By enhancing the body's electrical signaling process, wound healing can be accelerated by increasing the migration of repairing cells to the site of the wound. Zhao et al. demonstrated that the electric signal as a directional cue probably plays a far more important role in directing cell migration in wound healing of epithelium than previously believed. They showed that two proteins are important for electric field-induced cellular response. One is phosphatidylinositol 3-kinase (PI3K), steering the migration of human cells across an electrical gradient in a process called electrotaxis. Another is the lipid phosphatidylinositol 3,4,5-triphosphate (PIP3), a pivotal molecule concentrated at the leading edge of the cell, where signaling components bind to it. These signaling components, in turn, lead to the localized polymerization of actin to form a protrusion in the direction of migration. It was reported that the bioelectric field appeared to play an important role in controlling human fibroblast activity by either significantly increasing or decreasing gene expression of over 400 transcripts that were investigated. These included activity within specific cellular signaling pathways such as TGF-β, G-proteins, and inhibition of apoptosis. The epidermis generates a trans-epithelial potential and the charge inside is positive. Nuccitelli et al. measured the bioelectric wound current in human skin of two test subject groups to investigate the role of endogenous electric fields in wound healing of young and old human subjects. The lateral surface wound field was measured between the stratum corneum and epidermis near a lancet wound on the arm and leg in 40 adults. Ten women and ten men in the 18–29-year-old age group exhibited a mean electric field of 163 $\pm$ 59 mV/mm, whereas, ten women and ten men in the 65–80-year-old age range exhibited a mean field of only 78 $\pm$ 15 mV/mm. The mean electric field of individuals in the older age group is only half that of the younger group, demonstrating that the electric field at even minor skin wounds declines sharply with age. Since the wound electric potential appears to be proportional to healing rate, the reduced wound electric potential may be a contributing factor to the well-documented reduced tissue repair and decreased wound healing capacity among elderly. On the other hand, it is conceivable that if an external electric potential of the physiological magnitude, similar to the skin's own wound healing electrical signal were applied, the wound healing of elderly might be enhanced. Similarly, if a low-level electrical signal is applied to the aged skin in order to mimic the bioelectric signal associated with wound healing, tissue regeneration and rejuvenation processes may be enhanced for anti-aging benefits.

Therefore, it may be hypothesized that when intact aged skin is exposed to a biomimetic electrical signal, that is, an externally applied electric signal mimicking the skin's bioelectrical signal during wounding, the same skin repairing and rejuvenation mechanisms during wounding could be activated, leading to skin rejuvenation and noticeable anti-aging benefits.

Essential mineral ions and skin

Essential mineral ions are well known to play important roles in skin health, for example, zinc has a critical role in overall human physiology, and particularly as an important antioxidant for skin. Zinc concentration in the epidermis declines with aging: the average zinc concentration among test subjects older than 65 years of age is only about one half of that of test subjects younger than 35 years old, however, there is no significant difference in zinc concentrations in blister (interstitial) fluid between the two groups, indicating the absence of a correlation between plasma zinc and epidermal zinc. Both zinc and copper are involved in skin inflammation processes and age-related diseases.

Galvanic zinc-copper complex and biomimetic electricity for skin care

Bioelectricity and its relevance to skin care benefits, and the use of low-level electricity generated by galvanic couple particles to mimic bioelectricity have been reviewed recently. A galvanic bi-mineral complex composed of elemental zinc and copper has been reported for skin applications, such as reducing the appearance of the signs of photoaging. The galvanic action of elemental zinc-copper particles generates electrical potentials between the zinc and copper domains on the metal particle surfaces in the presence of moisture, and zinc ions are produced as a byproduct of the galvanic process.

Southall et al. reported the use of galvanic couple particles of elemental zinc and copper (Zn-Cu) to determine the effects of low-level electrical stimulation on intact skin physiology using a commercial Dermacorder device. Zn-Cu induced the electrical potential recorded on intact skin, enhanced H_2O_2 production and activated p38 MAPK and Hsp27 in primary keratinocytes. Treatment with Zn-Cu was also found to reduce pro-inflammatory cytokines, such as IL-1α, IL-2, NO and TNF-α in multiple cell types after stimulation with PHA or *Propionibacterium acnes* bacteria. The Zn-Cu complex led to a dose-dependent inhibition of TNF-α-induced NF-κB levels in keratinocytes as measured by a dual-luciferase promoter assay, and prevented p65 translocation to the nucleus observed via immunofluorescence. Suppression of NF-κB activity via cross-talk with p38 MAPK might be one of the potential pathways by which Zn-Cu exerts its inflammatory effects. Topical application of Zn-Cu successfully mitigated TPA-induced dermatitis and oxazolone-induced hypersensitivity in mice models of ear edema. Anti-inflammatory activity induced by the Zn-Cu galvanic couple appears to be mediated, at least in part, by production of low-level hydrogen peroxide since this activity is reversed by the addition of catalase enzyme. Collectively, these results show that a galvanic couple containing Zn-Cu strongly reduces the inflammatory and immune responses in intact skin, providing evidence for the role of electric stimulation in non-wounded skin.

Chantalat et al. conducted a randomized, double-blinded, placebo-controlled clinic trial to evaluate the efficacy and tolerability of the galvanic zinc-copper complex on photoaging parameters. In this eight-week study, women (aged 40–65 years) with mild to moderate photoaging were randomized to use placebo or one of three galvanic zinc-copper complex compositions (gel and activating moisturizer). Efficacy evaluations included clinical grading, specialized clinical imaging, and subject self-assessments performed at baseline, 15–30 minutes after treatment application and after 1, 2, 4, and 8 weeks. Tolerability was based on adverse events and clinical grading of irritation. Significance was set at $p < 0.05$ versus baseline and between treatment groups. The study was completed by 124 women. Compositions containing the galvanic zinc-copper complex showed statistically significant clinical improvements versus placebo and baseline rapidly (15–30 min) after application and through week 8. Clinical grading showed significant improvement versus placebo in skin radiance and under-eye dark circles 15–30 minutes after first application with continued improvement through week 8, and in overall photodamage, fine lines, lifted appearance of the eyes, and under-eye wrinkles starting after two weeks and continuing through week 8. Test compositions were well tolerated. This galvanic zinc-copper complex provided rapid and lasting improvements versus placebo in photoaged skin, supporting its use in topical anti-aging formulations. Figure 18.1 shows improvements over time in eyelid lifting /smoothing with placebo or premixed galvanic Zn-Cu formulation applied once daily.

Nollent et al. reported a clinical evaluation of the galvanic zinc-copper complex for anti-aging efficacy in the eye area of the skin. It is a non-interventional, open-label, baseline-controlled clinical study including 30-day washout period and eight-week treatment period with 34 healthy Caucasian female subjects with Fitzpatrick Skin Types I–IV, aged 35 years and older. The test Zn-Cu complex formula was applied each morning for eight weeks. Both subjective and objective assessments demonstrated significant improvements in the signs of facial photodamage during the eight-week treatment with the Zn-Cu complex. Results from clinical grading (Table 18.1) and self-assessments (Table 18.2) conducted at baseline, immediately after the first application (T imm), and at weeks 1, 4 (T4) and 8 (T8) indicate statistically significant ($p < 0.05$) improvements in several parameters including crow's feet, fine lines and wrinkles, under-eye fine lines and bags, eyelid puffiness and dark circles, and skin texture (i.e. skin radiance and tone). Objective methods showed a reduction in total wrinkle surface and mean length in skin replicas. The test formulation was well tolerated in the sensitive skin around the eyes throughout the 8-week treatment with no adverse events.

Bruning et al. described a clinical study using a topical lip composition containing the Zn-Cu complex for anti-aging benefits on human

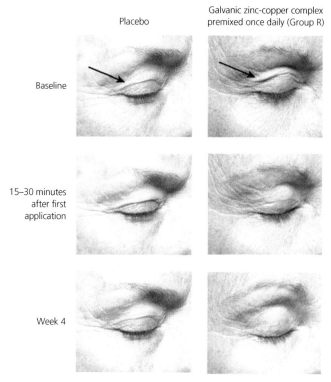

Figure 18.1 Clinical images of responder subjects treated with either the galvanic zinc-copper complex or placebo showing immediate and continuous improvement in lifting the eyelids.

lips. A small-scale, randomized, double-blind, placebo- and benchmark-controlled clinical study was conducted to evaluate the effect of compositions containing galvanic particulates on lip-related benefits such as anti-aging, lip beauty, and lip health. The study population consisted of females ages 40–65, Fitzpatrick Skin Types I–IV who at the time of enrollment (baseline), experienced the following based on expert grade and self-report: moderate to severe lines around lip contour, fine vertical lines on lips, lips that have lost color/look paler, lip edges that are less defined, lips that are thinner/less full, lips that experience lipstick bleeds and mild to moderate dry lips.

Four lip compositions in the form of lip balms/sticks having a common base formulation were used in the study. Two contained galvanic particulates (Product 1, Zn-Cu complex, Product 2, Benchmark + Zn-Cu complex) and two did not (Comparative Product A, Placebo, Comparative Product B, Benchmark). There were N = 11 subjects per lip composition, and the subjects used the products three times per day: in the morning, afternoon (after lunch meal), and in the evening.

Table 18.1 Clinical grading results showing percent improvement from baseline.

	T imm (%)	T4w (%)	T8w (%)
Wrinkles (crow's feet)	24	19	23
Fine lines (crow's feet)	37	31	40
Fine lines under the eye	34	28	39
Folds on the eyelids	17	23	23
Dark circles	21	33	69
Eye opening	5	14	16
Puffiness (upper eyelid)	58	45	70
Bags under the eye	34	31	43
Skin softness	68	43	49
Skin radiance	17	46	52
Yellowish complexion	52	40	82

Note: $p < 0.05$ vs placebo at all time points in all parameters, except at T imm for eye opening.

Table 18.2 Self-assessment results.

	(%) improved subjects*		
	T imm	T4	T8
Decrease in crow's-feet wrinkles	12.9	51.72	64.29
Decrease in crow's-feet fine lines	17.65	71.88	75.00
Decrease in under-eye fine lines	29.41	75.00	59.38
Decrease in under-eye bags	25.00	64.00	56.00
Decrease in under-eye dark circles	32.14	55.17	66.67
Decrease in folds on eyelids	16.67	53.85	58.62
Increase in eye opening	26.47	51.52	65.63
Decrease in upper eyelid puffiness	41.67	75.86	56.67
Increase in eye brightness	32.35	51.52	65.63
More radiant skin	35.29	63.64	75.00
More moisturized skin	91.18	93.94	96.88
Skin softened	97.06	96.97	96.88
Skin smoothed	70.59	87.88	87.50
Product well tolerated?	100.00	100.00	100.00

Note: * % subjects with self-assessment of "fully agree" or "rather agree."

The subjects were evaluated at Baseline, Week 1 and Week 8. At each of those time points subject self-assessment questionnaires were completed, high resolution digital images of the lips were taken, and spectral imaging of the lips was conducted.

The high resolution digital images were graded by an expert grader (blinded to the treatment groups) to provide an objective assessment of changes in the lips. The expert grader used eight visual grading parameters to grade the digital images.

The expert grading results indicated that the Product 1 (Zn-Cu complex) lip composition was significantly better ($p < 0.05$) versus the Comparative

Product A (placebo) in improving lines around the lips, and directionally better ($p < 0.10$) in definition and lines on lips at week 8. The
Product 2 (Benchmark + Zn-Cu complex) lip composition outperformed
the Comparative Product B (Benchmark alone) by showing significant
improvement versus baseline in fullness of lips and, even tone as well as
directional improvement in lines on lips, whereas the Comparative Product
B did not.

Overall, the digital images demonstrated visible lip improvements by
treating with both Product 1 and Product 2 in lip color, fine lines, and
fullness in just one week, with continuing efficacy in all parameters at
week 8.

Oxy-hemoglobin analysis was performed by spectral imaging (N = 7–9
subjects per treatment group). As shown in Figure 18.2, the Product
1 lip composition showed an almost 25% increase ($p = 0.05$) in oxy-
hemoglobin levels at week 8 versus baseline levels. Comparative Product
A did not show a significant change. This increase in oxy-hemoglobin level
is believed to have contributed to the observed visible improvement in lip
color demonstrated in the self-assessment and expert grading data.

The results of the subject self-assessment questionnaires indicated that
Product 2 consistently ranked higher than all other treatments, starting at
week 1. Product 2 also had the most between-treatment significance
and was the only lip composition that showed significant ($p < 0.05$)
improvement in the self-assessments versus baseline in all lip parameters
at week 8.

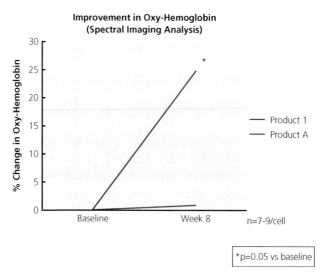

Figure 18.2 Oxy-hemoglobin analysis performed by spectral imaging show that the
Zn-Cu complex, Product 1 (upper line) yielded almost 25% increase ($p = 0.05$) in
oxy-hemoglobin at Week 8 over the Placebo, Comparative Product A (lower line).

Further reading

Bruning E, Chantalat J, Maitra P. Lip compositions comprising galvanic particulates. United States Patent Application US20110195100.

Chantalat J, Bruning E, Sun Y, Liu J-C. Application of a topical biomimetic electrical signaling technology to photo-aging: A randomized, double-blind, placebo-controlled trial of a galvanic zinc-copper complex. *J Drugs Dermatol* 2012; **11**(1): 30–37.

Dreno B. Evolution du zinc cutane au cours du vieillissement cutane [Changes in cutaneous zinc during skin aging]. *Ann Dermatol Venereol* 1992; **119**(4): 263–266.

Driban JB, Swanik CB, Huxel KC, Balsubramanian E. Transient electric changes immediately after surgical trauma. *J. Athletic Training* 2007; **42**: 524–529.

Encyclopedia Britannica. Bioelectricity. Available at: http://www.britannica.com/EBchecked/topic/65834/bioelectricity#ref=ref40797 (accessed August 27, 2009).

Encyclopedia Britannica. Cell. Available at: http://www.britannica.com/EBchecked/topic/101396/cell/37442/Cell-to-cell-communication-via-chemical-signaling#ref=ref313825 (accessed August 27, 2009).

Huttenlocher A, Horwitz AR. Wound healing with electric potential. *N Engl J Med* 2007; **356**: 303–304.

Jennings J, Chen D, Feldman D. Transcriptional response of dermal fibroblasts in direct current electric fields. *Bioelectromagnetics* 2008; **29**: 394–405.

Kaur S, Lyte P, Garay M, Liebel F, Sun Y, Liu J-C, Southall, M. Galvanic zinc-copper microparticles produce electrical stimulation that reduces the inflammatory and immune responses in skin. *Arch Dermatol Res* 2011; **303**(8): 551–562.

Lee BY, Wendell K, Butler G. Ultra-low microcurrent therapy: A novel approach for treatment of chronic resistant wounds. *Advances in Therapy* 2007; **24**: 1202–1209.

Martinsen OG, Grimnes S. *Bioimpedance and Bioelectricity Basics*. 2nd ed. St. Louis, MO: Elsevier Science & Technology Books, 2008.

New World Encyclopedia. Cell membrane. Available at: http://www.newworldencyclopedia.org/entry/Cell_membrane (accessed August 27, 2009).

Nollent V, Lanctin M, Nkengne A, Bertin C. Clinical evaluation of a zinc- and copper-based eye area anti-aging complex. *Cosmetics & Toiletries*, 2012; **127**(10): 718–725.

Nuccitelli R, Nuccitelli P, Li C, et al. The electric field at human skin wounds declines sharply with age. 18th Annual Meeting of the Wound Healing Society, San Diego, CA, April 24–27, 2008.

Ojingwa JC, Isseroff RR. Electric stimulation of wound healing. *J Invest Derm* 2003; **121**: 1–12.

Rostan EF, DeBuys HV, Madey DL, Pinnell SR. Evidence supporting zinc as an important antioxidant for skin. *Int J Dermatol* 2002; **41**: 606–611.

Schwartz JR, Marsh RG. Draelos ZD, Zinc and skin health: Overview of physiology and pharmacology. *Dermatol Surg* 2005; **31**(2): 837–847.

Sun Y, Liu J-C. Bioelectricity. In: Baran R, Maibach HI, *Textbook of Cosmetic Dermatology*, 4th ed. New York: Informa Healthcare, 2010, 466–481.

Vasto S, Mocchegiani E, Candore G, Listi F, Colonna-Rmano G, Lio D, Malavolta M, Giacconi R, Cipriano C, Caruso C. Inflammation, genes and zinc in ageing and age-related diseases. *Biogerontology* 2006; **7**(5–6): 315–327.

Zhao M, Song B, Pu J, et al. Electrical signals control wound healing through Phosphatidylinositol-3-OH Kinase-γ and PTEN. *Nature* 2006; **442**: 457–460.

CHAPTER 19

Stem Cell Cosmeceuticals

Mark V. Dahl

Mayo Clinic and Makucell, Inc., Scottsdale, AZ, USA

Aged skin differs from youthful skin. The aged epidermis lacks keratinocytes and is physically thinner. The rete ridges are flattened. The dermis also lacks normal numbers of cells and normal amounts of constituent tissues such as collagen, elastin, laminin, glycosaminoglycans, and fibronectin. The dermis also lacks elasticity, strength, vascularity, and ground substances such as hyaluronic acid. In addition to thinning and fragility, aged skin heals slowly. Epidermal turnover is prolonged, and the skin barrier is relatively defective. The skin appears thin, wrinkled, bruised, and rough.

To restore normal strength and function in a natural way, the skin needs to make more cells and tissue constituents to replenish cells and constituents lost as a consequence of normal wear-and-tear, sun damage, and aging. The stratum corneum must replace itself at more normal rates and the epidermis must thicken. The epidermis must establish and maintain orderly differentiation of basal cells into keratinocytes, granular cells, and corneocytes. Similarly, fibroblasts of the dermis must increase in number and increase synthesis of dermal matrix materials such as elastic fibers, collagen, and hyaluronic acid. Blood vessels must maintain normal numbers and functions. Nerves, hair follicles, sebaceous glands, and sweat glands must all be present in adequate numbers and produce appropriate and adequate products. Rejuvenated skin, by definition, must look and behave more like it did in youth.

Unfortunately, simple applications of dermal constituents to the skin surface do not sufficiently reconstitute normal dermis. They either do not pass through the epidermal barrier, or they pass it but do not effectively accumulate in the issues below it. Most applications simply add water to the epidermis, simply smooth the epidermis, or simply render it more pliant. A fully successful rejuvenation strategy should foster reestablishment of normal epidermis and normal dermis with normal cell numbers and normal cell functions, including normal production of the skin's normal cellular and normal chemical constituents.

Stem cells provide a reservoir of cells in the skin to rejuvenate or repair old or damaged skin. In the epidermis, stem cells reside in the bulge

---

region of hair follicles and in the interfollicular epidermis where they are indistinguishable morphologically from basal cells. In the dermis, stem cells reside around blood vessels, in the papillae of hair roots, and elsewhere. When activated by signals coming into their nuclei, stem cells divide and differentiate into lineage-specific cells such as keratinocytes, fibroblasts, melanocytes, adipocytes or other lines of cells. Some of these cells such as fibroblasts synthesize constituents of skin such as collagen.

Strategies to energize cells to rejuvenate skin

Cosmeceuticals could target living cells. Living cells not only can make constituent elements of skin, but also they can coordinate activities to place these elements in the right amounts in the right places, at the right times, in the right orientations and forms. Table 19.1 lists possible strategies to induce normal skin cells to maintain youthful function and increase synthesis of anatomic elements of skin.

Induce cells of the dermis to produce more extracellular structures and ground substance

Flogging cells in the dermis could make them work faster or better. In general, the flogging factors are cytokines generated by surrounding tissue cells and infiltrating inflammatory cells. A cytokine or small molecule of some kind could be the whip to jump-start synthesis of cells and their products. Cosmeceuticals purporting to stimulate collagen production include retinoids, vitamin C, copper peptides, transforming growth factor β, palmitoyl pentapeptide-3, certain oligopeptides, flavonoids, and estradiol. Injuring skin slightly with skin peeling agents or superficial laser treatments also seem to stimulate collagen production.

Table 19.1 Possible strategies to energize cells to rejuvenate skin.

Induce cells of the dermis to produce more extracellular structures and ground substance
Help skin organize remaining tissue elements to maintain function
Induce topically applied cells to enter the skin
Inject autologous differentiated cells into the dermis or hypodermis
Induce adult/stromal stem cells to migrate from blood into skin
Prolong cell life by inhibiting destruction (apoptosis) of cells
Induce stem cells of the skin to undergo proliferative (symmetric) divisions
Induce transient amplifying cells of the skin to undergo proliferative divisions
Induce stem cells in the skin to undergo differentiative (asymmetric) divisions

Help skin organize remaining tissue elements to maintain function

The epidermis contributes to the appearance of healthy, normal rejuvenated skin. Cosmetic and cosmeceutical moisturizers do help smooth and plump it up. Cosmeceuticals do a good job by supplying humectants, normalizing the disheveled stratum corneum, fostering release of natural moisturizing factor, and smoothing the skin with applications of grease or dimethicone, which mat down superficial scales. Cosmeceuticals have a harder job supplying normalizing factors to cells below the epidermis in the dermis and subcutaneous fat because the skin barrier and epidermis limit percutaneous absorption, and because the skin's lymphatic drainage tends to carry chemicals away.

Induce topically applied cells to enter the skin

This strategy seems like science fiction, but is it? Cells move randomly (chemokinesis) and directionally (chemotaxis). It might be possible to induce cells to migrate thorough the stratum corneum into the epidermis and dermis, just as leukocytes migrate into the epidermis from below in response to various infectious agents, allergens, and irritants. Could a fibroblast or a precursor (stem) cell be induced to migrate into skin from above? The stratum corneum presents a formidable barrier, but perhaps it could be removed by stripping it off with tapes or other maneuvers.

Inject autologous differentiated cells or stem cells into the dermis or hypodermis

Right now, injected autologous stem cells and differentiated cells mostly act as fillers, bulking up the tissues for a shorter or longer period of time. They add only temporary volume, unless the cells survive and subsequently replicate and/or synthesize fluids or tissue substances after injection. Stem cells and differentiated tissue cells need guidance from surrounding cells and structures in order to replicate and function normally. They need signals to work. Therefore, the success of cell injection strategies likely will require the assistance of cosmeceuticals to supply the needed signals or alter the stem cell niche. For example, fat cell-derived stem cells have been induced to form fibroblasts when supplied with a rye-based ingredient.

Induce adult/stromal stem cells to migrate from blood into skin

Bone marrow-derived stem cells can migrate into skin. Patients with recessively-inherited epidermolysis bullosa dystrophica genetically lack the anchoring fibrils that hold the epidermis onto the basement membrane zone of skin. They lack them because the patients genetically lack the ability to synthesize type VII collagen. Without anchoring fibers, the epidermis shears off from the dermis after even minor traumas. In some of these patients with eroded, wounded skin, allogeneic bone marrow-derived stem cells have migrated into skin and differentiated into cells that synthesized type VII collagen.

Under certain circumstances, stem cells from blood slowly migrate into skin to reconstitute skin stem cell populations. The numbers of stem cells in skin remain rather constant over normal life spans. Mostly this is due to infrequent divisions and the long lives of stem cells. However, after wounding, stem cells may undergo rapid symmetric divisions designed to rapidly heal the wound. If depleted, stem cells from blood may restore a population of stem cells in the healed skin.

Some products claim that stem cells seek out damaged skin and repair it. Supplying stem cell-specific chemotactic factors and cytokines in cosmeceuticals might help move stem cells from blood to skin. However, even if stem cells were to migrate into the skin from the blood, they might not rejuvenate the skin. Stem cells in unwounded, aged skin seem content to remain relatively quiescent, regardless of number. Only with proper signaling could recruited stem cells synthesize rejuvenating structures such as collagen I fibers and elastic tissue fibers.

Prolong cell life by inhibiting destruction (apoptosis) of cells

Apoptosis protects the organism from troubles such as cancer. Cells, including stem cells, can sense irreparable damage to their DNA and self-destruct. They also die when attacked by cytotoxic T cells or cytotoxic antibodies, such as happens when a cell becomes infected with a virus or other intercellular organisms, and also after a cell expresses certain tumor-specific antigens related to malignant growths. However, cosmeceuticals interfering with this normal apoptotic protective process could lead to dangerous side effects. If cosmeceuticals blunted the killing of infected cells or cancerous cells, clinical infections and cancers might result.

Induce stem cells of the skin to undergo proliferative (symmetric) divisions

Cells of epidermis and dermis have finite lives. As they die or exfoliate, they are replaced by new cells that differentiate from stem cells. A stem cell can divide in two ways: (1) with a symmetric, proliferative division; or (2) with an asymmetric, differentiative division. A symmetric, proliferative division produces either two stem cells or two transient amplifying cells that each undergo more symmetric divisions and then post-mitotic differentiation to form functional end-line cells such as fibroblasts, melanocytes, and keratinocytes. In contrast, an asymmetric, differentiative division produces one stem cell to replace itself, and one transient amplifying cell to divide and differentiate further. If stem cells were to replicate more often, the density of cells in skin should increase. If each differentiated progeny cell functioned normally, the density of cell products should increase as well (e.g. collagen, elastic fibers, ground substances).

With aging, the number of stem cells in the skin remains relatively constant and their function is mostly retained. With increasing age, stem cells replicate less often. Presumably, signaling or response to signaling fails to maintain normal proliferative and differentiative activities. Adding growth factors or boosting signal pathways could rejuvenate skin by restoring normal youthful proliferation and differentiation.

Cosmeceuticals designed to foster replication of skin cells face many potential hurdles. First, too much proliferation is bad. Hyperproliferative activity could produce excessive tissue, or skin tumors. Second, proliferative divisions of stem cells eventually deplete them, since the dividing stem cell is not renewed or preserved. Third, normal regulatory pathways may neutralize any strategy designed to increase stem cell numbers.

Growth factors must be at the right place at the right time, and overcome "fail safe" mechanisms used by cells to prevent unwanted cell divisions. The decision of a cell to leave a resting phase and enter the cell replicative cycle is a critical one. Too much proliferation causes excessive tissue or too many cells. Too little proliferation will not produce the needed effects. To decide to replicate, a skin stem cell monitors its environment taking into account space, cell polarity, cytokine milieu, available nutrients, oxygen tension, and perhaps hundreds of other factors. A cosmeceutical providing a signal to start cell replication might do so, but it might instead do nothing. Other signals favoring rest (nonproliferation, nondifferentiation) may trump effects of cosmeceuticals trying to foster cell divisions.

Induce transient amplifying cells of the skin to undergo proliferative divisions

Growth factors such as epidermal growth factor, transforming growth factor β, and nerve growth factor have been formulated into cosmeceuticals, and success in stimulating stem cells or transient amplifying cells has been claimed. Real data from in vivo use are mostly lacking. Most growth factors are large, and do not penetrate into skin. Incorporation of growth factors into liposomes or microspheres might overcome this problem. Most growth factors are also temperature-sensitive and unstable. However, a cosmeceutical that incorporates a small molecule with growth factor actions could be a successful product to reverse or minimize the changes associated with aging.

Induce stem cells in the skin to undergo differentiative (asymmetric) divisions

The name "stem cell factor" (a.k.a. SCF) is reserved for a particular molecule known also as "kit-ligand" or "steel factor." The molecule binds to the c-Kit receptor (CD117). Produced by fibroblasts and endothelial cells, this rather large molecule (MW 18 KDa) plays a role in hematopoiesis and stem cell maintenance. Its large size may limit absorption. Melanoblasts express the c-Kit receptor. Stem cell factor may help position melanocytes in tissues and also help govern melanocyte proliferation and survival.

Some cosmeceuticals contain components of stem cells ("stem cell-released molecules") alone or in addition to growth factors. These agents include liquefied placenta, unfertilized human eggs, bovine embryonic fluid, umbilical cord derivatives, cytokines, interleukins, antioxidants, molecular chaperones, and micro-RNA. Evidence of efficacy when applied topically in creams is sparse. Stem cells themselves (not contents of stem cells) produce transient amplifying cells and their more differentiated, lineage-specific skin cells. The contents of stem cells would seem irrelevant to the process of stem cell proliferation or differentiation. Even if they could get into the skin, stem cell-released factors might not possess growth factor or stem cell proliferative activity. Stem cell-released molecules are alleged to act as though they were secreted products with autocrine and paracrine activities designed to "nourish the stem cell niche."

Since plant stem cells repair damaged tissues, applications of plant stem cell extracts are claimed to foster repair of aging human skin. Known as "meristem cells" in plants such as apples, melons, tomatoes, trees, roses, or rice, these chemicals have antioxidant properties .

Cells derived from the argan tree (*Argania spinosa*) dedifferentiate in organ culture. Homogenates of these cells enhanced expression of Sox2 (a stem cell marker) in dermal cells derived from excised hair follicles compared to controls. Furthermore, passage of cells incubated with argan tree extracts increased the numbers of secondary spheres formed by dermal Sox2+ cells in culture, suggesting that the extracts "stimulate the vitality of dermal stem cells." A clinical trial of an emulsion of the extract in a cream base increased the echogenicity of the upper dermis compared to placebo (implying increased density), and decreased depth in crow's feet wrinkles.

An effective strategy might target events more downstream in signaling pathways. Signals favoring stem cell replication generally track down the Wnt (pronounced "wint") signaling pathway. As the cell monitors its environment, Wnt proteins bind to cell membrane receptors. If only a trickle of signal arrives, then the cell stays in its preferred resting, non-proliferative, nondifferentiative state and maintains its "stemness." Increasing the amount of signal favors a differentiative stem cell division. The stem cell divides to produce one stem cell (thus maintaining itself

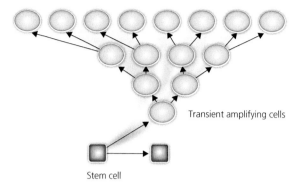

Figure 19.1 In an asymmetric (differentiative) division, a replicating stem cell divides into two types of cells. It renews itself to create a new stem cell, and it differentiates itself to create a transient amplifying cell. The transient amplifying cell will undergo symmetric divisions to produce myriad differentiated cells of a specific lineage, for example, fibroblasts. Source: Dahl MV. 2012. Reproduced with permission of John Wiley & Sons Ltd.

and pluripotency for future use) and one differentiated, less potent cell (a "transient amplifying cell"). The organism uses transient amplifying cells to produce functional differentiated cells of lineages such as keratinocytes and fibroblasts. When transient amplifying cells are relatively depleted, another asymmetric division of stem cells is required (Figure 19.1).

Stem cell numbers in skin do not generally decline with age. They do become less likely to undergo asymmetric divisions to differentiate into constituent cells of skin, such as fibroblasts and keratinocytes. Asymmtate™ is a cosmetic ingredient that fosters normal differentiative divisions of stem cells. Asymmtate encourages signals trickling down the Wnt pathway to bind (via β-catenin) to a coactivator protein called p300 rather than the structurally similar coactivator protein called CBP. This allows a stem cell to undergo differentiative (asymmetric) divisions. Asymmtate encourages stem cells to produce increased numbers of normal skin cells and increased amounts of normal skin cell products. The desirability of this strategy is obvious; asymmtate helps skin stem cells behave as they did at a younger age. The ingredient works to help restore normalcy. Asymmtate seems safe for topical use. Furthermore, the ingredient discourages proliferative symmetric divisions, which mitigates worries about excessive proliferation or induction of skin tumors.

Conclusion

Stem cells ultimately produce skin cells and their constituents. With aging, inadequate or improper signaling renders stem cells less likely to undergo the asymmetric, differentiative cell divisions necessary to maintain normal numbers of differentiated cells. Aged stem cells seem less responsive to signals coming down the Wnt pathway. Cosmeceuticals that work to boost and support normal stem cell differentiative divisions should stop and reverse changes associated with the appearance of aging skin.

Further reading

Dahl MV. Stem cells and the skin. *J Cosmetic Dermatol* 2012; **11**: 297–306.

Fenske NA, Lober CW. Structural and functional changes of normal aging skin. *J Am Acad Dermatol* 1986; **15**: 571–585.

Giangreco A, Qin M, Pintar JE, Watt FM. Epidermal stem cells are retained in vivo throughout skin aging. *Aging Cell* 2008; **7**: 250–259.

Kahn M. Symmetric division versus asymmetric division: A tale of two coactivators. *Future Med Chem* 2011; **3**: 1745–1763.

Kohl E, Steinbauer J, Landthaler M, Szeimies RM. Skin aging. *J Eur Acad Derm Venerol* 2011; **25**: 873–884.

Montano I. Dermal stem cells are the target of the latest treatments for deep-seated skin rejuvenation. info@mibellebiochemistry.com, www.mibellebiochemistry.com.

Pera MF, Tam PPL. Extrinsic regulation of pluripotent stem cells. *Nature* 2010; **465**: 713–720.

Sethi J, Videl-Puig A, Wnt signaling and the control of cellular metabolism. *Biochem J* 2010; **427**: 1–17.

Wu Y, Zhao RCH, Tredget EE. Concise review: Bone marrow-derived stem/progenitor cells in cutaneous repair and regeneration. *Stem Cells* 2010; **28**: 905–915.

Zouboulis CC, Adjaye J, Akamatsu H, et al. Human skin stem cells and the aging process. *Exp Gerontology* 2008; **43**: 986–991.

CHAPTER 20

Cosmeceutical Applications from Marine Organisms

Sung-Hwan Eom[1] and Se-Kwon Kim[1,2]

[1] Marine Bioprocess Research Center, Pukyong National University, Busan, Republic of Korea
[2] Marine Biochemistry Laboratory, Pukyong National University, Busan, Republic of Korea

Introduction

Cosmetics are commonly prescribed to use for improving the appearance of skin and maintaining skin care. Recently, cosmetic products with biologically active and natural ingredients have been produced to enhance the condition and beauty of our skin when treating various dermatologic conditions.

Marine natural products provide a rich source of chemical diversity that can be used to design and develop potentially useful therapeutic products. In addition, various marine compounds have been found to be promising cosmeceutical agents because of their antioxidant, anti-inflammatory, anti-allergic, anti-aging, anti-wrinkling, tyrosinase inhibitory, MMP inhibitory, and ultraviolet (UV)-protective activities. They are currently being investigated for therapeutic use as nutritional supplements and cosmeceutical products with clinical evaluation of efficacy and safety.

Among various marine-derived compounds, polyphenols, carotenoids, and mycosporine-like amino acids are well-known effective phytochemical agents. It is well known that these kind of biological effects are closely related to cosmeceutical applications. Thus, this chapter focuses on the current research on cosmeceutical effect of marine compounds and their therapeutic potential. It is hoped that this chapter will improve interest in the marine compounds-based cosmeceutical products with their potential application as functional and nutritional ingredients.

Marine-derived compounds from marine organisms

Phlorotannins

Marine algae have become an important source of pharmacologically active metabolites. Also, they are widely distributed and abundant throughout

Cosmeceuticals and Cosmetic Practice, First Edition. Edited by Patricia K. Farris.
© 2014 John Wiley & Sons, Ltd. Published 2014 by John Wiley & Sons, Ltd.

the coastal areas of many countries. In addition, they are a source of useful secondary metabolites such as agar, carrageenan and alginate with interesting pharmaceutical properties. Among the marine algae, brown algae have been reported to contain high phlorotannin contents as marine phenolic compounds. Phlorotannins consist of polymers of phloroglucinol (1,3,5 – tryhydroxybenzene) units, formed in the acetate-malonate pathway in marine algae. Furthermore, these phlorotannins are highly hydrophilic components with a wide range of molecular sizes (126 Da–650 kDa).

Furthermore, several phlorotannins purified from brown seaweeds such as *Ecklonia cava*, *E. kurome*, *E. stolonifera*, *Eisenia aborea*, *E. bicyclis*, *Ishige okamurae*, and *Pelvetia siliquosa* contain medicinal and pharmaceutical benefits and have shown strong anti-oxidant, anti-inflammatory, anti-viral, anti-tumor, anti-diabetes and anti-cancer properties. Eckol, dieckol, and phloroglucinol from *E. cava* have shown potential anti-hypertensive effects. In addition, *E. cava* contains other phlorotannins including 6,6′-bieckol, 8,8′-bieckol, 8,4‴-dieckol, dioxinodehydroeckol, fucodiphlorethol G, phlorofucofuroeckol-A, triphlorethol-A. In addition, *E. kurome* and *E. bicyclis* have reported phlorotannin compounds such as eckol, phlorofucofuroeckol A and dieckol, and 8,8′-bieckol was isolated. Phlorotannins in *E. Arborea* possessed a strong anti-allergic effect and their structures were elucidated as eckol, 6,6′-bieckol, 6,8′-bieckol, 8,8′-bieckol, phlorofucofuroeckol-A, and phlorofucofuroeckol-B. Moreover, 6,6′-bieckol, diphlorethohydroxycarmalol, and phloroglucinol have been isolated from brown algae *Ishige okamurae*. Collectively, phlorotannins can be used for functional ingredients in the cosmeceutical and pharmaceutical industries.

Carotenoids
Carotenoids are the most common pigment in nature and are synthesized by plants algae, fungi, and microorganisms. These properties depend on intense molecules such as yellow, orange, and red colors of various fruits, vegetables, flowers, birds, fish, and crustaceans. Carotenoids are known to be potent quenchers and to serve a protective role that prevents the generation of reactive oxygen species, and deactivates the generation of singlet oxygen. In particular, fucoxanthin and astaxanthin are major constituents of marine carotenoids which have been recognized as showing strong antioxidant activities (Figure 20.1).

Mycosporine-like amino acids
In nature, marine organisms have a range of photoprotective mechanisms to protect them from harmful ultraviolet radiation (UVR: 280–400 nm) by the synthesis of UV-absorbing compounds such as mycosporine-like

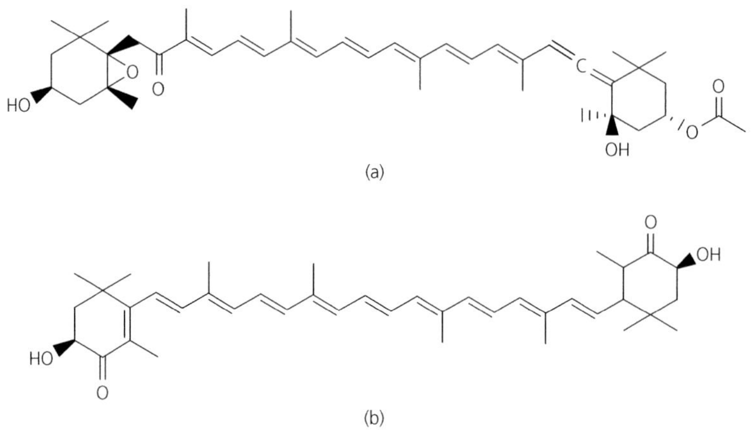

(a)

(b)

Figure 20.1 Chemical structure of fuxanthin (a) and astaxanthin (b).

amino acids (MAAs). Mycosporine-like amino acids (MAAs) are small (<400 kDa), colorless, and water-soluble compounds with cyclohexenone chromophore conjugated with the nitrogen moiety of an amino acid or imino alcohol. MAAs have high absorbances between 310 nm and 360 nm, and they are thus thought to have a protective function as UV-absorbers in marine organisms. Furthermore, UV-absorbing compounds like MAAs are resistant to abiotic stressors such as temperature, UV radiation, and pH. As a result of these properties, MAAs have been considered interesting candidates as UV sunscreens for cosmetic and pharmaceutical formulations.

Cosmeceutical potential of marine organism

Tyrosinase inhibitory activities (skin-whitening properties) of phlorotannins

The enzyme tyrosinase (polyphenols oxidase, EC 1.14.18.1) is a cosmetically important factor affecting the degree of melanin pigmentation and the oxidation of polyphenols. Therefore, tyrosinase inhibitors have an important role in the pharmaceutical industries for their skin-whitening effects and depigmentation. Mushroom tyrosinase (EC 1.14.18.1) is a copper-containing oxidase that catalyzes both the hydroxylation of tyrosine to dihydroxy-L-phenylalanine (L-DOPA) and the oxidation of the L-DOPA to dopaquinone into *o*-quinones. This *o*-quinone can be changed into brown melanin pigments in the browning process. This enzymatic browning reaction can be prevented by trapping the *o*-dopaquinone intermediate. Some tyrosinase agents, kojic acid, arbutin, catechins, hydroquinone (HQ) and azelaic acid are popularly used as skin-lightening and dermatologic agents. Some artificial preservatives and additives used in the cosmetic industry have been evaluated as toxic to various cells and organs, mutagens and tumor promoters over long-term use. Therefore, recently a great deal of interest has been devoted to searching for novel natural ingredients and these studies have shown that phlorotannins in brown algae can act as a potential tyrosinase agent in the cosmeceutical industry and pharmaceutical industries.

The isolated and characterized phlorotannins (**1–7**) from brown algae with tyrosinase inhibitory activity are presented in Figure 20.2, such as phloroglucinol (**1**), eckol (**2**), phlorofucofuroeckol-A (**3**), 6,6′-bieckol (**4**), dieckol (**5**), dioxinodehydroeckol (**6**), and 7-phloroeckol (**7**). In addition, triphloroethol A, 8,8′-bieckol and 8,4‴-dieckol have also been reported. These isolated phlorotannins have been shown to have a tyrosinase inhibitory role as a skin whitening and de-pigmenting effect (Table 20.1). In 2012, Kang et al. have revealed that dieckol purified from *E. cava* is responsible for tyrosinase inhibitory activity. Dieckol has shown a potent tyrosinase inhibitory activity with its binding and docking mode of receptor-ligand interaction. Kinetic analysis revealed that dieckol is a noncompetitive inhibitor. In the molecular modeling simulation, the binding residues of dieckol (His208, Met215, and Gly46) could interact with the active site of tyrosinase as the main contributor in the receptor-ligand interaction. In 2004, Kim et al. studied the inhibitory activities of phlorotannins from *Ecklonia cava*. From the ethyl acetate-soluble extract (EtOAc) of *E. cava*, phloroglucinol (**1**), eckol (**2**), phlorofucofuroeckol-A (**3**), 6,6′-bieckol (**4**), and dieckol (**5**) were isolated. The inhibition is expressed as a concentration necessary for 50% inhibition (IC_{50}). The results of tyrosinase inhibitory activity showed IC_{50} values of 20.00 ± 0.46, 7.60 ± 0.90, and $8.70 \pm 0.23\,\mu g/mL$ for **2**, **4**, and **5**, respectively (Table 20.1). They found inhibition activity to be comparable to arbutin (IC_{50} values of $65.00 \pm 0.61\,\mu g/mL$) and kojic acid (IC_{50} values of $1.10 \pm 0.53\,\mu g/mL$).

Furthermore, the methanolic extract of *E. stolonifera* showed tyrosinase inhibition activity (IC_{50} values of $354.00\,\mu g/mL$). From the EtOAc fraction, five compounds were isolated. Among them, dieckol (**5**) showed a strong tyrosinase inhibitory activity with an IC_{50} value of $2.16\,\mu g/mL$. Other compounds such as phloroglucinol (**1**), dioxinodehydroeckol (**6**), eckol (**2**), and phlorofucofuroeckol-A (**3**) exhibited IC_{50} values of 92.80, 126.00, 33.20, and $177.00\,\mu g/mL$, respectively. They were compared with arbutin and kojic acid (IC_{50} values of 112.00 and $6.32\,\mu g/mL$, respectively). Kinetic analysis by the Lineweaver-Burk plot revealed that phloroglucinol (**1**) and dioxinodehydroeckol (**6**) were competitive inhibitors of L-tyrosine of mushroom tyrosinase. In addition, eckol (**2**), dieckol (**5**) and phlorofucofuroeckol-A (**3**) acted as non-competitive

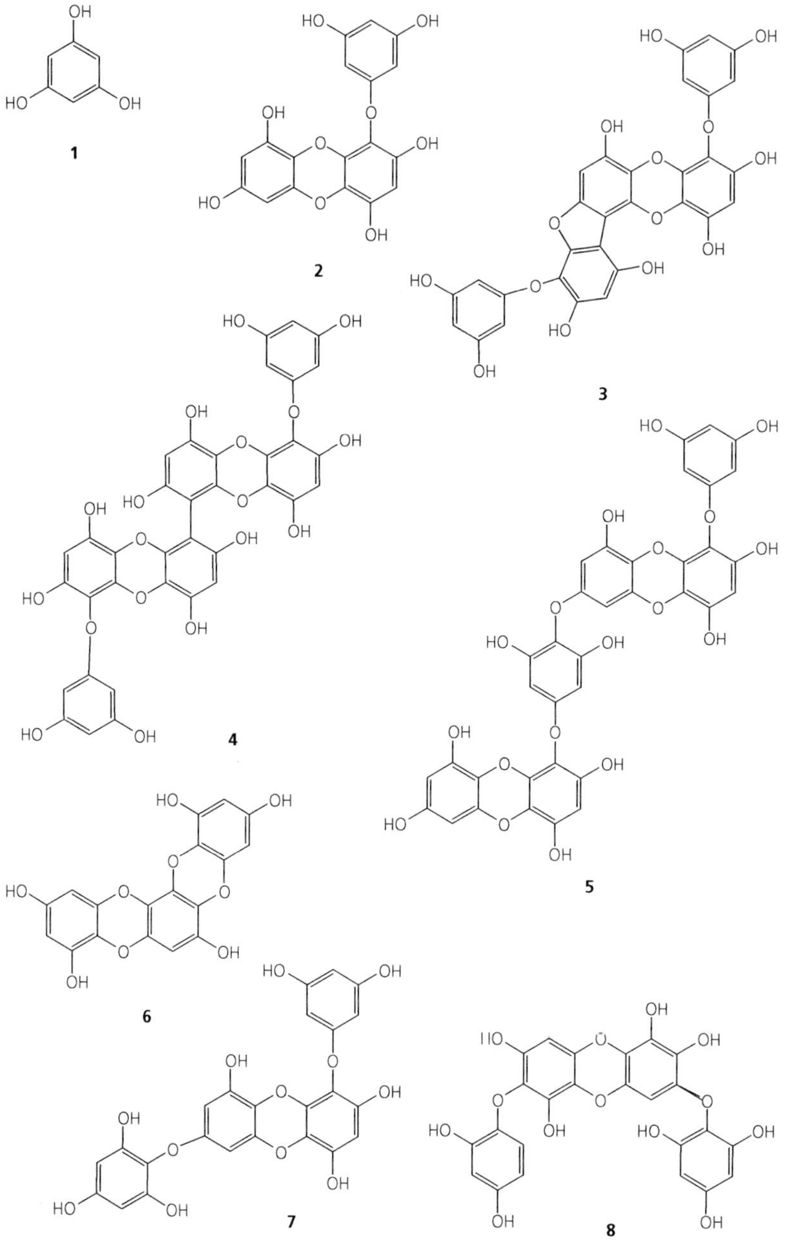

Figure 20.2 Structures of phlorotannins from brown algae (phloroglucinol (**1**), eckol (**2**), fucofuroeckol-A (**3**), dioxinodehydroeckol (**4**), 8,8′-bieckol (**5**), 7-phloroeckol (**6**), phlorofucofuroeckol-A (**7**), dieckol (**8**)).

Table 20.1 Phlorotannin compounds with tyrosinase inhibitory effect.

Source	Phlorotannin	Mode of inhibition	IC$_{50}$[a]	References
Ecklonia cava	Phloroglucinol (**1**)	–[b]	N.D.[c]	Kim et al. (2004)
	Eckol (**2**)	–	20 ± 0.46 μg/mL	
	Phlorofucofuroeckol-A (**3**)	–	N.D.	
	6,6′-Bieckol (**4**)	–	7.6 ± 0.90 μg/mL	
	Dieckol (**5**)	–	8.7 ± 0.23 μg/mL	
	Arbutin	–	65 ± 0.61 μg/mL	
	Kojic acid	–	1.1 ± 0.53 μg/mL	
Ecklonia cava	Phloroglucinol (**1**)	–	300 μg/mL	Yoon et al. (2009)
	Dioxinodehydroeckol (**6**)	–	222.94 μg/mL	
	7-phloroeckol (**7**)	Competitive	0.85 μg/mL	
	Arbutin	–	243.16 μg/mL	
	Kojic acid	–	40.28 μg/mL	
Ecklonia cava	Dieckol (**5**)	Competitive	about 20 μM	Kang et al. (2012)
	Arbutin	–	–	
Ecklonia stolonifera	Phloroglucinol (**1**)	Competitive	92.8 μg/mL	Kang et al. (2004)
	Dioxinodehydroeckol (**6**)	Competitive	126.0 μg/mL	
	Eckol (**2**)	Noncompetitive	33.2 μg/mL	
	Phlorofucofuroeckol-A(**7**)	Noncompetitive	177.0 μg/mL	
	Dieckol (**5**)	Noncompetitive	2.16 μg/mL	
	Arbutin	–	112.0 μg/mL	
	Kojic acid	–	6.32 μg/mL	
Ishige okamurae	Diphlorethohydroxycarmalol (**8**)	–	142.20 μM	Heo et al. (2010)
	Arbutin	–	342.82 μM	

Notes:

[a] IC$_{50}$ Inhibitory effect was expressed as 50% inhibitory concentration.

[b] – Not available.

[c] N.D. not detected.

inhibitors. Yoon et al. investigated the potential tyrosinase inhibitory activity of phloroglucinol (**1**), dioxinodehydroeckol (**6**), and 7-phloroeckol (**7**) isolated from *E. cava*. 7-phloroeckol (**7**) exhibited promising tyrosinase inhibitory activity with IC_{50} values of 0.85 μg/mL and competitive inhibitor. Other identified constituents such as phloroglucinol (**1**), dioxinodehydroeckol (**6**) showed IC_{50} values of 300.00 μg/mL and 222.94 μg/mL respectively, compared with arbutin (IC_{50} values of 243.16 μg/mL) and kojic acid (IC_{50} values of 40.28 μg/mL). In 2010, Heo et al. isolated diphlorethohydroxycarmalol from *Ishige okamurae* as tyrosinase inhibitor. The diphlorethohydroxycarmalol evaluated the tyrosinase inhibitory activity with an IC_{50} value of 142.20 μM, compared with arbutin (IC_{50} values of 342.82 μg/mL). Although the current knowledge related to the structure and activity of these active phlorotannins is limited, the physiological activity may depend on the degree of polymerization of phlorotannin derivatives. Therefore, the tyrosinase activity of phlorotannins might be related to the degree of polymerization phloroglucinol. In addition, according to the significant results of the tyrosinase inhibitory activity comparison to catechins-derivatives as terrestrial plant, it has been reported that the IC_{50} values of gallocatechin, *epi*-gallocatechin gallate, methyl gallate, and quercitrin from *Distylium racemosum* showed 4.80, 30.2, and 37.3 μg/mL. The tyrosinase inhibition activity of phlorotannins isolated edible brown algae was equal to those of catechins originated from terrestrial plants.

Therefore, it is thought that phlorotannins from brown algae would be very useful in the food and pharmaceutical industries as whitening agents. In addition, brown algae include various health-enhancing compounds such as fucoxanthin, sulphated polysaccharides, sterols, polyunsaturated fatty acids, and soluble fibers.

Antioxidant effects of fucoxanthins and astaxanthins

Fucoxanthin is one of the carotenoids found in marine bacteria, diatoms, brown seaweed and crustaceans, of which the distinctive feature is the presence of allene bond and oxygenic functional groups such as hydroxyl, carbonyl, epoxy and carboxyl moieties. According to Nomura et al., fucoxanthin from *Phaeodactylum tricornutum* was shown to have a stronger radical scavenging activity than the other tested carotenoids such as β-carotene, β-cryptoxanthin, zeaxanthin, licopen and lutein. Furthermore, Nishida et al. have shown that carotenoids exhibit higher singlet oxygen- quenching activities than α-tocopherol and L-ascorbic acid etc. Recently, Heo et al. (2008) reported that fucoxanthin can effectively inhibit intracellular ROS formation, DNA damage, and apoptosis induced by H_2O_2, and considerably reduced intracellular ROS generated by exposure to UV-B radiation in human fibroblast, as a promising skin-protective agent.

Astaxanthin also has higher antioxidant activities than β-carotene and α-tocopherol as potential clinical applications. Astaxanthin consists of two additional oxygenated groups on each ring structure. It has recently been shown that astaxanthin can prevent UVA-induced DNA alterations in human dermal fibroblasts, human melanocytes, and human intestinal cells. In addition, astaxanthin is more effective than α-tocopherol in inhibiting free radical-initiated lipid peroxidation in rat liver microsomes. Astaxanthin is 100 times higher than α-tocopherol in protecting rat mitochondria against lipid peroxidation.

Collectively, marine- derived carotenoids such as fucoxanthin and astaxanthin appear to be effective and safe candidates for industrial applications as cosmeceuticals.

Photoprotective effects of mycosporine-like amino acids

The protective effect of MAAs against UV radiation has been demonstrated on various cell lines and human skin. Three UV-absorbing compounds like shinorine, porphyra-334, and mycosporine-glycine from *Patinopecten yessoensis* can act as a UV protector on human fibroblast cells. Furthermore, the treatment of MAAs resulted in a concentration-dependent protection effect of UV-A irradiation on mouse fibroblasts 3T3. Similarly, Helioguard-365 isolated from *Porphyra umbilicalis* has a DNA-protecting effect on human fibroblast (IMR-90) and human keratinocytes (HaCaT) exposed to UV-A irradiation respectively. The cream containing MAAs from *P. umbilicalis* efficiently protects the skin against UV-induced photoaging. The daily use of MAAs seems to sustain skin smoothness and firmness effectively and to prevent premature skin aging. In the case of Collemin A isolated from *Collema cristatum*, its photo-protective effects were investigated in the human keratinocyte cell line (HaCaT) and human skin. It was found that Collemin A strongly prevented UV-B-induced cell destruction and partially prevented pyrimidine dimer formation. Some MAAs are known to protect the cell against UV radiation by scavenging reactive oxygen species such as singlet oxygen, superoxide anions, hydroperoxyl radicals, and hydroxyl radicals. The antioxidant activity of mycosporine-glycine from *Palythoa tuberculosa* was evaluated by measuring its peroxyl radical-trapping abilities. Suh et al. showed that mycosporine-glycine suppresses various detrimental effects of the Type-II photosensitization in biological systems, such as inactivation of mitochondrial electron transport, lipid peroxidation of microsomes, and hemolysis of erythrocytes. With these results, MAAs may have played a key role in protecting marine organisms against sunlight damage by eliminating reactive oxygen species. Furthermore, the photo-protective effects of MAAs from marine organisms have a high resistance to UV-B and UV-A regions of the solar spectrum. Thus, these compounds are recognized to be a preventive and therapeutic treatment of the free radicals' production and UV irradiation in human skin.

Conclusion

In this chapter, since marine-derived compounds provide a promising source of skin whitening, antioxidant, photoprotective effect, and low cytotoxicity, which can be used to develop potential, cosmeceutical and pharmacological agents. Recently, increasing consumer knowledge of the link between safety and health has raised the demand for novel health promotion and functional cosmetic products. Hence, marine organisms have attracted much attention as alternative agents. Thus, marine-derived compounds are one of the effective and alternative candidates as cosmeceuticals.

Further reading

Heo SJ, Ko SC, Kang SM, et al. Cytoprotective effect of fucoxanthin isolated from brown algae *Sargassum siliquastrum* against H_2O_2-induced cell damage. *European Food Research and Technology* 2008; **228**: 145–151.

Heo SJ, Ko SC, Kang SM, et al. Inhibitory effect of diphlorethohydroxycarmalol on melanogenesis and its protective effect against UV-B radiation-induced cell damage. *Food and Chemical Toxicology* 2010; **48**: 1355–1361.

Kang HS, Kim HR, Byun DS, et al. Tyrosinase inhibitors isolated from the edible brown alga *Ecklonia stolonifera*. *Archives of Pharmacol Research* 2004; **27**: 1226–1232.

Kang SM, Heo SJ, Kim KN, et al. Molecular docking studies of a phlorotannin, dieckol isolated from *Ecklonia cava* with tyrosinase inhibitory activity. *Bioorganic and Medicinal Chemistry* 2012; **20**: 311–316.

Kim JA, Lee JM, Shin DB, et al. The antioxidant activity and tyrosinase inhibitory activity of phloro-tannins in *Ecklonia cava*. *Food Science and Biotechnology* 2004; **13**: 476–480.

Ko RK, Kim GO, Hyun CG, et al. Compounds with tyrosinase inhibition, elastase inhibition and DPPH radical scavenging activities from the branches of *Distylium racemosum* Sieb. et Zucc. *Phytotherapy Research* 2011; **25**: 1451–1456.

Nishida Y, Yamashita E, Miki W. Quenching activities of common hydrophilic and lipophilic antioxidants against singlet oxygen using chemiluminescence detection system. *Carotenoid Science* 2007; **11**: 16–20.

Nomura T, Kikuchi M, Kubodera A, et al. Protondonative antioxidant activity of fucoxanthin with 1,1-diphenyl-2-picrylhydrazyl (DPPH). *Biochemistry and Molecular Biology International* 1997; **42**: 361–370.

Suh HW, Lee HW, Jung J. Mycosporine glycine protects biological systems against photodynamic damage by quenching singlet oxygen with a high efficiency. *Photochemistry and Photobiology* 2003; **78**: 109–113.

Yoon NY, Eom TK, Kim MM, et al. Inhibitory effect of phlorotannins isolated from *Ecklonia cava* on mushroom tyrosinase activity and melanin formation in mouse B16F10 melanoma cells. *Journal of Agricultural and Food Chemistry* 2009; **57**: 4124–4129.

PART III

Practical Applications for Cosmeceuticals

CHAPTER 21

Cosmeceuticals for the Treatment of Acne Vulgaris

Joshua A. Zeichner
Mount Sinai Medical Center, New York, NY, USA

Introduction

Acne vulgaris affects approximately 85% of people in the United States at some point in their lives, which translates to 40–50 million people. Combination therapy using prescription medications is the cornerstone of treating acne. Prescription products include topical and oral retinoids, topical and oral antibiotics, topical benzoyl peroxide (BPO), and topical dapsone. Over-the-counter (OTC) products are commonly used by acne patients alone or in combination with prescription medications. Many of these OTC products are categorized as cosmeceuticals, which have intended medical benefits but are not considered drugs. Several cosmeceuticals have been evaluated in treating acne vulgaris. These include minerals, botanicals, antioxidants, and hydroxy acids.

Clinical description: acne vulgaris

Acne vulgaris is a disease of the pilosebacous unit that commonly occurs in adolescents, but can continue into adulthood in some patients. Clinically, patients develop comedones, papules, pustules, and nodules of varying severity on the face and trunk. The pathogenesis of acne is multifactorial, due to a combination of follicular epidermal hyperproliferation, Propionibacterium acnes (P. acnes) growth, sebum production, and inflammation. Early, effective therapy is important to reduce the risk of permanent scarring.

Combination therapy using medicines with different mechanisms of action address multiple pathogenic factors at the same time. Topical retinoids normalize abnormal follicular desquamation and inhibit microcomedone development. Moreover, topical retinoids are anti-inflammatory through their effects on toll-like receptors, cytokines, and nitric oxide.

Cosmeceuticals and Cosmetic Practice, First Edition. Edited by Patricia K. Farris.
© 2014 John Wiley & Sons, Ltd. Published 2014 by John Wiley & Sons, Ltd.

Oral retinoids are used in severe cases and have the added benefit of reducing sebum production. Topical antibiotics are primarily anti-inflammatory by reduction of P. acnes on the skin and their pro-inflammatory effects. BPO has anti-inflammatory, anti-bacterial, and keratolytic properties. It is used frequently in combination with topical antibiotics to inhibit the development of bacterial resistance.

The role of cosmeceuticals in treating acne

Natural ingredients may be defined as products that are not artificial, are found in nature, or extracted from plants or animals. Natural remedies have been used for centuries to treat various skin ailments, and many natural ingredients are now being incorporated into mainstream cosmeceutical products. The efficacy of many of these ingredients has been evaluated in clinical trials, and their mechanisms of action are being studied. Patients turn towards these types of alternative treatments for several reasons, including intrigue, the desire for a more "natural" treatment, dissatisfaction with conventional therapies, or a wish to combine a natural-type treatment with their traditional medicines. Moreover, since these products are sold over-the-counter, patients have far greater access to these products than to physician-prescribed drugs. Below summarizes the list of cosmeceutical agents that have been studied for the treatment of acne vulgaris (Table 21.1).

Ascorbic acid

Ascorbic acid (vitamin C) is a water-soluble vitamin obtained from citrus fruits, tomatoes, and broccoli. It is an important co-factor needed for the production of healthy collagen. In addition, vitamin C has antioxidant properties, quenching free radical damage to DNA. Vitamin C has been shown to be a potential treatment for acne by addressing pathogenic factors involved in acne development. As an antioxidant, vitamin C may prevent

Table 21.1 Cosmeceutical Ingredients useful for treating acne.

Vitamin C
Tea tree oil
Niacinamide
Green tea extract
Resveratrol
Salicylic acid
Alpha hydroxy acids

the oxidation of sebum which contributes to inflammation and follicular keratinization. Vitamin C has been shown to prevent UVA-induced sebum oxidation up to 40%. Moreover, in vitro testing has demonstrated a strong antimicrobial effect against P. acnes.

Several clinical trials have demonstrated the efficacy of vitamin C in the treatment of acne. However, vitamin C itself is unstable and easily degrades in many cosmetic formulations. Sodium ascorbyl phosphate (SAP) is a stable vitamin C precursor that has been incorporated in several topical formulations. In one study, monotherapy with a SAP 5% lotion for 12 weeks showed statistically significant improvement in treating facial acne. Another randomized, double-blind clinical trial showed efficacy of topical SAP 5% for treating acne as both monotherapy and in combination with topical retinol 0.2% cream after both 4 and 8 weeks. A third study of 60 acne patients showed similar improvement with another SAP-containing lotion. Vitamin C is a non-antibiotic option that may be an effective monotherapy or part of a combination regimen for acne.

Zinc

Zinc is a trace element that serves as a co-factor in pathways for cellular development and homeostasis. It also has antioxidant and anti-inflammatory properties, as enzymes such as superoxide dismutase depend on copper and zinc for proper functioning. Two main factors may explain the positive effect of zinc in treating acne vulgaris. First, zinc has been shown to play a role in decreasing sebum production, and, second, it is bacteriostatic against P. acnes. Zinc has been reported to be more effective in studies of inflammatory and severe acne than in mild to moderate disease. Despite theoretical mechanisms of action, clinical data on its efficacy is modest, and more research needs to be done to evaluate the optimal zinc formulation, route of administration, and dosage.

Both oral zinc supplementation and topical application have been evaluated for the treatment of acne. Elemental zinc or zinc gluconate are the preferred forms of oral zinc supplementation, as they have superior tolerability to zinc sulfate. No clear-cut dosage has emerged as first line. Zinc gluconate 200 mg daily and 400–600 mg of zinc sulfate daily have been evaluated and were associated with nausea, vomiting, and diarrhea, which can be lessened by taking zinc directly after eating. In addition, chronic, high dose zinc supplementation (e.g. a chronic intake of greater than 100 mg/day) has been reported to lower copper levels, which is correctable by copper supplements.

In head-to-head studies against oral tetracycline antibiotics, oral zinc supplementation did help treat acne vulgaris. However, oral antibiotics outperformed zinc. In one study, 332 acne patients were randomized to receive 30 mg of elemental zinc or 100 mg of minocycline daily. At

12 weeks, 31.2% of patients in the zinc arm and 63.4% of patients in the minocycline arm achieved the study's success rate end point.

Several different topical zinc preparations have been evaluated in clinical trials for acne. Combination erythromycin 4%/zinc acetate 1.2% gel outperformed vehicle after 12 weeks. Without monotherapy arms for comparison, definite conclusions on the efficacy of zinc compared to erythromycin are unclear. A second study compared zinc sulfate 5% solution to a 2% tea lotion. Twice daily application of the products for 8 weeks resulted in a statistically significant improvement in the tea arm, and a trend towards improvement without statistical significance in the zinc arm.

Niacinamide

Niacinamide (also known as nicotinamide) is a water-soluble vitamin derived from Niacin (vitamin B3). Nicotinamide plays an important role in cellular function, as it is the precursor for nicotinamide adenine dinucleotide (NAD), a coenzyme needed for energy production.

Topical niacinamide has been incorporated into many OTC cosmetic products because of its soothing and anti-inflammatory properties. Niacinamide is used to treat acnes because of its inhibitory effect on inflammatory chemokines. P. acnes on the skin activates interleukin-8 (IL-8) via toll-like receptor 2 stimulation. In vitro, nicotinamide has been shown to significantly decrease IL-8 production in a dose-dependent manner. It is thought that niacinamide exerts this anti-inflammatory effect through regulation of NF-kappaB and MAPK pathways.

Nicotinamide 4% gel was evaluated in a head-to-head study against clindamycin 1% gel. After twice daily application for 8 weeks, both treatment arms provided reduction in acne severity, and there was no statistical significance between the treatment arms ($p = 0.19$). While more clinical trials must be performed to evaluate the efficacy of niacinamide, it may be an alternative anti-inflammatory therapy without the risk of bacterial resistance that antibiotics carry.

Tea tree oil

Tea tree oil (also referred to as melaleuca oil) is produced from the leaves of the *Melaleuca alternifolia* tree. In Australia, it has traditionally been used to treat infections, as it possesses antiseptic properties. Clinical trials have also demonstrated efficacy in treating acne. In a randomized, double-blind, controlled clinical trial, 60 patients were randomized 1:1 to receive either a tea tree oil gel or vehicle. After the 45-day study period, the group applying tea tree oil showed statistically significant improvement as compared to the vehicle arm.

In a single-blind clinical trial, 124 participants were randomized to receive either 5% tea tree oil or 5% benzoyl peroxide lotion. Both the tea tree oil and benzoyl peroxide significantly reduced both inflammatory and non-inflammatory acne lesions. The tea tree oil showed a slower onset of action, but patients experienced fewer cutaneous adverse events compared to benzoyl peroxide.

Green tea

Green tea is derived from the *Cammelia sinensis* plant and contains potent polyphenolic compounds called catechins that possess antioxidant and anti-inflammatory properties. For this reason, green tea extracts are commonly used in many OTC topical anti-aging products.

Few clinical trials have been performed to evaluate green tea to treat acne. Twenty patients with mild to moderate acne were enrolled into this open-label study, in which they applied a 2% green tea lotion twice daily for 6 weeks. The investigators found a statistically significant reduction in mean total lesion count (58.33%, $p < 0.0001$) and mean severity index ($p < 0.0001$). As previously mentioned, a 2% tea lotion was compared to zinc sulfate 5% solution in acne patients. The tea lotion showed statistically significant improvement, which the zinc solution did not.

Resveratrol

Resveratrol is a naturally occurring compound produced by several plants, such as grapes. It is found at high concentrations in red wine, and less so in white wine. Resveratrol has antioxidant and anti-inflammatory properties and is thought to be cardio-protective. It has also been shown to reduce keratinocyte hyperproliferation and suppress inflammation, two major pathogenic factors in the development of acne. Moreover, in vitro resveratrol has been demonstrated to inhibit P. acnes growth.

A clinical trial using a resveratrol-containing hydrogel improved acne severity. In a single-blind split-face study, 20 acne patients applied the active gel on one side and the vehicle on the other, once daily for 60 days. At the end of the study, the side treated with resveratrol demonstrated a 53.75% mean reduction in the global acne grading score compared with 6.10% on the vehicle-treated side. Moreover, cyanoacrylate follicular "biopsies" were performed pre- and post-treatment. This is a simple, noninvasive technique that removes dead cells from the skin's surface and allows evaluation of the stratum corneum. From cyanoacrylate biopsies, the investigators found a statistically significant difference in the mean reduction in the average area of comedones on the resveratrol versus vehicle-treated sides of the face.

Salicylic acid

Salicylic acid is a beta hydroxy acid that is chemically similar to amino salicylic acid, the active ingredient in aspirin. It is found in nature and was originally extracted from the bark of the white willow tree. Salicylic acid has been used for decades to treat acne and is commonly found in OTC products, including washes and leave-ons. It is a chemical exfoliator that dissolves the connections between keratinocytes of the stratum corneum, leading to desquamation of dead cells. Moreover, salicylic acid may have an anti-inflammatory effect in the skin. As a lipophilic molecule, it penetrates easily into the oily environment of the pilosebaceous unit, making it ideal for treating acne. It is comedolytic, but is generally accepted to be less potent than topical retinoids. So, salicylic acid is typically used when patients cannot tolerate topical retinoids.

Salicylic acid is frequently employed as adjuvant therapy with topical prescription medications. The maximum concentration of salicylic acid permitted in OTC products in the United States is 2%, although concentrations higher than that may be used by prescription or in the form of in-office chemical peels. A combination therapy of benzoyl peroxide with salicylic acid has been shown to give superior results in acne reduction at early time points (weeks 2–4) as compared to benzoyl peroxide alone, topical antibiotics alone, or benzoyl peroxide in combination with topical antibiotics.

Alpha hydroxy acids

Alpha hydroxy acids are weak acids found in fruits, milk sugars, and plants. Glycolic acid is one example of an alpha hydroxy acid which is naturally derived from sugar cane and is commonly incorporated into OTC products for acne and anti-aging. Alpha hydroxy acids weaken the strength of corneocyte intercellular bonds. They thereby reduce skin hyperkeratinization by increasing corneocyte desquamation. Besides thinning the stratum corneum, alpha hydroxy acids have been shown to disperse basal layer melanin and increase dermal collagen synthesis. By creating a controlled wound and allowing re-epithelialization, glycolic acid has been shown to reduce excessive pigmentation.

Over the counter, alpha hydroxy acids are available in concentrations up to 10% and have been formulated into various leave-ons, washes, and peels. They are available at higher concentrations as peels in physicians' offices. While salicylic acid has traditionally be used more commonly to treat acne because of its lipophilicity, a clinical trial comparing glycolic to salicylic acid peels showed comparable results in treating acne. In the double-blind, split-faced, randomized study, 20 patients received 30% glycolic acid to one side and 30% salicylic acid to the contralateral side. Patients received peels every two weeks for 6 treatments. By the second peel, both chemicals were significantly effective ($p < 0.05$), but there was no significant difference between them. In addition, glycolic acid monotherapy, topical combinations of glycolic acid with retinaldehyde have been shown to enhance the effects of benzoyl peroxide and topical antibiotics.

Conclusion

Acne patients frequently use OTC cosmeceutical products to treat their acne. To improve outcomes, it is important for consumers to use the right OTC products. Patients frequently turn to dermatologists for product and ingredient recommendations. In some cases, patients may even prefer OTC products over prescription ones and look for guidance on alternative therapies rather than prescription medications. Vitamin C, zinc, tea tree oil, niacinamide, green tea, resveratrol, salicylic acid, and glycolic acid are found in many OTC preparations and all have data to support their use in treating acne, either as monotherapy or as an adjunct to prescriptions medications.

Further reading

Bassett IB, Pannowitz DL, Barnetson RS. A comparative study of teatree oil versus benzoyl peroxide in the treatment of acne. *Med J Aust* 1990; **153**: 455–458.

Bowe WP, Patel N, Logan AC. Acne vulgaris: The role of oxidative stress and the potential therapeutic value of local and systemic antioxidants. *J Drugs Dermatol* 2012; **11**(6): 742–746.

Bowe WP, Shalita AR. Effective over-the-counter acne treatments. *Semin Cutan Med Surg* 2008; **27**: 170–176.

Dreno B, Moyse D, Alirezai M, et al. Multicenter randomized comparative double-blind controlled clinical trials of the safety and efficacy of zinc gluconate versus minocycline hydrochloride in the treatment of inflammatory acne vulgaris. *Dermatology* 2001; **203**(2): 135–140.

Elsaie ML, Abdelhamid MF, Elsaaiee LT, Enam HM. The efficacy of topical 2% green tea lotion in mild-to-moderate acne vulgaris. *J Drugs Dermatol* 2009; **8**(4): 358–364.

Fabbrocini G, Staibano S, De Rosa G, et al. Resveratrol-containing gel for the treatment of acne vulgaris: A single-blind, vehicle-controlled, pilot study. *Am J Clin Dermatol* 2011; **12**(2): 133–141.

Fowler JF, Woolery-Lloyd H, Waldorf H, Saini R. Innovations in natural ingredients and their use in skin care. *J Drugs Dermatol* 2010; **9**(6 Suppl.): S72–81.

Kessler E, Flanagan K, Chia C, et al. Comparison of alpha- and beta-hydroxy acid chemical peels in the treatment of mild to moderately severe facial acne vulgaris. *Dermatol Surg* 2008; **34**(1): 45–50.

Shalita AR, Smith JG, Parish LC, et al. Topical nicotinamide compared with clindamycin gel in the treatment of acne vulgaris. *Int J Dermatol* 1995; **34**(6): 434–437.

Woolery-Lloyd H, Baumann L, Ikeno H. Sodium L-ascorbyl-2-phosphate 5% lotion for the treatment of acne vulgaris: A randomized, double-blind, controlled trial. *J Cosmet Dermatol* 2010; **9**(1): 22–27.

CHAPTER 22

Cosmeceutical Skin Lighteners

Marta I. Rendon[1], Yvette Vazquez[2], and Suzanne Micciantuono[2]

[1]The Rendon Center for Dermatology and Aesthetic Medicine; University of Miami, Boca Raton, FL, USA

[2]Wellington Regional Medical Center, Boca Raton, FL, USA

Introduction

There are numerous treatment options for hyperpigmentation and hyperpigmented lesions. Cosmeceuticals are among these options and have been shown to be safe and effective. To date, hydroquinone seems to be the most useful topical agent. However, combination therapy is even more efficacious, as agents used concurrently can address each of the various steps in the melanin production pathway to prevent pigmentation.

Hyperpigmentation disorders and hyperpigmented lesions, such as melasma, postinflammatory hyperpigmentation, and solar lentigines can cause significant stress on patients and may have a profound impact on their quality of life. Because uniform skin color and texture are highly desirable in many cultures, hyperpigmentation disorders may cause patients psychosocial issues, such as low self-esteem and poor social interactions.

Various etiologies (Table 22.1), including genetic predisposition, chronic ultraviolet radiation exposure, hormonal influences, and inflammation, may contribute to hyperpigmentation development or exacerbation. Hyperpigmentation may also be a result of certain medications, including photosensitizing cosmetics or hormone replacement therapy. Additionally, hyperpigmentation may occur as the result of a postinflammatory response to any skin injury, including physical trauma or iatrogenic treatments, such as chemical peels or other resurfacing procedures.

Certain conditions, such as melasma and post-inflammatory hyperpigmentation, historically affect patients with ethnic skin, most frequently African Americans, Hispanics, and Asians, while lighter skin types are more often affected by other forms of hyperpigmentation, such as lentigines. Therefore, ethnic variability must be carefully considered when treating patients with these disorders.

Cosmeceuticals and Cosmetic Practice, First Edition. Edited by Patricia K. Farris.

Table 22.1 Causes of hyperpigmentation.

Exogenous causes	Skin disorders	Other diseases and conditions
Ultraviolet light (melasma, solar lentigines)	Melasma	Addison's disease
Photosensitizing agents (bergamot oil, furocoumarin)	Postinflammatory hyperpigmentation	Liver disease
Medications (estrogens, tetracyclines, amiodarone, phenytoin, sulfonamides)	Erythromelanosis follicularis	Hemochromatosis
	Linea fusca (Pellagra)	Pituitary tumors
	Poikiloderma of Civatte	
	Riehl's melanosis	Pregnancy

Multiple prescription and nonprescription skin-lightening agents are available on the market. Numerous studies support the use of topical agents, alone and in combination, for the treatment of hyperpigmentation. These agents include hydroquinone, tretinoin, mequinol, and azaleic acid.

The melanin production pathway

In order to comprehend the way in which skin-lightening agents function, one must first have an understanding of the melanin production pathway (Table 22.2). This pathway begins with the enzyme tyrosinase, which converts the amino acid tyrosine into dihydroxyphenylalanine (DOPA), and then converts DOPA to dopaquinone. Dopaquinone is then converted to dopachrome, and then to either dihydroxyindole or dihydroxyindole-2-carboxylic acid (DHICA). In the presence of dopachrome tautomerase and DHICA oxidase, dopaquinone becomes the black-brown pigment eumelanin. In the presence of cysteine or glutathione, dopamine is converted into the yellow-red pigment pheomelanin. Depigmentation may occur when a skin-lightening agent acts upon key steps of this pigmentation pathway.

Skin-lightening agents

The most widely and successfully utilized agent for hyperpigmentation is the phenolic compound, hydroquinone (HQ). It is available over the counter in the United States in strengths of up to 2%, and by prescription in strengths of up to 4%. Increased concentrations of HQ are available as a compounded product. Studies suggest that approximately 6–12 weeks of diligent treatment are generally needed to see a clinical

Table 22.2 The melanin production pathway.

Premelanin synthesis	During melanin synthesis	Postmelanin synthesis
Tretinoin (tyrosinase transcription)	Hydroquinone (tyrosinase inhibition)	Linoleic acid (tyrosinase degradation)
	4-hydroxyanisole (tyrosinase inhibition)	α-linoleic acid (tyrosinase degradation)
	Arbutin (tyrosinase inhibition)	Lecithins and neoglycoproteins (melanosome transfer inhibition)
	Aloesin (tyrosinase inhibition)	Soymilk extracts (melanosome transfer inhibition)
	Azelaic acid (tyrosinase inhibition)	Niacinamide (melanosome transfer inhibition)
	Kojic acid (tyrosinase inhibition)	Glycolic acid (skin turnover acceleration)
	Ascorbic acid (product reduction and reactive oxygen species scavengers)	Retinoic acid (skin turnover acceleration)
	Ascorbic acid palmitate (product reduction and reactive oxygen species scavengers)	

improvement in certain disorders of hyperpigmentation, such as melasma and postinflammatory hyperpigmentation.

The most common adverse effects associated with HQ are contact dermatitis and skin irritation, which can be treated with topical steroids. Patients with darker skin types are at highest risk for exogenous ochronosis due to HQ use. The accumulation of homogentisic acid in the dermis appears as hyperpigmentation. Ochronosis has not been common in the United States, but it continues to be reported in Africa and Asia, even when HQ is used at lower concentrations.

Using HQ in combination with other naturally derived depigmenting agents, such as glycolic acid, vitamin C, or aloesin, may help reduce side effects and improve efficacy. The most widely used combination is HQ with prescription compounds such as retinoids and steroids.

This chapter will review a variety of cosmeceutical ingredients that have been used in the treatment of hyperpigmentation, and their mechanisms of action (Table 22.3).

Cosmeceutical Ingredients for Skin Lightening

Aloesin is a natural derivative of aloe vera. Its depigmenting properties are attributed to the inhibition of tyrosinase activity. Aloesin acts as a competitive inhibitor of dopa oxidation and a non-competitive inhibitor of

Table 22.3 Depigmenting agents.

Aloesin
Arbutin
Azelaic acid
Glabridin (licorice extract)
Glycolic acid
Hydroquinone
Kojic acid
Lignin peroxidase
Melatonin
Mequinol
Niacinamide
Oligopeptide combination
Phenylethyl resorcinol
Paper mulberry
Retinoic acid
Soy-derived extracts
Vitamin C

tyrosine hydroxylase activity. It has also been shown to possess powerful antioxidant and anti-inflammatory properties.

Arbutin (hydroquinone-β-D-glucopyranoside) is a skin-lightening glucoside found in bearberry, pears, and other natural herbs. It is also a mild inhibitor of melanosomal tyrosinase activity.

Azelaic acid is a naturally occurring dicarboxylic acid derived from the yeast *Pityrosporum ovale*. It inhibits DNA synthesis, as well as tyrosinase activity. Azelaic acid has the greatest effect on heavily pigmented melanocytes and has also proven to be effective in the treatment of melasma, rosacea, and solar keratosis.

Glabridin is the principal component in licorice root extract. It inhibits tyrosinase activity and UVB-induced pigmentation and also exerts anti-inflammatory properties by inhibiting free radical formation. In one study, glabridin was shown to have greater skin- lightening effects and a faster-acting profile than HQ. It is available in concentrations of 10–40%, but in combination with betamethasone and retinoic acid it has demonstrated efficacy in concentrations as low as 0.4%.

Glycolic acid is an α-hydroxy acid derived from sugarcane. It can be used in lower concentrations for the rapid desquamation of pigmented keratinocytes. However, in higher concentrations, it causes epidermolysis. When used for postinflammatory hyperigmentation, glycolic acid peels should be initiated at lower concentrations. One study that compared a 70% glycolic acid peel with a 1% tretinoin peel revealed similar depigmentation results, but patients experienced more irritation with the glycolic acid peel. While this increased irritation did not cause post-inflammatory hyperpigmention in this study, it certainly has the potential to induce this condition in darker skin types. Glycolic acid peels can also be used in conjunction with topical therapies in patients with melasma, post-inflammatory hyperpigmentation, acne, and photoaging.

Kojic acid is a depigmenting agent derived from a species of fungi. It works by inhibiting the activity of tyrosinase. Kojic acid can be used together with HQ and glycolic acid for the treatment of hyperpigmentation. Using these agents together may reduce irritant contact dermatitis, which is one of the common side effects of kojic acid. Kojic acid has been banned in Japan due to its potential for causing irritation.

Lignin peroxidase is a relatively new product derived from the tree fungus, *Phanerochaete chrysosporium*. Lignin breaks down melanin, but it does not prevent pigment formation. Therefore, it should be used in combination with another skin-lightening product, such as HQ. However, a randomized, double-blinded study showed that lignin peroxidase was more effective at treating hyperpigmentation than placebo and 2% hydroquinone, demonstrating skin lightening within as few as eight days of use.

Newer combination skin-lightening systems containing multiple ingredients have recently been released. One such system contains 0.01% oligopeptide cream, 20% glycolic acid, and a moisturizing sunscreen. It effectively inhibits melanogenesis by reducing tyrosinase activity, without causing cytotoxicity to human melanocytes. This system has been used to treat hyperpigmentation disorders such as melasma and postinflammatory hyperpigmentation, and patients give it high satisfaction ratings. One study showed that applying concentrations of 0.01% daily provided a 50% improvement in hyperpigmentation within 16 weeks of use.

Another recently introduced skin-lightening system consists of phenylethyl resorcinol (a tyrosinase inhibitor), leucine (a precursor of melanin production), undecylenoyl phenylalanine (a compound that minimizes sun-induced melanin formation), and sodium glycerophosphate. When patients used this skin-lightening system twice daily for 12 weeks in combination with a sunscreen, it decreased the appearance of facial lentigines by up to 43%.

With regard to these newer products, it is important to note that the studies published thus far are few in number and include small sample sizes. Further studies with larger sample sizes are necessary to reach definitive conclusions about the efficacy of these products, and their potential role in our treatment armamentarium.

Melatonin is a hormone secreted by the pineal gland in response to sunlight. It has been shown to inhibit cyclic AMP-driven processes in melanocytes. The concentration of melatonin needed for effective cosmeceutical skin lightening in human skin has not yet been established. However, it is sold as an antioxidant in a cream formulation.

Mequinol (4-hydroxyanisol) is approved in concentrations of 2–20% for the treatment of solar lentigines. Although its exact mechanism of action is unknown, mequinol appears to competitively inhibit tyrosinase substrates. Mequinol is most frequently used in combination with tretinoin since this combination has superior depigmenting activity than either agent alone. The solution containing 2% mequinol and 0.01% tretinoin has been shown to be superior to 3% HQ in the treatment of solar lentigenes in 216 patients after 16 weeks with twice daily application. This combination product may also potentiate the action of pigment-specific lasers, possibly reduce the number of treatments required and prevent recurrences.

Niacinamide is a form of vitamin B_3 that is commonly found in cosmeceuticals. It reduces transepidermal water loss, improves barrier function and can be used to treat photodamage. Niacinamide has also been shown to inhibit the transfer of melanosomes to epidermal keratinocytes, making it a valuable depigmenting agent for all skin types. Multiple products containing niacinamide are available over the counter, and physicians can dispense formulations in concentrations of up to 5%. Although niacinamide has been shown to be less irritating than HQ, as evidenced in a study comparing 4% niacinamide to 4% HQ in the treatment of melasma, it requires a longer treatment duration to produce visible results, and the improvement in hyperpigmentation is not significantly better than with HQ.

Paper mulberry extract is a popular skin-lightening agent used in Europe and South America that is derived from the roots of the Broussonetia papyrifera tree. Its tyrosinase inhibiting activity, in one study, has been compared favorably to that of HQ and kojic acid. Paper mulberry produces little or no skin irritation, and is therefore appropriate for use in people with darker skin types and in those who cannot tolerate HQ. There are no clinical trials to date, however, demonstrating the use of this ingredient.

Vitamin A (retinol) and tretinoin can be used for treating melasma, postinflammatory hyperpigmentation, and lentigines. In animal studies, retinol has been shown to inhibit tyrosinase induction. Retinoids may also interfere with pigment transfer to keratinocytes and accelerate pigment loss by causing the epidermis to be shed more quickly. Retinoids have been shown to be effective both as monotherapy and in combination with other products. A prescription product containing 0.15% retinol plus 4% hydroquinone and sunscreen has been shown to be effective for the treatment of hyperpigmentary disorders and hyperpigmented lesions. When used together, corticosteroids, hydroquinone, and retinoic acid have a

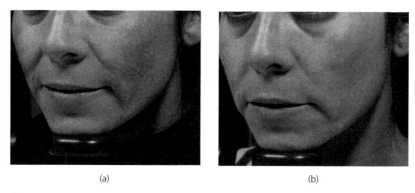

(a)   (b)

Figure 22.1 Melasma. (a) Baseline (b) After 6 months of treatment with a combination of 0.1% tretinoin and 4% HQ.

synergistic effect. Studies have demonstrated that using varying concentrations of retinoids and steroids in combination can clear melasma by up to 79% (Figure 22.1). Concentrations of the ingredients are dependent upon skin sensitivity, ethnicity, patient tolerance, and various other factors. Because of its success, this combination therapy has been an important and commonly utilized treatment method since Kligman and Willis introduced it in 1975.

Soy-derived extracts have been utilized in the treatment of mottled hyperpigmentation and solar lentigines. Unpasteurized soymilk contains Bowman-Birk and soybean trypsin inhibitors, two serine protease inhibitors that interfere with the protease-activated receptor-2 pathway. These inhibitors effectively reduce melanin transfer and induce depigmentation. Soy also has an added advantage of protecting against photodamage through its potent antioxidant activity.

Vitamin C interferes with pigment production at various oxidative steps in the melanin production pathway. It interacts with copper ions at the tyrosinase active site and reduces dopaquinone production. The stable derivative known as magnesium L-ascorbic acid 2-phosphate (MAP) has been shown to have skin-lightening activity. Topically applied vitamin C formulations may protect against ultraviolet-B radiation-induced phototoxicity and improve hyperpigmentation disorders, such as melasma and postinflammatory hyperpigmentation. Topical vitamin C is generally non-irritating, and thus is useful in dark-skinned ethnic groups in whom post-inflammatory hyperpigmentation is a concern.

Conclusion

Hyperpigmentation disorders are common dermatologic conditions. Although numerous treatment options exist, resolving hyperpigmentation continues to be a therapeutic challenge. Traditionally, HQ has been the most widely used and effective agent for the treatment of hyperpigmentation. A recent interest in natural ingredients has driven researchers to study other agents, but while these products have been shown to cause less irritation, they have not demonstrated the success of HQ. In our experience, as well as in the literature, combination therapy (especially when it contains HQ) is more effective than monotherapy with any single agent we have available today. The use of these products, along with proper skin care for these conditions, such as gentle cleansers and appropriate moisturization, can provide a safe and effective treatment regimen for many patients. As always, sun protection is of utmost importance in not only the overall condition and health of the skin, but also in the treatment and prevention of hyperpigmentation.

Further reading

Draelos ZD. Skin lightening preparations and the hydroquinone controversy. *Dermatol Ther* 2007; **20**(5): 308–313.

Faghihi G, Shahingohar A, Siadat AH. Comparison between 1% tretinoin peeling versus 70% glycolic acid peeling in the treatment of female patients with melasma. *J Drugs Dermatol* 2011; **10**: 1439–1442.

Gold MH, Biron J. Efficacy of a novel hydroquinone-free skin-brightening cream in patients with melasma. *J Cosmet Dermatol* 2011; **10**: 189–196.

Hantash BM, Jimenez F. A split-face, double-blind, randomized and placebo-controlled pilot evaluation of a novel oligopeptide for the treatment of recalcitrant melasma. *J Drugs Dermatol.* 2009; **8**: 732–735.

Mauricio T, Karmon Y, Khaiat A. A randomized and placebo-controlled study to compare the skin-lightening efficacy and safety of lignin peroxidase cream *vs.* 2% hydroquinone cream. *J Cosmet Dermatol* 2011; **10**: 253–259.

Navarrete-Solís J, Castanedo-Cázares JP, Torres-Álvarez B, et al. A double-blind, randomized clinical trial of niacinamide 4% versus hydroquinone 4% in the treatment of melasma. *Dermatol Res Pract* 2011; **2011**: 379173.

Rendon MI. Skin lightening agents. In: Grimes PE (ed.) *Aesthetics and Cosmetic Surgery for Darker Skin Types*. Philadelphia, PA: Lippincott, Williams & Wilkins, 2008, 73–81.

CHAPTER 23

Cosmeceuticals for Treating Cellulite

Doris Hexsel[1,2] and Camile L. Hexsel[2,3]

[1]Pontifícia Universidade Católica do Rio Grande do Sul (PUC-RS), Porto Alegre, RS, Brazil
[2]Brazilian Center for Studies in Dermatology, Porto Alegre, RS, Brazil
[3]The Methodist Hospital, Houston, TX, USA

Introduction

Cellulite results from alterations in the skin and subcutaneous tissue leading to irregular depressions and raised areas. Clinical morphological patterns vary between patients, and include an orange peel, cottage cheese or mattress appearance of the skin surface. Cellulite usually occurs on buttocks and thighs, but it can also affect other areas such as the abdomen, arms and back.

Clinical description of the challenge (disease pathogenesis and challenges in treatment)

Depressed lesions are due to the presence of fibrous septa that pull the skin surface down. Recently, a study demonstrated that significantly thicker subcutaneous fibrous septa are present in areas with cellulite depressions. On the other hand, raised areas result from the projection of underlying fat to the skin surface.

The anatomy of the subcutaneous tissue (fibrous septa and fat lobes) of males is different from that of females, elucidating why this condition is predominantly found in females. In females, the fibrous septae are oriented longitudinally between the dermis and the deep fascia. When there is accumulation of fat between these septae and the fat layer expands, there is formation of "pockets," and thus the fat is projected into the dermis in a way very similar to a quilt or mattress, resulting in the puckered appearance of the skin. In addition, women have bigger and more rectangular "pockets" of fat compared to men. In men, the connective tissue is

---

oriented in a criss-crossing pattern, which holds the fat layer and prevents the projection of the adipose tissue on the skin surface.

Other factors have been implicated in the pathogenesis of cellulite, such as hormonal, biochemical, inflammatory and circulatory factors. Furthermore, cellulite is aggravated by localized fat deposition, obesity, and progressive skin laxity or flaccidity that occurs with aging.

Therefore, cellulite is a condition that is very difficult to treat, given the deep anatomical structures involved in its pathogenesis and its multifactorial nature. Moreover, there is large clinical morphologic variability among different subjects. Treatment should be individualized depending on the clinical findings, and it often requires a combination of different modalities, including procedures and devices that target the fibrous septa, fat accumulation, flaccidity and circulation and lymphatic drainage. Even when combined, these treatment options often do not lead to the complete disappearance of the condition, but usually to improvement.

This chapter describes cosmeceuticals that may have a theoretical effect when topically applied to cellulite-affected areas, based on their mechanisms of action, whether they restore the dermis and subcutaneous tissue, affect the fatty tissue by potentially reducing lipogenesis or lipolysis, act as antioxidants, or affect the circulation.

The role of cosmeceuticals in treating this condition

Medical therapy for the treatment of cellulite despite weight loss, balanced diet and exercise is limited. Despite the fact that many topical cosmeceutical agents for the treatment of cellulite are marketed worldwide, little scientific evidence currently exists to attest the efficacy of most products. Furthermore, products have to undergo proper quality control measures, be dispensed in proper concentrations to achieve a clinical effect, and be able to reach the dermis and subcutaneous tissue to perform the desired action. Furthermore, certain morphological aspects of cellulite will not be affected by cosmeceuticals, such as lesions due to subcutaneous fibrous septae pulling down on the skin. Therefore, the role of cosmeceuticals in the treatment of cellulite is mainly their use in conjunction with other measures, such as weight loss, subcision™ and devices that target the fat and connective tissue.

Since cellulite is a condition that affects the skin morphologically down to the fat and fascia, the clinical efficacy of many cosmeceuticals is limited due to their inability to penetrate the skin barrier and the deep planes. For this reason, topical formulations must include the proper vehicle and possibly the presence of skin enhancers to augment cutaneous penetration. Chemical promoters or surfactants cause modifications in the lipid bilayer structure and alteration of the skin/vehicle partitioning coefficient. Physical promoters such as massage, electroporation and iontophoresis are useful for ionic molecules, large molecular weight actives and substances with very low potency. Transdermal systems, such as transdermal patches, have the ability to facilitate the administration of the exact dosage of effective drugs at the site of action. Multivesicular emulsion systems involve the creation of a two-phase emulsion system that produces concentric multilamellar spheres of oil and water. By this percutaneous delivery system, active ingredients can be controlled-released from their respective layers upon application to the skin.

Since cellulite affects large areas of the skin, concentration and penetration of the active ingredients should be known for safety reasons.

Cosmeceutical ingredients and actives appropriate for treating this condition

Agents that may affect the structure of the dermis

The appearance of cellulite may be improved by increasing the thickness of the dermis with a potential decrease in the fat herniation into the superficial tissue.

- *Topical retinoids* have been used for the treatment of cellulite. They increase dermal collagen deposition, promote the synthesis of dermal glycosaminoglycans, improve the contour of elastic fibers, increase the elasticity of the skin, improve the circulation and decrease the adipocyte size. A placebo-controlled study by Kligman investigated the topical use of *retinol 0.3%* on the thighs for six months in 19 patients, and it demonstrated improvement in cellulite on the treated side in 63.1% of the patients compared to the untreated side, by clinical dermatologic evaluation and laser Dopler velocimetry.
- Furthermore, *vitamin C* stabilizes collagen and stimulates collagen deposition. Because of this property of potentially strengthening the dermis, it can be used in cellulite creams but has not been tested in clinical trials for the treatment of cellulite.
- *Centella asiatica* extract, which is derived from an aquatic plant grown in India and Southeast Asia, stimulates fibroblastic activity and collagen synthesis in the extracellular matrix, and reduces the size of adipocytes. It also stimulates lymphatic drainage, and has anti-inflammatory activity. It may be used in concentrations from 2–5%.
- *Bladderwrack* (*Fucus vesiculosus*) is a brown marine algae reported to produce contraction of the dermal connective tissue via increased expression of integrin. It also stimulates vascular flow.

Agents that may affect localized fat

Agents that reduce the lipogenesis and promote lipolysis may reduce the size and volume of adipocytes, decreasing the tension of the surrounding connective tissue with a possible decrease in the clinical appearance of cellulite.

Adipose cell fat comes from plasma-circulating lipoproteins. During lipolysis, the fat is hydrolyzed and eliminated back to the plasma as free fatty acids and glycerol. Different enzymes, such as insulin, cyclic adenosine monophosphate (cAMP) and especially triglyceride lipase, participate in the process.

Furthermore, adipose cell fat expresses receptors that promote the storage of fat and lipogenesis, such as neuropeptide Y and peptide YY. On the other hand, other surface receptors, such as β1 and β2, promote lipolysis and the elimination of fat.

- *Phosphatidylcholine* (soybean lecithin extract) causes lipolysis via activation of β adrenoreceptors, and it induces a mixed septal and lobular panniculitis with abundant fat necrosis and lipoatrophy. In a randomized controlled, double-blind study, nine healthy female volunteers with Grade II–III thigh cellulite were treated with a phosphatidylcholine-based, cosmeceutical anti-cellulite gel. Twice weekly, each thigh was exposed to treatment with light-emitting diode (LED) array at 660 nm and 950 nm for 24 treatments. Eight of nine thighs treated were downgraded to a lower cellulite grade by clinical examination, digital photography, and pinch test assessment. Digital ultrasound at the dermal-adipose interface demonstrated a statistically significant reduction of immediate hypodermal depth and echo-like intrusions into the dermal layer, confirmed by three biopsies. In nine placebo and LED-treated thighs and one of the actively treated thighs, minimal clinical changes were observed. At the month-18 evaluation period for the eight responsive thighs, five thighs reverted back to their original cellulite grading, indicating a need for maintenance treatment.
- *Methylxanthines*, such as *caffeine, aminophylline, theophylline, and theobromine* are β-agonists that reduce lipogenesis and promote lipolysis. They are the most frequently used active ingredients in anti-cellulite products.
- *Caffeine*, which is extracted from the coffee beans of the *Coffea arabica* (L) plant, is normally used in concentrations of 1–2%. It offers good skin penetration and absorption. Caffeine acts on the adipose cells, promoting lipolysis and activates the triglyceride lipase enzyme that breaks down triglycerides into free fatty acids and glycerol. It also has a stimulating effect on the cutaneous microcirculation. Lupi et al. published a controlled clinical study (N = 134) using a 7% caffeine

solution, showing a reduction of 2.1 cm in the thigh circumference in >80% of treated patients. No specific measurement of effect on the appearance of cellulite was assessed. There are reports of allergic reactions to topical products containing caffeine as well as reports of cases of dermatitis in the workers who handle the coffee grains. Lesser et al. also demonstrated reduction of the thickness of adipose tissue in a double-blind, single-center, placebo-controlled study (N = 41).

- *Aminophylline* also has lipolytic effects. Collis et al. evaluated the effectiveness of topical aminophylline gel in combination with 10% glycolic acid and concluded that it failed to improve cellulite in a randomized controlled trial in 52 women. No statistically significant difference existed in the measurements between affected areas for any of the treatment groups.
- Other agents that have been shown to have lipolytic activity include β-adrenergic agonists such as *isoprotenerol* and *adrenaline*, and α-adrenergic antagonist such as *phentolamine, dihydroergotamine, yohimbine* and *piperoxan*. Greenway and Bray, in a double-blind, placebo-controlled study, demonstrated a statistically significant reduction in the medial thigh antropometric measurements with the use of topical isoprotenerol, aminophylline, and yohimbine. The reduction was greatest with the use of all active drugs. Of the agents used separately, aminophylline gave the best results.
- *Coenzyme A* and the amino acid *L-carnitine* simulate the mobilization and destruction of free fatty acids, preventing the negative feedback on lipolysis and stimulating adipocyte lipase activity. They also increase the lipolytic effect of methylxanthines.
- *Petroselinic acid* and *conjugated linolenic acid* improve epidermal differentiation, reduce inflammation, increase extracellular matrix components and induce skin tightening. Furthermore, in vitro studies have shown that conjugated linolenic acid can prevent lipid accumulation in adipocytes, and a randomized controlled clinical trial showed clinical improvement in cellulite in 75% of patients, as well as an average reduction in thigh circumference of 2.2 cm, when used orally in a dose of 800 mg in conjunction with a herbal anticellulite pill. The herbal anticellulite pill alone had minimal effect on cellulite.

Antioxidant agents

Antioxidant agents can protect the dermal and subcutaneous fat cell membranes from free radical toxicity membrane lipid peroxidation. Examples include vitamin C, vitamin E, green tea extract, and flavonoids, among many others.

Agents that may stimulate local circulation and lymphatic drainage

Adipose tissue is very vascular, which leads to the theory that cellulite may worsen in predisposed areas where circulation and lymphatic drainage are decreased, potentially due to injury or inflammation. Furthermore, impairment in microvascular circulation can lead to increased microedema in the subcutaneous fat layer. Therefore, many treatments for cellulite target improving circulation and lymphatic drainage, based on this theory.

- *Ginko biloba* contains flavonoids, biflavones and terpenes that reduce blood viscosity, inhibit platelet-activating factor, improve vascular tone, and thus lead to improvement in microcirculation. Flavonoids also act as antioxidants. The recommended concentration is 1–3%. There have been reports in the literature of cases of hypersensitivity to the ginkgo-containing products.
- *Red grapes* (*Vitis vinifera*) have antioxidant properties, stimulate lymphatic drainage, and inhibit elastase and collagenase. It is used in concentrations of 2–7%. There have been reports of hand dermatitis in workers who squeeze the fruit to obtain the juice.
- The fruit and the leaves of the *papaya* (*Carica Papaya*) and of the *pineapple* (*Ananas sativus*) have anti-inflammatory properties. The recommended concentration is 2–5%. Dermatitis can rarely occur.
- *Artichoke* or *chophytol* (*Cynara scolymyus*) stimulates the circulation and has a diuretic and anti-edema effect.
- *Pentoxyphylline* improves microcirculation by inhibiting platelet aggregation and affecting the plasmatic concentration of fibrinogen.
- *Ground ivy* (*Glechoma hederacea*) is used in concentrations of 2–5%. It contains coumarin, which reduces lymphatic edema and diminishes capillary permeability.
- *Common ivy* (*Hedera helix*) improves capillary permeability, venous and lymphatic drainage and has anti-inflammatory, antiedema and analgesic effects. Allergic reactions have been reported.
- *Butcher's broom* (*Ruscus aculeatus*) is a venous constrictor that decreases vascular permeability and edema, improving lymphatic drainage. It also activates cutaneous circulation, allowing better oxidation and cellular metabolism. It is frequently used in concentrations of 1–3%.
- *Sillicium* modifies venous and lymphatic capillary permability.
- *Indian* or *horse chestnut* (*Aesculus hippocastanum*) has mild peripheral vasoconstriction properties, decreases capillary permeability and reduces lysosomatic enzymes activity by up to 30%.

Combination agents

Many products consist of a combination of multiple active ingredients with the goal of increasing efficacy by combining different mechanisms of action. However, the number of scientific studies published in the literature assessing such products is limited.

Bertin et al. performed a placebo-controlled double-blind study evaluating an anti-cellulite product that combined *retinol, caffeine, Asiatic centella, L-carnitine, esculoside* (to improve local microcirculation), and *ruscogenine* (which inhibits elastase activity). The combination product was more effective than the placebo in reducing cellulite appearance.

A double-blind randomized placebo-controlled study by Rao and Goldman assessed the efficacy of a combination topical anti-cellulite cream containing *caffeine, green tea extract, black pepper seed extract, citrus extract, ginger root extract, cinnamon bark extract* and *capsicum annum resin* with and without occlusion with bioceramic-coated neoprene shorts (N = 17). There was an overall clinical improvement in cellulite by photographic assessment in 65% of the treated legs with occlusion and 59% of the treated legs without occlusion. Another multicenter, randomized, placebo-controlled study by Rao et al. tested the same combination anti-cellulite cream under occlusion with bioceramic-coated neoprene shorts and showed clinical improvement on photographs in 68% of the subjects.

On the other hand, a study by Lis-Balchin showed lack of effect of the combination product *Cellasene*, which contains *ginkgo biloba, sweet clover, seaweed, grape seed oil, lecithins* and *primrose oil* in a placebo-controlled clinical trail. There was an increase in cellulite, which could be attributed to weight gain in both groups.

Adverse effects

Many cosmeceutical products used for the treatment of cellulite can cause allergic reaction and contact dermatitis. Sainio et al. investigated 32 anti-cellulite products, mostly botanicals and emollients, each containing an average of 22 ingredients, finding that 25% of the substances have been shown to cause allergy.

Conclusion

Many cosmeceutical products are available on the market. Considering that cellulite is directly linked to the subcutaneous structures, cosmeceuticals can be used in patients presenting mild cellulite as well as adjuvant treatment of other therapeutic modalities.

Further reading

Birnbaum L. Addition of conjugated linoleic acid to a herbal anticellulite pill. *Adv Ther* 2001; **18**(5): 225–229.

Hexsel D, Orlandi C, Zechmeister do Prado D. Botanical extracts used in the treatment of cellulite. Dermatol Surg 2005; **31**(7 Pt 2): 866–872 (discussion 872).

Hexsel D, Soirefmann M. Cosmeceuticals for cellulite. *Semin Cutan Med Surg* 2011; **30**(3): 167–170.

Hexsel D, Zechmeister do Prado D, Goldman MP. Topical management of cellulite. In: Goldman MP, Hexsel D, eds. *Cellulite Pathophysiology and Treatment*. New York: Taylor & Francis, 2010, 13–23.

Lesser T, Ritvo E, Moy LS. Modification of subcutaneous adipose tissue by a methylxanthine formulation: A double-blind controlled study. *Dermatol Surg* 1999; **25**(6): 455–462.

Lis-Balchin M. Parallel placebo-controlled clinical study of a mixture of herbs sold as a remedy for cellulite. *Phytother Res* 1999; **13**(7): 627–629.

Rao J GM, Goldman MP. A two-center double-blinded randomized trial testing the tolerability and efficacy of a novel therapeutic agent for cellulite reduction. *Am J Cosm Surg* 2005; **4**: 93–102.

Rao J, Paabo KE, Goldman MP. A double-blinded randomized trial testing the tolerability and efficacy of a novel topical agent with and without occlusion for the treatment of cellulite: A study and review of the literature. *J Drugs Dermatol* 2004; **3**(4): 417–425.

Sainio EL, Rantanen T, Kanerva L. Ingredients and safety of cellulite creams. *Eur J Dermatol* 2000; **10**(8): 596–603.

Sasaki GH, Oberg K, Tucker B, Gaston M. The effectiveness and safety of topical PhotoActif phosphatidylcholine-based anti-cellulite gel and LED (red and infrared) light on Grade II–III thigh cellulite: A randomized. double-blinded study. *J Cosmet Laser Ther* 2007; **9**(2): 87–96.

CHAPTER 24

Cosmeceuticals for Hair Loss and Hair Care

Nicole E. Rogers

Tulane University School of Medicine, New Orleans, LA, USA

Introduction

For both men and women, hair is a powerful indicator of health and fertility. Up to 40% of women and 50% of men are affected by thinning hair over the course of their lifetime. The most common cause of hair loss is inherited androgenetic alopecia, also known as male or female pattern hair loss (Figures 24.1 and 24.2). The cosmeceutical industry has literally exploded in recent years, as manufacturers have incorporated various plant extracts into products for hair care and hair loss. In this chapter we will focus on active ingredients with scientific data supporting their role in hair growth or hair care.

At present, there are only two FDA-approved medications for hair loss and one medical device that has FDA 510 K approval. These include topical minoxidil, sold under the trade name Rogaine® (for men and women), oral finasteride (trade name Propecia®, approved for men only) and the Hairmax Lasercomb, which is a handheld device emitting a 655 nm low-level laser beam (for men and women). In this chapter we will examine the data available on other plant-based ingredients to see how they may have potential for further incorporation into hair products. Table 24.1 provides a summary of some of the proposed plant-based mechanisms of action on hair growth.

Polyphenols: grape seed, apple extract, barley, and raspberry

Antioxidants such as polyphenols (including flavonoids) are known for their abilities to scavenge free radicals, and thus reduce oxidative stress from ultraviolet radiation and environmental pollution. Japanese researchers demonstrated the growth-promoting effects of proanthocyani-dins from *grape seeds* (Chardonnay variety). The effects were seen both in

Cosmeceuticals and Cosmetic Practice, First Edition. Edited by Patricia K. Farris.

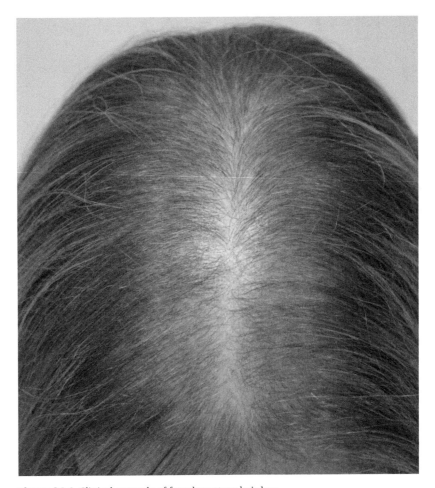

Figure 24.1 Clinical example of female pattern hair loss.

Table 24.1 Summary of plant-based mechanisms for hair growth.

Inhibition of 5α-reductase[7]
Inhibition of TGF-β[2]
Up-regulation of IGF-1[4]
Inhibition of protein kinase C[3]

vitro and in vivo, where 3% proanthocyanidin extract was as effective as 1% minoxidil in converting mouse hair follicles from telogen to anagen phase. Procyanidin B-2 (an epicatechin dimer) exhibited the greatest in vitro growth-promoting activity for hair epithelial cells.

In 2001, the first clinical trial tested the topical application of a 1% procyanidin B-2 tonic for hair growth in humans. In this double-blind,

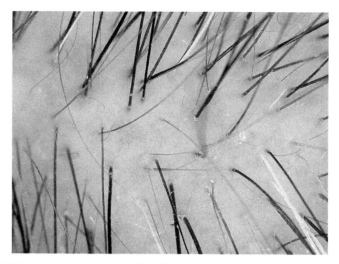

Figure 24.2 Dermatoscopic image of female pattern hair loss.

placebo-controlled study involving 29 male subjects with androgenetic alopecia (19 treated, 10 placebo), 78.9% of the treatment group showed an increase in mean hair diameter, while only 30% of the placebo group showed any increase. In a second double-blind clinical trial, 0.7% *apple (Malus pumila)* procyanidine oligomers were applied to the scalps of men with androgenetic alopecia. At 6 and 12 months, the treatment group (N = 21) had a significant increase in hair density versus the placebo group (N = 22). Several commercially available products contain procyanidins of apple extract (Figure 24.3).

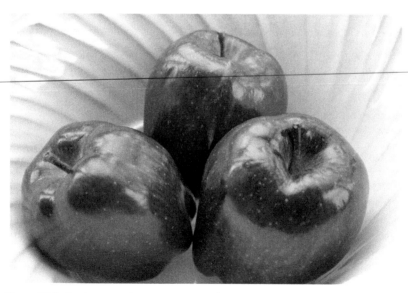

Figure 24.3 Apples are an important source of procyanidin extract.

Procyanidin studies have helped provide a better understanding of the mechanisms involved in regulating hair growth. The growth factors TGF-β, FGF-5, TNF-α, IL-1α, and IL-1β are known to negatively regulate hair growth. Based on this evidence, procyanidin B-3, isolated from the seed husks of *barley* (*Hordeum vulgare* L. var *distichon* Alefeld), was found to counteract the inhibitory effects of TGF-β1 on hair growth. Procyanidin B-2 also was shown to reduce the expression of protein kinase C, a known inhibitor of hair growth.

Raspberry may also have a role in treating hair loss. Based on previous work showing that capsaicin could promote hair growth, researchers tested raspberry ketone (RK), a structurally similar aromatic compound contained in red raspberries (*Rubus idaeus*) for similar effects (Figure 24.4). When applied to the scalp, .01% RK promoted hair growth in 50% of humans with alopecia areata (N = 10) after 5 months. This effect appears to occur as a result of sensory neuron activation, resulting in increased levels of dermal insulin-like growth factor I (IGF-I).

Isoflavones and soy

Isoflavones are organic compounds that have biologic activities similar to estrogens, hence their other name phytoestrogens. In one study, dietary isoflavones increased both the number of hair follicles and IGF-I expression within the follicles of wild-type C57BL/6 mice, whereas this effect was not seen in control mice. In another study, both isoflavone (75 mg/day) and capsaicin (6 mg/day) were administered to 31 human volunteers.

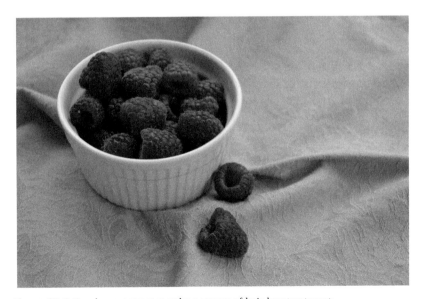

Figure 24.4 Raspberry extract may be a source of hair loss treatment.

Significantly more hair growth was seen in the treatment group (20/31, 64.5%) than was seen in the placebo group (2/17, 11.8%).

An oral soy peptide derivative called soymetide-4 was shown to prevent chemotherapy-induced alopecia in rats. In another study, dietary soy was given to C3H/HeJ rats grafted with skin from alopecia areata rats, and found to have a dose-dependent protective effect on the hair follicles, with lower rates of alopecia observed in the 5% and 20% groups versus the 1% soy diet groups. However, some controversy exists because one older study suggested that protease inhibitors derived from soymilk could actually *reduce* unwanted hair growth.

Ginseng, gingko and relatives

Ginseng has been investigated extensively for its role in potentially treating male and female pattern hair loss. The active ingredients are believed to be saponins, of which 26 have been isolated and identified. Red ginseng was shown to have superior efficacy over white ginseng in promoting hair growth in cultured mouse vibrissal hair follicles. Part of its mechanism of action may be through the inhibition of 5A-reductase enzyme. At present, only one human clinical trial exists showing that oral consumption of Korean red ginseng extract (3000 mg/day) for 24 weeks effectively increased hair density and thickness in patients with androgenetic alopecia. Interestingly, Ginkgo biloba has also been shown to regrow hair when applied as a 70% ethanolic extract to mice.

Plant-derived 5-alpha-reductase inhibitors

Finasteride is presently the most effective 5-alpha reductase (5-AR) inhibitor available today. However, its side effect profile has prompted many researchers to investigate plant-based alternatives to finasteride. A number of these are listed in Table 24.2.

Saw palmetto (*Serenoa repens*) has been suggested as an alternative to finasteride in treating urinary symptoms of benign prostatic hypertrophy in men. Its active ingredients, liposterolic extract and β-sitosterol, have 5-AR inhibiting properties. However, the only data we have examining its role in treating hair loss is a small trial from 1999 wherein 6/10 men treated with oral saw palmetto were subjectively improved after oral intake of softgels containing saw palmetto extract for 5 months. Although it was a randomized, double-blind, placebo-controlled trial, no objective measures were used to assess hair follicle diameter or density.

Green tea was identified as a 5-AR inhibitor in 1995, and it was suggested as a treatment for androgenetic alopecia in 2002. Researchers observed

Table 24.2 Summary of plant-derived 5-alpha reductase inhibitors.

Plant	Latin name	Active ingredient(s)
Saw Palmetto, American dwarf palm	*Serenoa repens* *Sabal serrutala*	Oleic acid Lauric acid Myristic acid γ-linoleic acid β-sitosterol
Black pepper	*Piper nigrum leaf*	Active lignin 1* Active lignin 2* Piperine (high in linoleic, oleic, and palmitic acids)
Green Tea Extract Japanese False Nettle	*Epicatechin-* *Boehmeria nipononivea*	With palmitic acid α-linoleic acid Elaidic acid Stearic acid
Safflower	*Carthamus tinctorius L.*	Carthamin Carthamidin Isocarthamidin
Lingzhi mushroom Red bayberry bark	*Ganoderma lucidum* *Murica rubra*	Triterpenoids Myricanol Myricanone
White cedar seed Japanese climbing fern Puereria flower	*Thuja occidentalis* *Lygodium japonicum* *Puerariae flos*	unknown Oleic, linoleic, and palmitic acids Soyasaponin I Kaikasaponin III
Rosemary Red Ginseng	*Rosmarinus officialis* *Ginseng rhizome and Ginsenoside Ro*	unknown Triterpine saponins Ginsenoside Rg1
Dried root of plant	*Sophora flavescens*	unknown

Note: *Interestingly, these two lignans also demonstrated stimulation of melanogenesis, a property that could be applied in the treatment of gray hair.

that its ability to inhibit 5-AR increased when the gallate ester in EGCG was replaced with a long-chain fatty acids, such as lauric (10 carbon chain), myristic (12 chain carbon), and stearic acid (16 carbon chain). The most potent inhibitor of 5-AR was formed with the addition of palmitic acid (14 carbon chain).

Another plant investigated for its ability to block 5-AR is *Sophora flavescens*. This plant has been widely used in Chinese medicine for the treatment of cancers and inflammation. When it was applied to the backs of C57BL/6 mice, the anagen cycle was initiated earlier than in control groups, but it did not affect dermal papillae cells in culture. It specifically induced mRNA levels of growth factors such as insulin-like growth factor and keratinocyte growth factor, and was found to significantly inhibit 5-AR levels in comparison with controls.

Essential oils

Scientists in Korea demonstrated the hair growth-promoting effects of *Zizyphus jujuba* essential oil. This comes from a thorny rhamnaceous plant that is already used as an analgesic as well as to prevent pregnancy and diabetes. Researchers applied 0.1%, 1%, and 10% concentrations of the essential oil to the backs of shaved BALB/c mice and observed their growth over 21 days. They found that the mice treated with the 1% and 10% solution had significantly longer hair (9.96 and 10.02 mm) than the control group (8.94 mm).

In India, the seeds of the teak tree (*Tectona grandis*) have been used by ancient tribesmen to prevent hair loss. Their hair-growth promoting activity was recently demonstrated to be on par with and slightly more effective than minoxidil 2% solution. Researchers in India tested 5% and 10% petroleum ether extract on shaved denuded skin of albino mice. They found that the treatment groups had a greater number of follicles entering the anagen phase (64% and 51%) than minoxidil treated follicles (49%).

Vitamin C

Vitamin C has long been known for its antioxidant effects, but its use in cosmetics has been made more difficult by its lack of stability. Therefore, researchers investigated the use of a more stable vitamin C derivative, L-ascorbic acid 2-phosphate, to stimulate hair growth. They found that it induced an earlier telogen to anagen conversion in C57BL/6 mice as compared with the control group, and prompted a greater elongation of hair shafts in treated cultures. This and a subsequent study both found a significant increase in mRNA expression of insulin-like growth factor (IGF-1) in treated cell lines, specifically mediated by phosphatidylinositol 3-kinase (PI3K). It may also work by attenuating DHT-induced dickkopf-1 expression in dermal papilla cells. So far, no clinical trials using this compound in humans have been conducted.

Amino acids and their derivatives

Taurine is a naturally occurring β-amino acid produced by methionine and cysteine metabolism. Its production by mammals is limited, so dietary intake is crucial. When human hair follicles were treated with taurine in vitro, there was significantly greater hair elongation in the treated groups versus the control. When follicles were exposed to TGF-β1, their growth was compromised, but taurine was found to have a protective effect.

L-carnitine is an amino acid necessary for the transport of fatty acids to the mitochondria for subsequent β-oxidation and energy production. It has been shown to increase hair shaft elongation in vitro as well as to prolong anagen by up-regulating proliferation and down-regulating apoptosis in organ-cultured human scalp hair follicles. L-carnitine-L-tartrate was also shown to promote human hair growth when applied topically in a prospective, randomized, placebo-controlled observational study of human volunteers (N $=$ 26, placebo $=$ 25).

Products for hair coloring

Since the ancient Egyptian days of Cleopatra, women have used various plant extracts and vegetable dyes to darken and color their hair. One of the most common of these is henna, a plant with leaves that render a burgundy-colored compound called lawsone. It is primarily concentrated in the leaves and has an affinity for protein. When the lawsone is dissolved in an acidic liquid such as lemon juice, it can be applied to the hair and will bind to the proteins after several hours of leave-in. The widespread use of henna is somewhat limited by availability and the risk of contact dermatitis. Most modern hair dyes contain manufactured ingredients such as para-phenylene diamine.

Recently, researchers have investigated other plant compounds for possible sources of hair coloring. Typically, the hair coloring process involves the application of dye precursers (usually p-diamines and p-aminophenols) followed by an oxidizing agent (usually H_2O_2). This is done at an alkaline pH because the hair swells, the cuticle lifts, and it becomes easier for dyes to penetrate the hair shaft. However, this alkaline pH can cause damaging side-reactions to the hair follicle.

Therefore, different researchers have investigated the use of laccase, an enzyme produced by various fungi, plants, bacteria, and insects as an alternative oxidizing agent. One group used the laccase enzyme from *Trametes versicolor* (also called the Turkey tail for its resemblance to the tail of a wild turkey) to oxidize natural plant-derived phenolic compounds. A second group used laccase from the Japanese mushroom, *Flammulina velutipes*. Both groups had excellent results achieving optimum coloring and withstanding subsequent shampooing.

Products for hair care and hair protection

Peptides

Black African hair can be extremely difficult to style due to its tight curl. As a result, many people resort to chemical straighteners or repeated application of flat irons or curling irons to smooth the hair and make it more manageable. However, this can result in a further compromise in the hair strength and leave it even more brittle and prone to breakage. Hair surface tends to be negatively charged, and becomes even more negatively charged when it is damaged. Therefore, peptides that have a positive charge are used to coat and repair the cuticle. There is evidence that the location of the positive charge (on the C-terminal end, which is smaller than the N-terminal end) allows for better penetration of the peptide component.

One group developed a keratin-based peptide, which contains 13 amino acids and mimics a fragment of the human keratin type II cuticular protein, that is encoded by the KRT85 gene. When applied to black relaxed hair, it was found to improve both mechanical and thermal properties. This corroborated previous results showing the same keratin peptide could also restore properties of over-bleached, damaged hair.

Cassia plant

Recent studies have demonstrated that extract from the plant *Cassia tora* and *Cassia obtusifolia* can provide an alternative to the chemical cationic polymers traditionally used in the conditioning process. The endosperm of the Cassia plant contains a quaternized galactomannan, which has a positive charge that binds to anionic surfactants to form a water-insoluble complex called coacervate. This complex helps reduce friction from the combing of wet hair and thus reduce breakage. Researchers found that the ability to use this plant extract reduced the amount of chemical polymer needed. This is an advantage because the chemical polymer can negatively affect the lather and stability.

Honeydew

The cotton honeydew also offers smoothing and protective effects on the hair shaft (Figure 24.5). It contains a number of oligosaccharides such as fructose, glucose, inositol, and trehalose, among others. One half-head study showed that patients treated with a 1% honeydew extract had increased smoothness compared with the control side. Also, scanning electron microscopy showed that the cuticle scales of treated hair appeared to lie more smoothly and were less prone to chipping. Honeydew is already available in several shampoos and conditioners.

Eucalyptus

Varying concentrations of scalp lotions with eucalyptus were applied in half-head studies in a period over 2.5–5 months, and found to increase

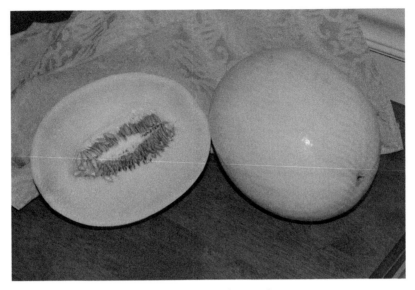

Figure 24.5 Honeydew elements may improve hair quality.

both hair elasticity and hair gloss intensity. More than 70% of the participants subjectively felt that the treated hair fibers had improved physical properties. One explanation may be an observed increase in the fraction of beta-sheets in the hair cortex, which are believed to lend strength to the hair fiber. On histologic examination, there was no noticeable change in hair caliber (thickness) between the treated and untreated hair fibers. Eucalyptus is presently available in commercial "root awakening" formulas.

Conclusion

Male and female pattern hair loss can be heartbreaking both for patients and for the physicians who treat them. We are presently quite limited with only two FDA-approved medications for treating hair loss. The cosmeceutical market for hair loss products will be exciting to watch as more plant-based products are introduced and more viable alternatives are available to patients.

Further reading

Collin C, Gautier B, Gaillard O, et al. Protective effects of taurine on human hair follicle grown *in vitro*. *Int J Cosm Sci* 2006; **28**: 289–298.
Foitzik K, Hoting E, Pertile P, et al. L-Carnitine tartrate promotes human hair growth in vitro. *J Inves Dermatol* 2006; **126**: s27 (P146).
Hiipakka RA, Zhang HZ, Dai W, et al. Structure-activity relationships for inhibition of human 5α-reductases by polyphenols. *Biochem Pharmacol* 2002; **63**: 1165–1176.

Kamimura A, Takahashi T. Procyanidin B-3, isolated from barley and identified as a hair-growth stimulant, has the potential to counteract inhibitory regulation by TGF-β1. *Exp Dermatology* 2002; **11**: 532–541.

Kamimura A, Takahashi T. Procyanidin B-2, extracted from apples, promotes hair growth: A laboratory study. *Br J Dermatol* 2002; **146**: 41–51.

Kobayashi N, Suzuki R, Koide C, et al. Effect of leaves of Ginkgo biloba on hair regrowth in C3H strain mice. *Yakagaku Zasshi* 1993: **113**: 718–724.

Kwack MH, Shin SH, Kim SR, et al. L-Ascorbic acid 2-phosphate promotes elongation of hair shafts via the secretion of insulin-like growth factor-1 from dermal papilla cells through phosphatidylinositol 3-kinase. *Br J Dermatol* 2009; **160**: 1157–1162.

Matsuda H, Yamazaki M, Asanuma Y, et al. Promotion of hair growth by *Ginsenz Radix* on cultured mouse vibrissal hair follicles. *Phytother Res* 2003; **17**: 797–800.

Takahashi T, Kamiya T, Yokoo Y. Proanthocyanidins from grape seeds promote proliferation of mouse hair follicle cells *in vitro* and convert hair cycle *in vivo*. *Acta Derm Venereol* 1998; **78**: 428–432.

Zhao J, Harada N, Kurihara K, et al. Dietary isoflavone increases insulin-like growth factor-I production, thereby promoting hair growth in mice. *J Nutr Biochem* 2011; **22**: 227–233.

CHAPTER 25

Cosmeceuticals for Treating and Preventing Scars

Ellen Marmur and Katherine Nolan
Icahn School of Medicine at Mount Sinai, New York, NY, USA

Introduction

Cutaneous scarring is one of the most common concerns of patients visiting dermatologists. Every year over 100 million patients in the developed world develop scars as a result of 25 million operations after trauma and 55 million elective operations. Moreover, there are approximately 4 million burn scars, 70% of which occur in children, and 11 million keloid scars. Individuals with skin scarring may face substantial physical and psychosocial consequences. We will describe many of the most commonly used actives in scar treatments as well as some natural remedies that are becoming increasingly popular.

Pathogenesis

Normal wound healing is composed of three phases. The first phase is inflammation which is followed by the proliferative or granulation phase, and finally the maturation or remodeling phase. Many signaling molecules, including growth factors, matrix metalloproteinases, mitogen-activated protein kinases, and tissue inhibitors of metalloproteinases, regulate this complex process of wound healing. Abnormalities in this complex process lead to the development of hypertrophic scars and keloids.

Normally in the maturation phase, concurrent collagen synthesis and degradation cause the wound to soften and flatten and the connective tissue elements normally decrease after the third week. However, in keloids, the collagen synthesis is 20 times higher than in normal skin and three times higher than in hypertrophic scars. Moreover, the ratio of type I to type III collagen is also high in hypertrophic scars and keloids.

Cosmeceuticals and Cosmetic Practice, First Edition. Edited by Patricia K. Farris.
© 2014 John Wiley & Sons, Ltd. Published 2014 by John Wiley & Sons, Ltd.

Risk factors

There are several known risk factors for the development of hypertrophic scars and keloids. The most important risk factor is genetic predisposition. For example, keloids are 15 times more likely to occur in darker-skinned individuals. Also, tension in wounds has also been strongly associated in the development of hypertrophic scars and keloids. For this reason, wounds that cross joints are more likely to form hypertrophic scars due to constant tension forces that disrupt normal healing. Keloids and hypertrophic scars are also less likely to occur in certain areas like acral surfaces and mucous membranes. Finally, formation of abnormal scars seems to be influenced by hormones, especially in women. Keloids tend to develop more commonly during and after puberty while the menopause seems to induce recession of these scars. Similarly, women report keloid onset and enlargement during pregnancy.

Cosmeceutical actives that are most commonly used in the prevention and treatment of scars

Table 25.1 shows the cosmeceutical actives and their effects on the treatment of scars.

Onion extract

Onion extract or *Allium cepa* is a commonly used ingredient in over-the-counter scar treatments. This is the main active in many over-the-counter scar remedies. These products are popular with patients due to their availability, low cost, and appealing reputation as a natural product. Onion extracts were once thought of as a promising new treatment modality due to their in vitro effects which suggest that onion extracts accelerate wound healing through their effect on mast cells and fibroblasts. In these studies, onion extract acts as an anti-inflammatory and down-regulates collagen production. Quercetin and onion extract also up-regulate matrix metalloproteinase-1 expression. Unfortunately, this promising in vitro data has not been well replicated in the clinical setting. Several clinical studies failed to demonstrate any added benefit with onion extract compared to plain petrolatum in patients with post-surgical scars. Most recently, two studies showed that a gel containing onion, when used in combination with intralesional corticosteroids or alone, improved the overall appearance of hypertrophic scars. However, these studies were small and not randomized or double-blinded. Overall, more clinical research needs to be done to fully elucidate the efficacy of onion extracts in scar treatment.

Table 25.1 Cosmeceutical actives and their effects.

Active	Evidence
Onion extract	In vitro studies showed that onion extracts accelerate wound healing through their effect on mast cells and fibroblasts in the inflammatory cascade, as well as their anti-inflammatory effects. Also, they decrease expression of fibroblasts in vitro. Two small clinical studies showed improvement in the overall appearance of hypertrophic scars.
Vitamin A	Daily topical application of retinoic acid has also been shown to reduce the size and pruritis associated with hypertrophic and keloid scars. A large randomized, double-blind study showed that 0.05% retinoic acid showed a significant reduction in the size of scars.
Vitamin E	Large clinical studies failed to show an improvement in the appearance of scars. However, some more recent smaller studies have shown more positive results for the use of vitamin E in the prevention and treatment of surgical scars.
Imiquimod	Randomized, double-blind studies have shown the efficacy of 5% imiquimod cream in the prevention of hypertrophic scars. Imiquimod was found to significantly improve scar appearance particularly color and elevation.
Silicone	Studies support the efficacy of both silicone sheeting and gels in the prevention and treatment of scars. However, silicone sheeting has been shown to be significantly more effective than silicone gels.
Antibiotic ointment	Polymyxin B sulfate-bacitracin zinc-neomycin sulfate helped minimize scarring associated with abrasion-type wounds. In particular, the use of this antibiotic ointment had a most pronounced effect on reducing pigmentary changes.
Mango butter	A study of a cream composed of mango butter, olein and vitamin E in a rat model found that the cream allowed for better wound closure and significantly decreased scarring.
Honey	Clinical trials involving patients with superficial burns showed the anti-inflammatory effects of honey. Studies have also demonstrated the honey's ability to retain moisture in the wound.
Aloe	Extracts have shown significant activity in the repair of pressure ulcers, radiation damage and other types of wounds. Also, aloe can help increase proliferation of human fibroblasts and increase intracellular communication.

Topical vitamin A

Vitamin A and the synthetic retinoids are common ingredients in widely available cosmeceuticals. Studies show that topical vitamin A helps to improve the appearance of scars, especially those that are hypertrophic or keloidal. Topical retinoic acid flattens, softens and reduces hyperpigmentation in scars. A large randomized, double-blind study in 1986 by Daly et al. showed that 0.05% retinoic acid cream significantly reduced the size of scars. A smaller but more recent study by Mizutani et al. showed that 0.25% tocoretinate ointment, a vitamin A derivative, significantly reduced the size, erythema, stiffness, and pruritis associated with mature hyper-trophic scars. This author finds retinoic acid 0.1% works moderately to reduce scar pain on the scalp post operatively or for post herpetic (zoster) neuropathic pain. While studies seem to support the efficacy of vitamin A in the treatment of scars, disadvantages include possible systemic absorption and teratogenicity in pregnant women as well as skin irritation and photosensitivity.

Topical vitamin E

Vitamin E, also known as tocopherol, is another common ingredient found in over-the-counter anti-scarring products. Vitamin E is a lipid soluable antioxidant that may penetrate into the reticular dermis where it theoretically reduces the formation of oxygen radicals which impair healing and damage cellular membranes, lipids, and DNA. Also, vitamin E alters glycosaminoglycan and collagen production and inhibits the peroxidation of lipids and thus vitamin E may stabilize cell membranes.

While anecdotal reports have suggested Vitamin E accelerates wound healing and improves the appearance of scars, clinical studies have not supported these claims. In a study of burn patients who had undergone surgical reconstruction, vitamin E failed to show an improvement in the appearance, range of motion and thickness of scars. In fact, the use of vitamin E was associated with a higher rate of local reactions that contributed to a worsened appearance of the scars. However, more recent studies have shown more positive results for the use of vitamin E in the prevention and treatment of surgical scars as well as for systemic sclerosis related digital ulcers. It seems that more research is needed before vitamin E can be recommended as an effective treatment for scars.

Imiquimod

Topical imiquimod, an immune response modifier, has a variety of uses in dermatology. This popular dermatologic therapy is used to treatactinic keratoses, superficial basal cell andsquamous cell carcinomas, genital warts and molluscum contagiousum. Imiquimod 5% cream has been shown in one study to prevent the recurrence of keloids after surgical excision. Most recently, Prado et al. conducted a randomized, double-blind study of 5% imiquimod cream in the prevention of hypertrophic scars following breast surgery. Imiquimod 5% cream was found to significantly improve scar appearance, particularly color and elevation, when evaluated at 24 weeks post-surgery. Of great interest, there was an absence of keloids and hypertrophic scars in the treatment group. Side effects seen in the imiquimod group included pinpoint bleeding, local pain and erythema.

Overall, 5% imiquimod cream seems to be an effective treatment for the prevention of hypertrophic scars and keloids.

Silicone ointment, gel and sheeting

Since their introduction 30 years ago, silicone topicals and sheeting are some of the most commonly used treatments for the prevention and reduction of hypertrophic scars. While the mechanism of silicone gel sheeting is still not completely understood, it is thought that silicone helps create an occluded, hydrated environment that decreases capillary activity which helps reduce fibroblast-induced scar hypertrophy. The efficacy of silicone gel sheeting in reducing erythema, pruritis, induration and the size of scars is well documented. There have also been numerous studies supporting the efficacy of silicone gel in the treatment of scars. However, studies have shown that silicone gel may not be as effective as silicone sheeting. Sawada et al. showed that the use of silicone cream alone showed 22% improvement in scarring while silicone cream used in conjunction with an occlusive dressing showed an 82% improvement. Overall, studies support the efficacy of both silicone sheeting and gels in the prevention and treatment of scars. Anecdotal observations suggest the occlusion effect in scar reduction is temporary.

Antibiotic ointment and petrolatum

For clean, sterile wounds, petrolatum is equivalent to antibiotic ointment for wound healing. If infection is a concern, for example, a wound caused by laceration or abrasion from an unclean surface, then wound healing is compromised and the risk of scar formation increases. In fact, one randomized study by Berger et al. showed polymyxin B sulfate-bacitracin zinc-neomycin sulfate helped minimize scarring associated with abrasion type wounds. This study found triple antibiotic ointment was superior to gauze dressings alone in minimizing scarring. In particular, the use of this antibiotic ointment had a most pronounced effect on reducing pigmentary changes. The mechanism of action may be simply the vehicle, petrolatum, optimizes wound healing and avoids scar formation, where gauze is a dry agent and may not allow optimal healing. Another study showed that blisters treated with the triple antibiotic ointment had significantly faster healing than wounds treated with any antiseptic and those receiving no treatment. These studies seem to support the idea that the use of triple antibiotic ointment helps reduce scarring though eliminating microbial contamination in wounds. These ointments are commonly used in over-the-counter preparations but can sometimes be associated with irritation and contact dermatitis in sensitive individuals.

Natural therapies

Mango butter

Exotic lipids from the shea, mango, kokum tree and others have become increasingly popular as emollients. Accordingly, a foot cream containing mango butter and its olein fraction fortified with vitamin E was tested on human volunteers with a variety of foot ailments including cracked skin. The mango butter cream healed cracked skin in all participants with no irritancy or contact sensitivity. Furthermore, the same test cream exhibited significant healing response in incision and excision wound models in animals. Further studies on the wound healing properties of botanical emollients are warranted.

Honey

Honey is thought to be one of the most ancient treatments for wounds. Honey is known to have antimicrobial and anti-inflammatory activity Studies have also demonstrated honey's ability to retain moisture in the wound. Finally, honey has angiogenic activity and aids in the formation of granulation tissue and reepithelialization.

Aloe

Aloe vera (*Aloe barbadensis*) has been used since antiquity for various dermatologic ailments and has been used especially to treat wounds and burns. Several studies support aloe's beneficial role in wound healing. Extracts have shown significant activity in the repair of pressure ulcers, radiation damage and other types of wounds. Also, aloe increases the proliferation of human fibroblasts and increases intracellular communication. Aloe's role in the treatment of burns is thought to be related to its ability to reduce tissue loss from ischemia by decreasing thromboxane A2, prostaglandin 2α, and thromboxane B2, which cause vasoconstriction and platelet aggregation.

Conclusion

Overall, there are a great variety of treatments available for the treatment of scars. In addition to the topical treatments described, other therapies like intralesional corticosteroids, laser therapy, and cryosurgery are also used to prevent and treat scars. Of the treatments described, silicone gel sheeting and imiquimod have the most clinical evidence to support their efficacy, especially in hypertrophic scars and keloids. Both vitamin A and antibiotic ointment have proven efficacy as well, but their effects are subtler and may not be suitable as a monotherapy for hypertrophic scars and keloids. While onion extract and vitamin E are common ingredients in popular scar treatments, more clinical evidence is needed to support their efficacy. Vitamin E has been associated with contact dermatitis and worsening of scar appearance and therefore should be used with caution. Popular natural remedies like aloe, honey and mango butter show promise and are associated with few side effects, but larger, controlled studies are needed to ascertain their efficacy.

Further reading

Ahn ST, Monafo WW, Mustoe TA. Topical silicone gel for the prevention and treatment of hypertrophic scar. *Arch Surg* 1991; **126**: 499–504.

Bayat A, McGrouther DA, Ferguson MW. Skin scarring. *BMJ* 2003; **326**: 88–92.

Bedi MK, Shenefelt PD. Herbal therapy in dermatology. *Archives of Dermatology* 2002; **138**: 232–242.

Berger RS, Pappert AS, Van Zile PS, Cetnarowski WE. A newly formulated topical triple-antibiotic ointment minimizes scarring. *Cutis: Cutaneous Medicine for the Practitioner* 2000; **65**: 401–404.

Daly TJ, Golitz LE, Weston WL. A double-blind placebo-controlled efficacy study of tretinoin cream 0.05% in the treatment of keloids and hypertrophic scars. *J Invest Dermatol* 1986; **86**: 470.

Jackson BA, Shelton AJ. Pilot study evaluating topical onion extract as treatment for postsurgical scars. *Dermatologic Surgery: Official Publication for American Society for Dermatologic Surgery* [et al] 1999; **25**: 267–269.

Martin A. The use of antioxidants in healing. *Dermatologic Surgery: Official Publication for American Society for Dermatologic Surgery* [et al.] 1996; **22**: 156–160.

Mizutani H, Yoshida T, Nouchi N, Hamanaka H, Shimizu M. Topical tocoretinate improved hypertrophic scar, skin sclerosis in systemic sclerosis and morphea. *J Dermatol* 1999; **26**(1): 11–17.

Prado A, Andrades P, Benitez S, Umana M. Scar management after breast surgery: Preliminary results of a prospective, randomized, and double-blind clinical study with aldara cream 5% (imiquimod). *Plastic and Reconstructive Surgery* 2005; **115**: 966–972.

Sawada Y, Sone K. Treatment of scars and keloids with a cream containing silicone oil. *Br J Plast Surg* 1990; **43**(6): 683–688.

Sund B. *New Developments in Wound Care*. London: PJB Publications, 2000.

Zurada JM, Kriegel D, Davis IC. Topical treatments for hypertrophic scars. *Journal of the American Academy of Dermatology* 2006; **55**: 1024–1031.

CHAPTER 26

Sun Protection and Self-Tanners

Darrell S. Rigel
New York University School of Medicine, New York, NY, USA

Introduction

The importance of effective protection against exposure to ultraviolet radiation (UVR) energy cannot be overstated. UVR plays a key role in increased risk for the development of skin cancer and accelerated photoaging changes. At current rates, 1 in 5 Americans will develop a skin cancer of some sort during their lifetime, with over 2,000,000 new cases appearing in 2012 in the US. The incidence of malignant melanoma is increasing faster than any other cancer in the United States. In 1935, the lifetime risk for an American developing invasive melanoma was 1 in 1500. In 2012, this risk was 1 in 52 for invasive melanomas and 1 in 27 if in-situ melanomas are included. The economic magnitude of this public health problem is illustrated by the fact that costs associated with the treatment of skin cancers are over 500 million dollars annually in the US alone. Therefore, the development and implementation of effective mechanisms that protect the skin from cancer-causing UV rays are critical.

UVR was recently upgraded to the highest cancer risk category by the International Agency for Research on Cancer (IARC). UVR is linked to more cancers worldwide than any other carcinogen. Although skin cancer is preventable, rates of unprotected sun exposure remain high. Given the rapid rise in skin cancer incidence, the need for protection from UVR exposure and for the use of safer alternatives to achieve a "tanned" look for those who are insistent upon doing so is increasingly important.

Spectral differences related to UV photocarcinogenesis

Most of the cutaneous damage resulting from radiation exposure occurs from the ultraviolet (UV) band. The shortest of the ultraviolet rays, Ultraviolet C (UVC, 100–280 nm), fails to penetrate the Earth's ozone layer and

Cosmeceuticals and Cosmetic Practice, First Edition. Edited by Patricia K. Farris.
© 2014 John Wiley & Sons, Ltd. Published 2014 by John Wiley & Sons, Ltd.

thus exerts little damage. Ultraviolet B (UVB, 290–320 nm) is responsible for most of the cutaneous changes induced by exposure to the sun. Known biochemical changes induced by UVB include alterations in DNA, RNA, and protein synthesis, induction of cyclobutyl pyrimidine dimers, and production of various cytokines.

In the past, UVA was believed to play less of a role in the pathogenesis of skin cancer and sun damage. The longer wavelengths of UVA (320–400 nm) allow deeper penetration into the skin. UVA induces an immediate pigment-darkening reaction and new melanin pigment formation. Earlier sun protection focused primarily on eliminating UVB exposure to the skin. UVA is now known to contribute to skin cancers by inducting DNA mutations directly as well as by augmenting damage incurred by UVB. Human skin exposed to UVA has altered expression of the p53 tumor suppressor protein . These mutations can be reduced by using UVA sunscreens, demonstrating that there is less p53 accumulation with better UVA protection.

Topical photoprotection

Topical photoprotection works primarily through two mechanisms: (1) scattering and reflection of UV energy; and (2) absorption of UV energy. Many current sunscreens contain ingredients that work through both mechanisms in terms of UV protection.

The most important assay for determining the effectiveness of a sunscreen is the sun protection factor (SPF). The SPF measures a sunscreen's ability to prevent development of erythema upon exposure to UV radiation, primarily UVB. The SPF value is defined as the ratio of the UV energy required to produce minimal erythema on protected skin to that required to produce the same erythema on unprotected skin in the same individual. For example, an individual using a sunscreen SPF 4 will take four times as long to develop cutaneous erythema when exposed to UVB radiation, as compared to when that individual has no protection. The FDA, which oversees the marketing and distribution of sunscreen products in the United States, mandates that a sunscreen agent must provide at least an SPF value of 2. Most commercially available sunscreen products have SPF values that exceed the minimum protection.

Despite attempts by the FDA to educate consumers and promote appropriate branding by manufacturers, sunscreen labeling has its limitations. The complicated names, as well as the variations in names for any given agent, may be overwhelming for the average consumer. The photostability of sunscreens is not quantified or labeled, and varies according to the chemical agent. The SPF value primarily measures a sunscreen's ability to protect against UVB radiation and does not adequately address the effects of UVA. In addition, SPF readings may also vary for a given agent depending on the light source.

As of the time of writing of this chapter, the FDA is preparing for the adoption of new sunscreen labeling regulations designed to enhance consumer understanding. The term "broad spectrum" will only be able to be used when both SPF 15 or higher are present and a UVA protection threshold is reached. The term "Waterproof" will be banned and only "Water resistant" (40 or 80 minutes) will be allowed. Confusing terminology such as "sunblock" and "all-day protection" is prohibited. A proposed SPF cap of 50+ has been deferred pending the results of several ongoing studies.

Sunscreening agents and mechanisms of action

Sunscreen use began in the early 20th century. Salicylates were the first agents used in sunscreen preparations, with the first reported sunscreen containing benzyl salicylate and benzyl cinnamate. In the 1940s, p-Aminobenzoic acid (PABA) was patented and incorporated into sunscreen formulations. Since its debut, various formulations and derivates of PABA have been introduced onto the sunscreen market.

The Food and Drug Administration (FDA) approves the use of 19 chemicals as defined sunscreen agents. Since no single agent effectively provides adequate protection from both UVA and UVB radiation, nearly all commercially available sunscreen products contain agents from both groups. Two or more sunscreen active ingredients may be combined with each other in a single product when used in the concentrations approved by the FDA for each agent. Each individual active ingredient must contribute a minimum SPF at least 2 to the finished product, with the finished product having a minimum SPF of not less than the number of sunscreen active ingredients used in the combination multiplied by 2.

Sunscreen agents are classified based on their method of protection. Organic sunscreens ("chemical sunscreens") absorb ultraviolet radiation while inorganic sunscreens ("physical blockers") act as particulate matter that reflect and scatter incident light and UVR.

Organic sunscreens

Organic sunscreen agents protect the skin by absorbing UV energy and transforming it into heat energy. These compounds absorb ultraviolet radiation and convert the energy into longer wave radiation. The sunscreen chemical is excited to a higher energy state from its ground state. As the excited molecule returns to the ground state, energy is emitted that is lower in magnitude than the energy initially absorbed. This energy is emitted in

Table 26.1 Sunscreen agents and their UV protective wavelengths.

Sunscreen	Range of protection (nm)	Maximal effect of protection (nm)
PABA and PABA esters		
PABA	260–313	283
Padimate O	290–315	311
Padimate A	290–315	309
Glycerol aminobenzoate	260–313	297
Cinnamates		
Octyl methoxycinnamate	280–310	311
Cinoxate	270–328	290
Salicylates		
Homosalicylate	290–315	306
Octyl salicylate	260–310	307
Triethanolamine salicylate	269–320	298
Octocrylene	287–323	303
Etocrylene	296–383	303
Benzophenones		
Oxybenzone	270–350	290–325
Dioxybenzone	206–380	284–327
Sulisobenzone	250–380	286–324
Menthylanthranilate	200–380	336
Dibenzoylmethanes		
Tert-butylmethoxy dibenzoylmethane (Parsol)	310–400	358
4-isopropyldibenzoyl-methane (Eusolex)	310–400	345
Trometrizole trisiloxane, terephthalylidene dicamphor sulfonic acid (Mexoryl XL)	300–400	328

the form of longer wavelengths, typically as very weak red light or mild infrared radiation.

Sunscreening agents are generally aromatic compounds conjugated with a carbonyl group. These synthetically derived compounds can be broadly categorized into two groups: UVB (290–320 nm) and UVA (320–400 nm) absorbing agents. Sunscreen agents can be classified based on their chemical properties, and each class has its own characteristic absorption spectra (Table 26.1).

p-Aminobenzoic acid (PABA) was a widely used sunscreen in the 1950s and 1960s. Several of the properties pertaining to the limitations of PABA can be attributed to its chemical structure: amino and carboxylic acid groups in a *para* orientation on a benzene nucleus. The highly polar nature of PABA made this agent extremely water-soluble, but the increased hydrogen bonding between molecules also promoted a crystalline physical state. This led to some difficulty in manufacturing a solvent that ensured continuous dissolution of PABA. The amine and carboxyl groups also made the PABA molecule sensitive to pH changes, and therefore somewhat labile in its effectiveness as a UV chemical absorbing agent. The molecule's lack of stability also led to changes in the color of the product when exposed to air.

Glycerol PABA was subsequently developed to protect the carboxylic acid group from pH changes and therefore was slightly more stable than the original PABA formulation. Other preparations attempted to protect both the carboxyl and the amine group. Padimate O (N, N-dimethyl PABA octyl ester) addressed many of the original structure's limitations and became a widely used sunscreen agent. Both the amino and the carboxyl groups are protected, making Padimate O less sensitive to pH changes. This new chemical structure also resulted in decreased intermolecular hydrogen bonding, resulting in a sunscreen agent that is a liquid instead of a crystalline solid.

The original PABA fell out of favor largely because of staining and allergic contact reactions. There is a much higher presence of contact and photocontact allergy to PABA than to other sunscreening agents. The PABA derivates also were reported to induce contact sensitization. Sensitization to PABA showed strong reactions to benzocaine, suggesting that reports of glycerol PABA allergy may in fact have been due to impurities in glyceryl PABA preparations. Other PABA derivates such as Padimate A, and to a lesser extent, Padimate O, have also been reported to cause sensitization or photocontact sensitization. Padimate A was also found to cause phototoxicity and is no longer used in the United States.

Salicylates were the first UV chemical absorbers used in commercially available sunscreen preparations. In contrast to the *para* distribution of the carboxyl and amine groups, the salicylates are *ortho*-distributed (the carboxyl and amine groups are on neighboring carbon atoms on the benzene ring). This spatial arrangement allows hydrogen bonding within the molecule itself, leading to a UV absorbance of about 300 nm. This intramolecular hydrogen bonding results in increased molecule stability, less interaction with other compounds, and good overall safety record. The salicylate group of sunscreen agents includes octyl salicylate and homomenthyl salicylate.

Cinnamates are effective sunscreen agents with a peak absorption wavelength of about 305 nm. They are chemically related to balsam of Peru, coca leaves, cinnamic aldehyde and cinnamic oil. The chemical structure of the cinnamates, as a group, makes the molecule insoluble to water, requiring more frequent reapplication of the preparation. Contact dermatitis to the cinnamates and cross-sensitization to structurally related products have been reported.

Benzophenone derivates and anthranilates are effective at absorbing UVA radiation. Although the primary protective range for benzophenone is in the UVA range, a secondary protective band is also noted in the UVB range. The most commonly used benzophenone agents are oxybenzone and dioxybenzone. Although these ingredients are much less allergenic than PABA, they do nonetheless still carry a risk of photocontact and contact allergy. Anthranilates, such as menthylanthranilate, provide low-level, yet broad-spectrum coverage. They are commonly added to sunscreens to augment protection. Camphor is an agent widely used in Europe, but not approved for use in the United States. They are effective UVB absorbing agents.

Dibenzoylmenthanes are a group of sunscreen agents and are especially effective at offering protection against UVA radiation. Tert-butylmethoxydibenzoylmethane (Avobenzone, Parsol 1789) is approved for use in the United States, while isopropyldebenzoylmethane (Eusolex 8020) has been widely used in Europe. The latter has been associated with a high incidence of contact dermatitis, and has not been approved in the United States. In a study of 19 patients with positive photopatch tests to sunscreens, eight showed positive reactions to butyl methoxy dibenzoylmethane.

Tert-butylmethoxydibenzoylmethane has been reported to have photo-stability issues after exposure to small amounts of UVA. Several formulations have been developed to extend the stability of this agent, including the use octocrylene and diethylhexyl 2,6-naphthalate (DEHN).

Inorganic sunscreens

Inorganic sunscreens are particles that scatter and reflect UV energy back into the environment. In sufficient quantities, they will serve as a physical barrier to incident ultraviolet and visible light. Their popularity has grown in recent years due primarily to their low toxicity profile. These agents are fairly photostable and have not been shown to induce phototoxic or photoallergic reactions. They are also extremely effective in protecting against both UVA and UVB. The most common particulate sunscreen agents are titanium dioxide and zinc oxide.

Early formulations of physical sunscreen agents were not widely accepted because the particulate matters had to be incorporated in high concentrations, resulting in an opaque film on the skin in order to achieve adequate protection. This was often not cosmetically acceptable. Newer formulations provide "micronized" formulations that give rise to a more translucent appearance, and allow for adequate protection with improved cosmetic results. Comparison between zinc oxide and titanium dioxide showed that zinc oxide is superior for UVA protection in the 340–380 nm range and tends to be less pasty on the skin.

Effectiveness of photoprotection

Primary prevention programs for skin cancer that are focused on lowering UV exposure appear to be having a positive effect in lowering skin cancer

Table 26.2 Studies evaluating protective effects of sunscreens on melanoma.

Interval of sunscreen use examined	Findings
1974–75	Increased MM in users
1974–80	NS
1977–79	NS
1978–83	Increased MM in a subset of users
1979–80	Protective for MM
1980–82	NS
1981–85	NS
1981–86	Protective for MM
1988–90	Increased MM in users
1989–93	Protective for MM
1991–92	Increased MM in users
1994–97	Protective for MM
1994–98	NS
1995–97	Increased MM in a subset of users
1996–2008	Prospective study protective for MM

Note: NS, not significant.

incidence. Persons with a prior history of BCC had fewer subsequent BCCs develop if they protected themselves from UV exposure. Reduction in sun exposure by daily use of a sunscreen may reduce risk of SCC.

A meta-analysis of 11 studies of melanoma risk and sunscreen usage showed only a small protective advantage. However, when evaluating only the more recent studies where high SPF sunscreens were available, there appeared to be a protective effect and other inherent flaws associated with retrospective studies may be responsible for protection not being noted (Table 26.2). A 2011 prospective study by Green et al. showed a significant decrease in melanoma risk in persons who regularly used sunscreen daily versus those who only used sunscreen occasionally or less.

Sunless tanning

An alternative for those who desire the "tanned" look to their skin is to promote sunless tanning products which do not rely on actual UVR exposure to provide that tanned skin tone. These products use a substance called dihydroxyacetone (DHA), a colorless vegetable-derived sugar that interacts with dead surface cells in the epidermis to stain the skin. DHA is a 3-carbon sugar moiety that forms the active ingredient in sunless tanning preparations which was approved by the U.S. Food and Drug Administration (FDA) as a color additive for cosmetics in 1973. DHA reacts preferentially with basic amino acids found in abundance in the keratinized stratum corneum to form brown-black compounds called melanoidins. This interaction, also known as the Maillard or browning reaction, is a common occurrence between carbohydrates and amines and is the cause of browning of sugar-containing foods kept in storage. When applied topically, DHA works at the level of the stratum corneum, as evidenced by its inability to induce tanning in areas that lack a stratum corneum (e.g, mucous membranes), and its deeper tanning of areas with a thickened stratum corneum (e.g, palms, soles, elbows, knees, ankles, and hyperkeratotic lesions). Sunless tanning preparations typically contain 3–5% DHA. Persons using sunless tanning preparations without added UV filters should be cautioned that DHA and its melanoidin by-products afford only minimal UV protection: DHA alone provides an SPF of 3 or 4. Color change should be apparent within 1 hour, with maximal darkening between 8 and 24 hours. Most individuals report the disappearance of color over 5 to 7 days.

The prevalence of self-reported use of sunless tanning products in 2010 among US adolescents was 10.8%. Adolescent users of these products were more likely to be older and female, to perceive a tanned appearance as desirable, to have a parent or caregiver who used sunless tanning products, and to hold positive beliefs or attitudes about these products. Use of sunless tanning products was independently associated with indoor tanning and higher frequency of sunburn but not with use of sunscreen.

The data on whether sunless tanning is a helpful or harmful sun safety recommendation are scant. The safety of DHA application has recently been questioned and further studies may need to be performed to verify safety. However, several studies have shown a decline in UVR tanning when sunless tanners are used. A randomized trial that followed college students for one month after an intervention that included both sunless tanning and UV imaging found significant increases in self-efficacy and intentions to use sunscreen, and a non-significant trend toward less sunbathing and greater sun protection compared to a control group, suggesting no evidence of harm in promoting sunless tanning. Almost three-quarters (73%) of people receiving a sunless spray tan reported that they had decreased their indoor tanning since they began sunless tanning, while only 7% reported having increased their indoor tanning. These data suggest that the use of sunless tanning might be an effective way to enhance skin cancer prevention efforts.

Future outlook

Based upon the best current information available, a regimen of overall photoprotection which includes protective clothing, avoiding midday sun, and regular use of broad-spectrum high SPF sunscreen should provide significant protection and appears to be reducing melanoma incidence rates. This is the current recommendation of the American Academy of Dermatology, Skin Cancer Foundation and other major international organizations and it is also the recommendation that is best supported by the existing data. Sunless tanners are a reasonable alternative but more studies need to be performed to assure safety. Hopefully, we will have even more definitive answers to questions related to the optimization of effectiveness of sunscreens and other forms of photoprotection and on reducing the risk from exposure to UV radiation as improved photo-protective agents, strategies and methods are developed in the future.

Further reading

Cokkinides VE, Bandi P, Weinstock MA, Ward E. Use of sunless tanning products among US adolescents aged 11 to 18 years. *Arch Dermatol* 2010; **146**(9): 987–992.

Draelos ZD, et al. (*eds.*) *Cosmetic Formulation of Skin Care Products* (Cosmetic Science and Technology Series Vol. 30). New York: Taylor and Francis, 2006.

Draelos ZD. Self-tanning lotions: Are they a healthy way to achieve a tan? *Am J Clin Psychol* 2002; **3**(5): 317–318.

Huncharek M, Kupelnick B. Use of topical sunscreens and the risk of malignant melanoma: A meta-analysis of 9067 patients from 11 case-control studies. *Am J Public Health* 2002; **92**(7): 1173–1177.

Palm MD, O'Donoghue MN. Update on photoprotection. *Dermatologic Therapy* 2007; **20**(5): 360–376.

Pagoto SL, Schneider KL, Oleski J, Bodenlos JS, Ma Y. The sunless study: A beach randomized trial of a skin cancer prevention intervention promoting sunless tanning. *Arch Dermatol* 2010; **146**(9): 979–984.

Shaath, NA. Evolution of modern sunscreen chemicals. In: Lowe NJ, Shaath NA, Pathak MA (eds.) *Sunscreens: Development, Evaluation, and Regulatory Aspects*. New York: Marcel Dekker, 1997.

Sheehan DJ, Lesher JL., Jr The effect of sunless tanning on behavior in the sun: A pilot study. *South Med J* 2005; **98**(12): 1192–1195.

Vainio H, Miller AB, Bianchini F. An international evaluation of the cancer-preventive potential of sunscreens. *Int J Cancer* 2000; **88**(5): 838–842.

Westerdahl J, Ingvar C, Masback A, Olsson H. Sunscreen use and malignant melanoma. *Int J Cancer* 2000; **87**(1): 145–150.

CHAPTER 27

Cosmeceuticals for Rosacea and Facial Redness

Doris Day
New York University Medical Center, New York, NY, USA

Introduction

Rosacea is a common and chronic inflammatory skin disease that affects over 14 million Americans. Facial redness presenting as transient flushing or persistent erythema is a common early sign of rosacea. Additional features associated with this chronic cutaneous disorder include papules, pustules and telangiectasias, typically in a central facial distribution. For affected individuals, facial redness can cause embarrassment and adversely affect self-esteem and quality of life.

Carefully considered skin care regimens have been used as adjuvant treatments to therapeutic agents for rosacea, helping to ameliorate the symptoms of the condition. Cosmetic skin care treatments have traditionally been most effectively used in treating the least severe (and most common) subtype of rosacea: erythematotelangiectatic rosacea, characterized by diffuse, episodic reddening of the skin accompanied, in many cases, by the presence of superficially obvious blood vessels beneath the skin, as well as the common issues of impaired barrier function and the not uncommonly associated dryness, scaling and hyperirritability. Recent advances in the understanding of the pathophysiology of this group of skin conditions have sparked significant research in identifying new effective agents that work across multiple pathways.

Biochemical pathways

The pathophysiology of rosacea involves interrelated vascular and inflammatory pathways which have been the focus of research to find an appropriate treatment. Erythema results from increased blood circulation in the skin microvasculature in response to inflammatory signals. Prostaglandin E_2 (PGE_2) plays a major role in cutaneous blood circulation

---

Cosmeceuticals and Cosmetic Practice, First Edition. Edited by Patricia K. Farris.
© 2014 John Wiley & Sons, Ltd. Published 2014 by John Wiley & Sons, Ltd.

by producing vasodilation in response to external stimuli such as chemical exposure, physical damage and UV exposure. Elevated expression of vascular endothelial growth factor (VEGF) is observed in the skin of patients with rosacea, possibly leading to telangiectasia. UV exposure increases VEGF expression and reactive oxygen species (ROS, free radicals) exacerbate inflammation, both of which could lead to increased flares of rosacea. Microorganisms such as *Demodex folliculorum* and *Helicobacter pylori* are thought to stimulate immune response. Many of the above triggers involve pathways linked to increased expression of Toll-like Receptor 2 (TLR2), a major component of the innate immune system. TLR2 expression is altered in rosacea skin, which enhances skin's susceptibility to innate immune stimuli.

Basic skin care needs for rosacea management

The inflammatory and barrier-disruptive etiological aspects of rosacea frequently result in a patient having sensitive skin, with a greater propensity for irritation, burning, stinging and itching. Therefore, the most appropriate cleansers and skin care products for rosacea patients would have formulations that are minimally irritating and preferably are designed for sensitive skin. These would be formulas based on lipid-free or high levels of non-ionic or amphoteric surfactants with an acidic pH closer to the natural pH of skin. Regular use of facial moisturizer provides a protective environment for skin, helping to promote the skin's own healing processes, including the restoration of barrier function, stratum corneum lipid composition and structure and desquamatory enzyme activity. Several studies have been published demonstrating the beneficial effect of specially selected moisturizers in rosacea therapy. Rosacea is thought to be aggravated by photoexposure, so consistent use of an effective broad-spectrum sunscreen product (SPF 15 or higher) is recommended for rosacea patients.

Role of cosmeceuticals in managing rosacea

In recent years, as the development of so-called cosmeceutical products for skin care has grown, the impact of such products as adjunct treatments in rosacea has also expanded beyond reduction of symptoms to having a greater influence on mechanistic attributes associated with the condition. Topical skin care products containing ingredients that improve barrier function or have anti-inflammatory or anti-oxidant properties, especially those of botanical origin, are being shown to be beneficial in rosacea treatment.

Combining actives that modulate the properties of capillary vasculature with those that control inflammation is the first step in creating an effective cosmeceutical product. Reducing pathogens and eliminating the effects of potential triggers further strengthens product efficacy. Typical regimens include a treatment product with one or more anti-inflammatory and antioxidant agents, a moisturizer that improves barrier function, a sunscreen that provides sun protection, and color camouflage with green tint to compensate for red facial overtones. Cosmeceutical regimens may also be combined with prescription treatments for rosacea to improve treatment outcome.

Advances in cosmetic actives

A wide variety of cosmetic actives are available to influence the treatment outcome based on the known biochemical pathways of rosacea. Niacinamide and its derivatives, licorice extracts and selected benzaldehyde derivatives have supporting clinical efficacy results in rosacea patients from controlled and published studies. Several other ingredients such as feverfew, licorice extract, green tea and aloe have published clinical data in other skin conditions or have data on file with product manufacturers. Table 27.1 lists selected ingredients classified by their proposed mechanisms of action.

Barrier repair and skin protection actives
Topical treatment with niacinamide has been shown to improve the stratum corneum barrier function and also improved red blotchiness in

Table 27.1 Cosmeceutical ingredients used in topical rosacea treatment.

Ingredient	Ingredient Benefit
Niacinamide Colloidal oatmeal Hydroxypropyl chitosan	Barrier improvement/protection
Licochalcone A Feverfew Quassia amara	Anti-Inflammatory
Vitamin C Coffeeberry Ginko biloba Tea polyphenols	Anti-Oxidants

photoaged (non-rosacea) patients. Improving barrier function reduces both the potential impact of topical triggers of flares and the susceptibility of the skin to subsequent external insults that could cause irritation or sensory negatives. In one study, the treatment of patients with subtype 1 or 2 rosacea, erythematotelangectatic and papulopusular rosacea respectively, with a moisturizer containing niacinamide for 4 weeks improved barrier function (trans-epidermal water loss) and also mitigated the signs and symptoms of rosacea based on both investigator and subjects' assessments.

Hydroxypropyl chitosan, a film-forming agent that provides a protective barrier, delivered benefits against rosacea as part of a combination treatment. Colloidal oatmeal has a long history of beneficial use in dermatology by virtue of its physical protection of the skin as well as the presence of avenanthramides that can inhibit the activity of nuclear factor kappa-b (NF-κb) and the release of pro-inflammatory factors.

Anti-inflammatory actives

Research has demonstrated that the innate immune system in rosacea-prone facial skin is hyper-responsive to signaling of inflammatory pathways. Skin inflammation can be controlled using many established interrelated pathways including enzymes such as cyclooxygenase (COX), lipooxygenase (LOX), metalloproteinases (MMP), elastase and hyaluronidase, nuclear transcription factors, such as AP1 and NF-κb, neuromodulators, such as substance P and reduction in TLR-2. Anti-inflammatory agents, including many natural products, constitute the largest category of cosmeceutical actives for rosacea. For example, a moisturizer containing licochalcone A isolated from licorice root was found in an 8-week clinical study to improve erythema in a patient population that included rosacea sufferers. A purified extract from the medicinal herb feverfew has been shown to have benefits against facial redness induced by UV exposure or shaving. An extract from the plant *Quassia amara*, used in homeopathic medicine, has shown benefits in treating rosacea topically.

Sensory nerves are closely associated with blood vessels and immune cells and are increased in erythematous rosacea with the up-regulation of genes involved in vasoregulation and neurogenic inflammation. Palmitoyl tripeptide-8 has been shown to reduce substance-P-mediated increases in capillary permeability.

Antioxidants

The generation and release of ROS in the skin can occur in rosacea as a consequence of inflammation and can also be exacerbated by UV exposure with a compromised barrier. Reduction of ROS through the use of topical anti-oxidants can therefore be of benefit in rosacea treatment. For example, a topical preparation of 5% vitamin C has been tested in a small study in rosacea patients and shown to improve the associated erythema. Natural agents with evidence of activity include various tea extracts (green, red, white, black), coffeeberry extract and caffeine, aloe vera, turmeric, chamomile (bisabolol) and mushrooms.

Actives controlling vascular diameter, permeability, and growth

Topical α1-adrenergic agonist drugs such as oxymetazoline have been successfully used to instantly control facial redness by producing vaso-constriction. Topical brimonidine is under development as a prescription treatment for rosacea and early clinical efficacy looks promising. For cosmeceutical use topical caffeine may produce some vasoconstriction but it may also be irritating for rosacea patients. A combination of glycosides of caffeic acid and gallic acid has shown some benefit in reducing erythema.

Most inflammatory pathways lead to an increase in PGE2, a key mediator of capillary vasodilation. Topical application of agents specifically designed to reduce PGE2 may therefore help normalize capillary diameter without vasoconstriction. 4-Ethoxybenzaldehyde was shown to reduce facial redness in patients with rosacea (Figure 27.1), most likely due to suppression of PGE2.

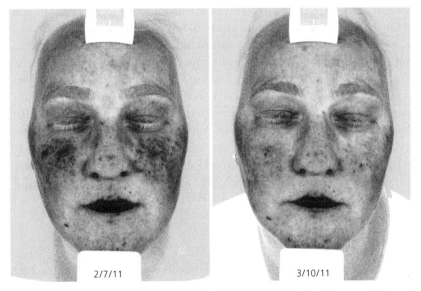

2/7/11   3/10/11

Figure 27.1 Changes in erythema assessed by monitoring red fraction of reflected light using a Visia image analysis at baseline and after 4 weeks of treatment with 4-ethoxybenzaldehyde and niacinamide containing cream (Redness Relief CalmPlex, SkinMedica Inc, Carlsbad, CA). Source: Courtesy of Dr. Mona Foad, Cincinnati, OH, USA.

Suppression of angiogenic growth factors such as fibroblast growth factor (FGF) and vascular endothelial growth factors (VEGF) with dobesilate has been shown to produce clinical improvement in erythema and telangiectasia. Active extracts of natural substances such as propolis, a resin-like material obtained from cone-bearing trees found in bee products and goji berry have been shown to produce anti-angiogenic effects.

Antimicrobial peptides and the innate immune system

Within the cutaneous innate immunity system, the production of antimicrobial peptides (AMPs) is a primary mechanism for protection against infection. AMPs are now known to have two distinct functions: (1) they have direct antimicrobial activity; and (2) they initiate a host cellular response resulting in cytokine release, inflammation and angiogenesis. Individuals with rosacea express abnormally high levels of cathelicidin and other AMPs due to altered TLR-2 profile. Derivatives of isoprenylcysteine and peptides from quinoa grains have shown a reduction in TLR-2 expression in preclinical studies.

Conclusion

Carefully prescribed skin care regimens including clinically proven cosmeceuticals have been used successfully for rosacea. Improved understanding of the pathophysiology of rosacea now allows us to design new cosmeceutical actives that provide benefits against biochemical pathways of rosacea. Anti-inflammatory agents and antioxidants designed to reduce inflammation resulting from a number of diverse stimuli represent a major class of cosmeceutical actives. Agents that help strengthen stratum corneum barrier constitute another important class of actives. Actives that reduce vascular permeability and flow help reduce inflammation and erythema. With improved understanding of the role of the innate immune system in the etiology of rosacea, it is expected that newer actives will target the way skin responds to inflammatory stimuli and provide better control of the symptoms of rosacea and related erythema.

Further reading

Ahn MR, Kunimasa K, Kumazawa S, et al. Correlation between antiangiogenic activity and antioxidant activity of various components from propolis. *Mol Nutr Food Res* 2009; **53**: 643–651.

Berardesca E, Iorizzo M, Abril E, Guglielmini G, Caserini M, Palmieri R, Piérard GE. Clinical and instrumental assessment of the effects of a new product based on hydroxypropyl chitosan and potassium azeloyl diglycinate in the management of rosacea. *J Cosmet Dermatol* 2012; **11**: 37–41.

Carlin RB, Carlin CA. Topical vitamin C preparation reduces erythema of rosacea. *Cosmet Dermatol* 2001; **14**: 35–38.

Cerio R, Dohil M, Jeanine D, et al. Mechanism of action and clinical benefits of colloidal oatmeal for dermatologic practice. *J Drugs Dermatol* 2010; **9**: 1116–1120.

Cuevas P, Arrazola JM. Therapeutic response of rosacea to dobesilate. *Eur J Med Res* 2005; **10**: 454–456.

Draelos ZD, Ertel K, Berge C. Niacinamide-containing facial moisturizer improves skin barrier and benefits subjects with rosacea. *Cutis* 2005; **76**: 135–141.

Draelos ZD, Fuller BB. Efficacy of 1% 4-ethoxylbenzaldehyde in reducing facial erythema. *Dermatol Surg* 2005; **31**: 881–885.

Emer J, Waldorf H, Berson D. Botanicals and anti-inflammatories: Natural ingredients for rosacea. *Semin Cutan Med Surg* 2011; **30**: 148–155.

Farris P: Idebenone, green tea, and coffeeberry extract: New and innovative antioxidants. *Dermatol Ther* 2007; **20**: 322–329.

Ferrari A, Diehl C. Evaluation of the efficacy and tolerance of a topical gel with 4% quassia extract in the treatment of rosacea. *J Clin Pharmacol* 2011; **52**(1): 84–88.

Fowler J, Jarratt M, Moore A, et al. Once-daily topical brimonidine tartrate gel 0·5% is a novel treatment for moderate to severe facial erythema of rosacea: Results of two multicentre, randomized and vehicle-controlled studies. *Br J Dermatol* 2012; **166**: 633–641.

Levin J, Miller R. A guide to the ingredients and potential benefits of over-the-counter cleansers and moisturizers for rosacea patients. *J Clin Aesthet Dermatol* 2011; **4**: 31–49.

Martin K, Sur R, Liebel F, et al. Parthenolide-depleted Feverfew (Tanacetum parthenium) protects skin from UV irradiation and external aggression. *Arch Dermatol Res* 2008; **300**: 69–80.

Shanler SD, Ondo AL. Successful treatment of the erythema and flushing of rosacea using a topically applied selective alpha1-adrenergic receptor agonist, oxymetazoline. *Arch Dermatol* 2007; **143**: 1369–1371.

Sonti S, Holtz R, Mehta R. Mechanistic studies on novel anti-inflammatory molecule used in the treatment of facial redness. *J Invest Dermat* 2012; **131**: S85–S96.

Weber TM, Ceilley RI, Buerger A, Kolbe L, Trookman NS, Rizer RL, Schoelermann A. Skin tolerance, efficacy, and quality of life of patients with red facial skin using a skin care regimen containing Licochalcone A. *J Cosmet Dermatol* 2006; **5**(3):227–232.

Wu WB, Hung DK, Chang FW, et al. Anti-inflammatory and anti-angiogenic effects of flavonoids isolated from Lycium barbarum Linnaeus on human umbilical vein endothelial cells. *Food Funct* 2012, Jul 3. [Epub ahead of print.]

CHAPTER 28

Cosmeceuticals for Enhancing Cosmetic Procedures

Mary Lupo and Leah Jacob
Tulane University School of Medicine, New Orleans, LA, USA

Introduction

Minimally invasive cosmetic procedures are utilized to treat a plethora of dermatologic conditions, including unwanted pigmentation, uneven skin tone, volume loss, and photoaging. Incorporating effective cosmeceutical formulations into the perioperative skin care regimen can improve overall cosmetic outcomes. In addition to synergistically enhancing overall skin rejuvenation, using a combination of topical cosmeceutical agents with cosmetic procedures can hasten postoperative healing, minimize unwanted complications, and prolong procedural results. This chapter describes the commonly used combination protocols, focusing on those with the most robust scientific evidence to support their use.

General considerations

Any and all cosmetic procedures should be accompanied by a daily morning and evening skin care regimen to optimize overall skin health. Morning treatment protocols should center on environmental protection for the prevention of photo-induced aging and carcinogenesis, using broad-spectrum sunscreens combined with antioxidants. The addition of antioxidants, specifically vitamin C, has been shown to synergistically enhance the photoprotective effects of sunscreen. Evening skin care should focus on epidermal barrier repair and collagen regeneration; retinoids, topical peptides, topical growth factors and moisturizers can all be utilized for this purpose. For patients with pigmentary disturbances and for those with darker skin types, a skin-lightening agent should be added daily to enhance procedures aimed at correcting the dyspigmentation and to prevent post-inflammatory hyperpigmentation.

The initial consultation is the perfect time to introduce the patient to a topical skin care regimen targeting their specific needs. Often, patients

Cosmeceuticals and Cosmetic Practice, First Edition. Edited by Patricia K. Farris.
© 2014 John Wiley & Sons, Ltd. Published 2014 by John Wiley & Sons, Ltd.

are initially hesitant to undergo more invasive cosmetic procedures due to their significant costs and downtime. Beginning the rejuvenation process with topical agents can be a less intimidating and more affordable initial step, easing the transition to more invasive, albeit more effective procedures. With time, patients will feel more comfortable and willing to add procedure-based solutions to their topical treatments. In addition to promoting overall skin heath, establishing a daily routine will prepare the patient for the post-operative skin care needed after resurfacing procedures. Patients unwilling to actively participate in daily skin care measures may not be optimum candidates for procedures with intensive post-operative wound care requirements and are best treated with more conservative approaches.

Synergistically enhancing procedural outcomes

The addition of properly selected topical cosmeceutical agents to minor cosmetic procedures can synergistically enhance the results obtained with either treatment alone, leading to faster and more noticeable clinical improvements. Synergistic combinations of various topical agents with chemical peels, ablative laser resurfacing, nonablative technologies and injectable agents are discussed below.

Chemical peels

Chemical peels continue to be one of the most commonly performed in-office cosmetic procedures. While deeper peels have largely been replaced by newer laser-based ablative treatments, superficial to medium-depth peels are still commonly utilized for the treatment of fine lines, uneven skin tone and texture, and pigmentary disturbances. Beneficial adjunctive agents that can enhance in-office chemical peels include alpha and beta hydroxy acids, retinoids, and skin-lightening preparations.

Alpha and beta hydroxy acids are beneficial when used as preparatory agents before chemical peels. Moisturizers containing alpha hydroxy acids and beta hydroxy acids can be used for two to three weeks prior to in-office superficial or medium depth chemical peels. Pretreatment with these superficial exfoliating agents thins the stratum corneum and creates a more uniform cutaneous surface, enhancing the evenness of the peel. The thinner stratum corneum also allows for deeper penetration of the peeling agent, enhancing results. Moisturizers containing salicylic acid are thought to be excellent pre-peel treatments, due to their ability to exfoliate better in oilier regions such as the nose. Retinoids are also excellent pretreatment agents. Several studies have evaluated the effects of retinoid pretreatment prior to chemical peeling, showing faster healing times in pretreated skin.

However, caution should be taken as the use of retinoids can increase the likelihood of excessive irritation; discontinuing retinoids for one week following peels can help to minimize this.

When used for the treatment of hyperpigmentation, a combination of chemical peels and topical skin-lightening agents has been shown in several well-designed studies to result in greater improvement than that seen with either treatment alone. The superficial exfoliation obtained with chemical peels increases the depth of penetration of the lightening agent, allowing access to deeper pigmented keratinocytes for enhanced lightening effects. Although hydroquinone is the most commonly used lightening agent, several other cosmeceutical ingredients possess skin lightening properties, such as kojic acid, ascorbic acid, and licorice extract, to name a few. The addition of these agents to hydroquinone and superficial peels may enhance overall skin lightening; this was demonstrated in a split-face study that showed more pigmentary improvement when kojic acid was added to glycolic acid and hydroquinone in patients with melasma. Another study demonstrated improved and longer responses of melasma with the addition of vitamin C to a trichloroacetic acid peel compared with TCA peel alone.

Ablative laser resurfacing and nonablative technologies

Ablative laser resurfacing remains the most effective and dramatic treatment for severely photodamaged skin. Rejuvenation is a result of thermally-induced full-thickness epidermal and dermal denudation, followed by cytokine-induced dermal collagen formation and re-epithelialization. As the epidermis is compromised following treatment, post-operative wound care with topical emollients is essential until re-epithelialization is complete. The impaired epidermal barrier may enhance dermal delivery of topical agents whose size would otherwise limit their penetration past the epidermis. Various nonablative technologies can also be used for cutaneous rejuvenation of photoaged skin; these are summarized in Table 28.1. As the epidermis is unaffected by

Table 28.1 Commonly used nonablative technologies.

Infrared (IR) lasers
Intense pulsed light
Radiofrequency
Ultrasound
Light-emitting diodes
Photodynamic therapy
KTP/PDL
1320 nm Nd:YAG
long-pulsed Er:YAG

these nonablative treatments, the cumbersome wound care and extensive downtime required with ablative resurfacing treatments are eliminated. However, clinical improvement is less dramatic than that seen after ablative resurfacing procedures. Combining nonablative treatments with topical cosmeceuticals allows for greater overall rejuvenation than that seen with either therapy alone (Figures 28.1 and 28.2).

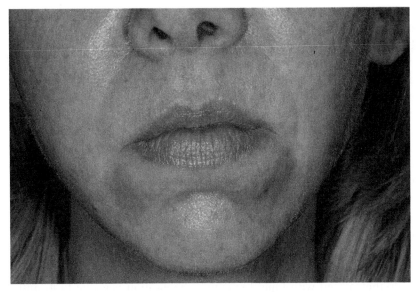

Figure 28.1 40-year-old female with photo-induced pigmentary changes and rosacea.

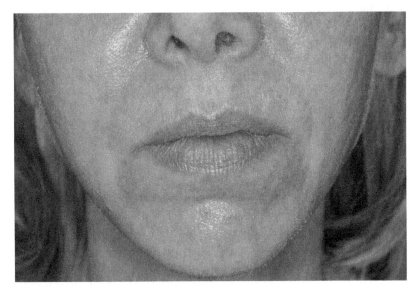

Figure 28.2 Improvement in dyspigmentation and erythema following combination treatment with IPL and topical retinoids.

Topical retinoids can be used preoperatively prior to both ablative and nonablative laser treatments. Several studies have confirmed that pretreatment with topical retinoids results in significantly faster healing and quicker re-epithelialization following ablative laser resurfacing procedures. Pretreatment with retinoids has been shown to result in increased dermal thickness and faster resolution of erythema following nonablative laser treatment. Additional proposed benefits to preoperative retinoid use include a decreased risk of postoperative milia development, decreased postoperative hyperpigmentation rates, and better penetration of the laser beam due to a thinner stratum corneum. Preoperative use can begin anywhere from months to weeks prior to the procedure; most physicians employ an approximately 2–4-week pretreatment regimen. After ablative resurfacing, retinoid use should be discontinued for several weeks to allow re-epithelialization and skin maturation.

Incorporating topical antioxidants into periprocedural skin care can serve to minimize post-procedural inflammation and erythema. Pretreatment with a topical formulation containing vitamin C has been shown to decrease post-procedural erythema, commonly seen after ablative laser resurfacing. One well-designed split-face study compared a 2-week pretreatment with topical vitamin C to placebo in 21 patients undergoing facial carbon dioxide laser resurfacing. Significantly decreased erythema was seen in skin treated with topical 10% L-ascorbic acid compared to skin treated with placebo. Researchers hypothesized that the reduction in erythema seen with topical vitamin C application was due to its anti-inflammatory effects. Further enhancement of these anti-inflammatory effects may be potentiated by laser treatment itself, as topical uptake of ascorbic acid was shown to be enhanced by ablative lasers and microdermabrasion devices. Another study demonstrated greater improvements in skin hydration, texture, and pore size following the addition of polyphenolic antioxidants to an intense pulsed light (IPL) treatment regimen compared with IPL treatment alone. Exactly how and when to begin topical antioxidant formulations is not well defined; many dermatologic surgeons will delay postoperative use until re-epithelialization is complete as it may cause burning upon application. One suggestion is to begin with an every other day application of a vitamin C solution approximately 14 days after resurfacing procedures and slowly advance to daily application by the third or fourth post-operative week in order to assist in reducing erythema.

Growth factors are regulatory proteins that act as signaling agents between and within cells. Topically applied growth factors have been shown to accelerate wound healing and improve the appearance of photoaged skin, due to their ability to initiate collagen and fibronectin synthesis and fibroblast production of glycosaminoglycans. Several anecdotal reports exist to support the benefits of topical growth factors used in conjunction with laser resurfacing, including faster re-epithelialization and less erythema. Following ablative laser resurfacing procedures, the lack of an effective epidermal barrier may allow for greater penetration of active ingredients, as their large protein size and charge somewhat prohibit their penetration past the epidermis. However, as keratinocytes have been shown to express receptors for growth factors, topical application following nonablative resurfacing procedures may also be beneficial, due to growth factor-mediated communications between the epidermis and dermis. Further studies are needed assessing the application of topical growth factors with laser resurfacing; however, these cosmeceutical agents represent an exciting and promising additional therapeutic domain.

Injectable treatments

Botulinum toxin injections and soft tissue augmentation with injectable dermal fillers are highly effective for the treatment of hyperkinetic rhytides and age-related volume loss. Wrinkles and volume loss are often accompanied by environmentally-induced textural changes and discoloration, resulting in an aged appearance. Combining botulinum toxin and dermal filler injections with cutaneous resurfacing procedures can maximize overall aesthetic improvement (Figures 28.3 and 28.4). Furthermore, daily use of collagen-stimulating topical agents, such as retinoids, topical peptides, and topical growth factors enhances overall wrinkle reduction. The

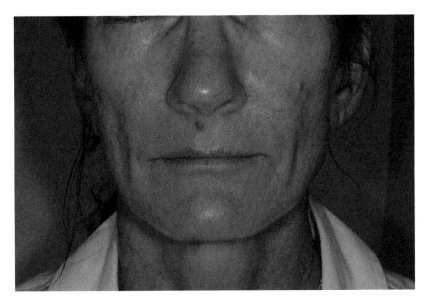

Figure 28.3 55-year-old female with age-related volume loss and environmentally-induced skin changes.

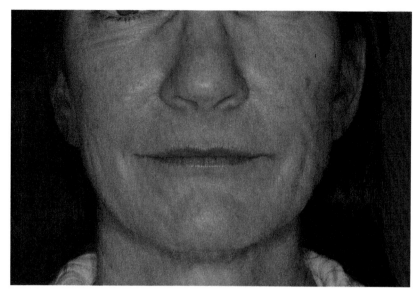

Figure 28.4 Results following treatment with fractionated CO_2 resurfacing and volume replacement using Sculptra®.

addition of antioxidants is beneficial as well. As oxidative stress is known to cause weakening of dermal connective tissue, contributing to wrinkle formation and volume loss, the addition of topical formulations containing antioxidants will prevent further damage and wrinkle formation. There are innumerable products containing various antioxidant combinations, and it is up to the cosmetic surgeon to select stable formulations with data supporting their clinical efficacy.

Minimizing procedural complications

Every procedure is associated with its own potential complications and inherent side effects. Bruising and hyperpigmentation deserve particular attention, as cosmeceutical ingredients can be used to minimize these unwanted events and help to hasten their resolution.

Bruising
Injections of dermal fillers and neurotoxins and treatments with vascular lasers are often associated with post-procedural bruising that can be upsetting for patients and slow to resolve. Although definitive data is sparse, cosmeceuticals containing arnica and vitamin K may be helpful in minimizing the severity of bruising and in hastening its resolution.

Most studies examining the effects of topical arnica on bruising have been equivocal; however, this may be due to lower concentrations of arnica in the tested products. One blinded randomized controlled trial demonstrated accelerated resolution of laser-induced bruises treated with topical 20% arnica ointment compared to those treated with placebo. Topical formulations containing vitamin K have been shown in placebo-controlled trials to lead to faster resolution of iatrogenic forearm bruising and actinic purpura. Several studies have demonstrated faster resolution and decreased severity of vascular laser-induced purpura when topical vitamin K preparations were used for several days following laser treatment. As such, the use of topical vitamin K following treatment with vascular lasers may be beneficial.

Post-inflammatory hyperpigmentation

One of the most common adverse events following resurfacing procedures is postinflammatory hyperpigmentation. Post-procedural inflammation causes the release of melanocyte-activating inflammatory mediators such as cytokines and chemokines, leading to increased production and dispersion of melanin by melanocytes. Those patients with darker skin types (Fitzpatrick IV–VI) are more prone to developing this complication, but lighter skin types are at risk as well. The risk of postoperative hyperpigmentation is increased when injury extends to the papillary dermis, such as that seen with medium-depth peels and ablative resurfacing lasers.

Preoperative treatment with skin-lightening agents can decrease the risk of postoperative hyperpigmentation. Hydroquinone is most commonly used as a pretreatment agent; preparations containing kojic acid, ascorbic acid, licorice extract or azelaic acid can be beneficial as well. These agents all act by inhibiting tyrosinase, the main enzyme involved in melanin synthesis. Additionally, hydroquinone is cytotoxic to melanocytes. Advocates of pretreatment regimens hypothesize that these lightening agents will decrease the melanin content of melanocytes and suppress the production of new melanin, thus decreasing the risk of postoperative hyperpigmentation. Commonly employed regimens include daily to twice-daily application of a skin-lightening agent for three to four weeks prior to the procedure; some surgeons will limit pretreatment to those patients with skin types III or higher as these patients are more likely to develop post-procedural hyperpigmentation. Should postoperative hyperpigmentation occur, a combination of topical bleaching agents, mild peeling agents, and sunblock can be used to hasten resolution.

Conclusion

In addition to synergistically enhancing overall skin rejuvenation and improving cosmetic outcomes, incorporating cosmeceuticals into peri-procedural skin care can minimize unwanted outcomes, hasten postoperative healing, and improve overall patient satisfaction. Choosing an overall treatment plan that combines topical agents with cosmetic procedures ensures the best outcomes for our patients. Most importantly, suggesting a daily skin care regimen encourages patients to actively contribute to the optimal health of their skin through prevention and repair.

Further reading

Alster TS, West TB. Effect of topical vitamin C on postoperative carbon dioxide laser resurfacing erythema. *Dermatol Surg* 1998; **24**(3): 331–334.

Brightman LA, Brauer JA, Anolik R, et al. Ablative and fractional ablative lasers. *Dermatol Clin* 2009; **27**: 479–489.

Elson ML. Topical phytonadione (vitamin K1) in the treatment of actinic and traumatic purpura. *Cosmet Dermatol* 1995; **8**: 25–27.

Freedman BM. Topical antioxidant application augments the effects of intense pulsed light therapy. *J Cosmet Dermatol* 2009; **8**(4): 254–259.

Goldman MP. The use of hydroquinone with facial laser resurfacing. *J Cutan Laser Ther* 2000; **2**(2): 73–77.

Hevia O, Nemeth AJ, Taylor JR. Tretinoin accelerates healing after trichloroacetic acid chemical peel. *Arch Dermatol* 1991; **127**(5): 678–682.

Lee WR, Shen SC, Kuo-Hsien W, Hu CH, Fang JY. Lasers and microdermabrasion enhance and control topical delivery of vitamin C. *J Invest Dermatol* 2003;**121**(5): 1118–1125.

Leu S, Havey J, White LE, Martin N, Yoo SS, Rademaker AW, et al. Accelerated resolution of laser-induced bruising with topical 20% arnica: A rater-blinded randomized controlled trial. *Br J Dermatol* 2010; **163**(3): 557–563.

Lim JT. Treatment of melasma using kojic acid in a gel containing hydroquinone and glycolic acid. *Dermatol Surg* 1999; **25**(4): 282–284.

Soliman MM, Ramadan SA, Bassiouny DA, Abdelmalek M. Combined trichloroacetic acid peel and topical ascorbic acid versus trichloroacetic acid peel alone in the treatment of melasma: A comparative study. *J Cosmet Dermatol* 2007; **6**(2): 89–94.

CHAPTER 29

The Future of Cosmeceuticals

Patricia K. Farris
Tulane University School of Medicine, New Orleans, LA, USA

Introduction

Today, consumers are looking for science-driven skin care that can improve and prevent skin aging, protect skin from environmental damage and provide therapeutic options for a myriad of skin problems. They want products that are natural, non-irritating, preservative-free, green and fully tested. This is a tall order for manufacturers who have to balance product safety, stability, consistency and efficacy while at the same time meeting consumer demands. The future of cosmeceuticals depends on innovation. Identifying product niches, new actives and more effective delivery systems will no doubt give way to a plethora of cosmeceutical products with broader clinical applications.

In spite of industry's best efforts, consumers remain skeptical about cosmeceuticals. They are confused about ingredients and distrust product claims leaving them to wonder if these products are really worth the money. When shopping for cosmeceuticals consumers are confused by ambiguous package labeling that lacks specific information including the concentration of key active ingredients. Many of these concerns could be addressed if stricter regulations were in place for cosmeceutical products. There are also significant challenges that must be met in order for cosmeceuticals to be legitimized in the eyes of physicians. Many dermatologists state that they do not believe in the validity of cosmeceuticals since they lack the scientific rigor that is applied to pharmaceuticals. This is a valid complaint that can only be addressed if manufacturers test products in an objective manner in order to substantiate claims. It is encouraging that some of the newer cosmeceuticals have been tested in double-blind vehicle-controlled studies designed to confirm their efficacy. In order to assist physician members in gathering credible information about cosmeceuticals, the American Academy of Dermatology (AAD) has convened the Work Group on Complementary and Alternative Medicine. This group includes dermatologists and members of the governing bodies that regulate cosmetics. Through this group we hope to provide AAD members with

Cosmeceuticals and Cosmetic Practice, First Edition. Edited by Patricia K. Farris.

easy access to safety and efficacy data on cosmeceutical products and other alternative treatments.

Challenges for the Future

Formulations: active ingredients and delivery systems

Identification and development of new active ingredients are essential to expand the cosmeceutical marketplace. The study of the pathogenesis of skin aging plays a pivotal role in finding new actives. These studies, many of which are conducted by manufacturers, are used to identify points in the aging process where novel cosmeceutical ingredients might be used to intervene. Using gene array analysis, cosmetic chemists can now screen potential actives and quickly determine their biologic profile and potential applications. Many of the newer actives have multiple biologic effects such as lightening pigmentation, boosting collagen production and down-regulating inflammation. These ingredients, referred to as multi-tasking actives, are sought after since they improve skin's appearance using a multi-mechanism approach. Natural and synthetic ingredients can be used in this regard and research and development are underway to identify new compounds that have multiple mechanisms of action.

In view of the continuing interest by consumers in actives that are viewed as natural, we are certain to see more skin care products touting ingredients from botanical sources. Plants can now be grown and culti-vated in a way that optimizes desired ingredients. Plant stem cells can be used to generate biologically active compounds, and hold promise as a resource for natural ingredients. Marine-based cosmeceuticals are an emerging category of naturals that represent an exciting new frontier for cosmeceutical manufacturers. Algae are a particularly rich resource, con-taining many biologically active compounds. Marine-derived antioxidants, polysaccharides, collagen, bioactive peptides and chitin are promising func-tional ingredients for cosmeceuticals. New synthetic ingredients will also play a role in this evolving market. One of the fastest growing categories of cosmeceuticals includes those containing biologically active peptides which have diverse biologic effects. These synthetic ingredients mimic peptides found in human skin and offer unique benefits. And finally, autologous skin care products will offer the ultimate for those who desire natural skin care. These cosmeceuticals use an individuals own cells to produce growth factors and other skin rejuvenating compounds. We are certain to see more research and development in this promising area of skin biology.

The skin is a formidable barrier to the penetration of topically applied ingredients. This has limited the effectiveness of cosmeceuticals in the past and remains a core concern in the industry. Delivery systems are essential for stabilizing ingredients, precise local targeting and reducing side effects, including irritation. Formulators are challenged by molecular size, charge and whether the active ingredient is lipophilic or hydrophilic in nature. Some of these concerns have been addressed by newer delivery systems that create water channels in the stratum corneum, allowing delivery of both hydrophilic and lipophilic molecules. In addition, since most cosmeceuticals today contain a combination of active ingredients, how these actives influence one another in terms of stability and skin penetration presents an additional challenge to the cosmetic chemist. No doubt new encapsulation technologies will be used to stabilize and deliver unique combinations of ingredients to the skin over time, increasing product efficacy while improving tolerability. In view of these significant advances in delivery systems, cosmeceutical efficacy can now be attributed to both the active ingredients and the delivery system. Finally, the safety of some delivery systems such as nanoparticles continues to be a lingering question. Only through long-term safety studies can we reassure consumers that these delivery systems are safe for continued use in personal care products.

Moving forward, cosmetic companies are well positioned to utilize at-home devices to enhance the delivery of skin care ingredients. At-home electrical devices, including those emitting galvanic charges, have already been marketed by cosmetic companies in combination with cosmeceuticals. Micro-needling has attracted interest and is now being offered by major cosmeceutical companies to facilitate product penetration. Lasers, light sources and other device-based technologies are currently being evaluated by cosmetic manufacturers for their use as penetration enhancers. These devices will be co-marketed with cosmeceuticals to provide the consumer with cutting-edge technologies that were previously available only the office or spa setting.

Sustainable practices

The notion of sustainability is affecting all consumer goods including health and beauty products. The goal of sustainable manufacturing is to ensure that everything put into the process gets returned to the environment in a positive way. In the case of cosmeceuticals sustainability applies to both the formulation and packaging. Good agricultural practices (GAPs) are essential for sustainability. Cultivating sustainable crops that can be used as a botanical resource for cosmeceuticals requires knowledge, skill and commitment. In general, Western agriculture has an advantage over agriculture in other parts of the world since there has been increasing legislation that has resulted in agricultural practices that are more sustainable.

In addition to growing practices, the processing of botanicals must also be done in a sustainable way. Solvents used during the extraction process may also leave a footprint on the environment and have been abandoned by some manufacturers. And finally, there is a growing concern about the impact of plastic derived from personal care products and other packaged goods on our environment. Package design, choice of material, recycling and reusing packaging components will all play a role as sustainable packaging moves into the skin care industry.

Beyond cosmeceuticals: nutraceuticals

Nutricosmetics is an emerging area of anti-aging medicine that is of growing interest to dermatologists. Science linking nutrition, skin aging and skin health has given rise to a growing demand for foods and supplements that can be used as part of a comprehensive program to improve appearance. Already taking hold of countries like Japan and China, the concept of beauty from within is still evolving in the US and Europe. Consumers in Japan and other Asian countries have embraced the notion that skin health and appearance are dependent on good nutrition. Sales of nutricosmetics including foods and beauty supplements were reported to be $1.3 billion dollars in Japan in 2010 compared to $60 million dollars in the US. The global market is projected to reach $4.24 billion dollars by 2017, according to Global Industry Analysts Inc. Beauty foods and drinks are among the most popular nutricosmetics in Japan. These products contain ingredients such as antioxidants, seaweed and collagen, and there are some studies confirming skin benefits. The acceptance of these products is at least in part due to the fact that Japan has a process whereby it approves of certain food-based products as Foods for Specific Health Use (FOSHU). In order for a product to be approved as FOSHU, manufacturers must complete an application process providing scientific documentation demonstrating the medical or nutritional basis for the health claim. This information includes dosing, safety, information on the ingredient and any relevant scientific papers. After approval is granted, specifically approved health claims can be made. In the US, most nutricosmetics are categorized by the FDA as dietary supplements which until recently have remained largely unregulated. In 2011, the FDA initiated requirements as part of the Food Safety Modernization Act (FSMA) whereby manufacturers must notify the agency when using a new dietary ingredient (NDI). The notification must include information that is the basis upon which manufacturers have concluded that a dietary supplement containing this new ingredient will be expected to be safe under the conditions of use recommended or suggested in the labeling. This type of requirement provides transparency to bring new ingredients into the market and will give consumers an added level of confidence in nutraceutical products. Nutricosmetics remain a forefront in the beauty, health and wellness category with tremendous growth potential in the US, Europe and around the world.

Conclusion

Cosmeceuticals continue to be a growing segment of the personal care market. Although demand is growing, competition is also increasing. Challenges, including finding new ingredients, better delivery systems and making products more green, face manufacturers worldwide. New horizons include the use of functional foods, nutritional supplements and at-home devices coupled with cosmeceuticals as a comprehensive approach to overall health maintenance.

Further reading

Anuciato TP, et al. Carotenoids and polyphenols in nutricosmetics, nutraceuticals and cosmeceuticals. *J Cosm Derm* 2012; **11**: 51–54.

Cosgrove MC, Franco OH, Granger SP, et al. Dietary nutrient intakes and skin-aging appearance among middle-aged women. *Am J Clin Nutr* 2007; **86**: 1225–1231.

Draelos ZD. Cosmeceuticals: Un-defined, unclassified and un-regulated. *Clin Dermatol* 2009; **27**: 431–434.

Dreno B. New assessment methods applied to a patented lacto-lycopene, soy isoflavones and vitamin C in the correction of skin aging. *Nouv Dermatol* 2003; **22**: 1–6.

Izumi T, Saito M, Obata A, et al. Oral intake of soy isoflavone aglycone improves the aged skin in adult women. *J Nutr Sci Vitaminol* 2007; **53**: 57–62.

Nino M, Calabro G, Santoianni P. Topical delivery of active principles: The field of dermatological research. *Dermatol Online J* 2010; **16**(1):6.

Piccardi N, Manissier P. Nutrition and nutritional supplementation: Impact on skin health and beauty. *Dermato-Endo* 2001; **5**: 271–274.

Thornfeld CR. Cosmeceuticals: Separating fact from voodoo science. *SkinMed* 2005; **4**(4): 214–220.

Yamakoshi J, Sano A, Taokutake S, et al. Oral intake of proanthrocyandin-rich extract from grape seeds improves chloasma. *Phytotherapy Research* 2004; **18**: 895–899.

Index

Note: Page references in *italics* refer to Figures; those in **bold** refer to Tables

---

Cosmeceuticals and Cosmetic Practice, First Edition. Edited by Patricia K. Farris.
© 2014 John Wiley & Sons, Ltd. Published 2014 by John Wiley & Sons, Ltd.

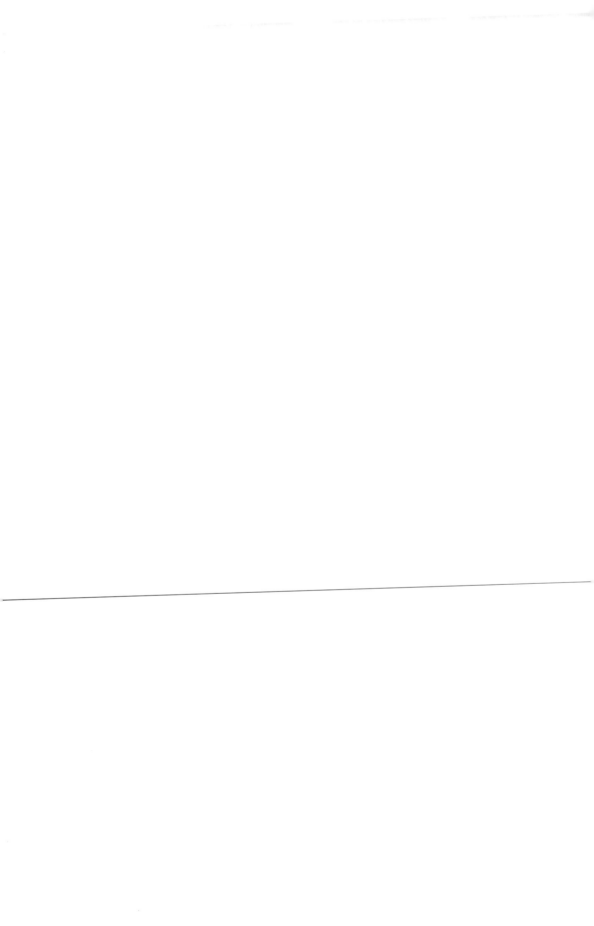

Printed and bound by CPI Group (UK) Ltd, Croydon, CR0 4YY

16/04/2025

14658553-0002

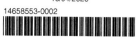